METHODS IN MOLECULAR BIOLOGY™

Series Editor
John M. Walker
School of Life Sciences
University of Hertfordshire
Hatfield, Hertfordshire, AL10 9AB, UK

For other titles published in this series, go to
www.springer.com/series/7651

Drug Design and Discovery

Methods and Protocols

Edited by

Seetharama D. Satyanarayanajois

Department of Basic Pharmaceutical Sciences, College of Pharmacy, University of Louisiana at Monroe, Monroe, LA, USA

Humana Press

Editor
Seetharama D. Satyanarayanajois, Ph.D.
Department of Basic Pharmaceutical Sciences
College of Pharmacy
University of Louisiana at Monroe
Monroe, LA
USA
jois@ulm.edu

ISSN 1064-3745 e-ISSN 1940-6029
ISBN 978-1-4939-5824-5 ISBN 978-1-61779-012-6 (eBook)
DOI 10.1007/978-1-61779-012-6
Springer New York Dordrecht Heidelberg London

Softcover re-print of the Hardcover 1st edition 2011

Printed on acid-free paper

Humana Press is part of Springer Science+Business Media (www.springer.com)

Preface

In a rational drug discovery approach, it is necessary to identify the cause of the disease and its mechanism at the molecular level. Protein molecules that are the basic cause of the disease are identified first. Altering or modifying the protein–protein interaction could lead to therapeutic agents. The state-of-the-art methodology in drug discovery demands rational drug design, which will lower side effects and enhance therapeutic effects. Research in the pharmaceutical sciences and medicinal chemistry has taken an important new direction in the past two decades with a focus on large molecules, especially peptides and proteins, and DNA therapeutics. Protein and peptide drugs are currently the most rapidly expanding class of drugs. At present, more than 130 different proteins or peptides have been approved for clinical use. Whether it is peptide/protein-based drugs or organic molecules, the process of drug discovery involves several steps. The first is target identification and lead optimization. In the former process, molecules that bind a drug target and modulate the biological activity are identified using an in vitro assay, while in the latter potential drug molecules are optimized with respect to in vitro potency and other important parameters reflecting bioavailability and pharmacokinetic or toxicological properties. When a therapeutic target has been identified and validated, the next stage in drug discovery is to conduct high-throughput screening based on target binding or cellular assay to identify a lead compound. Once a lead compound is identified, the compound is modified chemically for higher activity and less toxicity. This involves the synthesis of a large number of analogs of the lead compound and testing them for biological activity. With several hundred protein targets available, screening thousands of compounds for biological activity and toxicity is a tedious and time-consuming process. In recent years, there has been an interest in disrupting protein–protein interactions using small molecules and peptides. With this interest in protein–protein interactions for targeting drugs, the number of drug targets will increase from hundreds to thousands. Once the drug-like molecule enters preclinical and clinical trials, it becomes an extremely expensive task to study each target. Hence, several methods have been discovered to screen compounds that may have drug-like properties. These methods involve computational, spectroscopic, analytical, and purification methods, cellular assays, and molecular biology methods. In this particular volume of *Methods in Molecular Biology*, we present 16 chapters related to drug discovery and screening. It is impossible to cover all the methods related to drug discovery in a single volume. Our intent is to give an in-depth view of some protocols that are commonly used in drug discovery laboratories. Some of these techniques may be old and some are relatively new. They include computational docking, quantitative structure–activity relationship (QSAR), peptide synthesis, labeling of peptides and proteins with fluorescent labels, DNA-microarray, zebrafish model for drug screening, and other analytical screening and biological assays that are routinely used during the drug discovery process. With the availability of three-dimensional structures of protein/DNA target molecules, computational methods have played a key role in designing and screening thousands of compounds as possible candidates for druggable molecules. Hence, we have covered computational methods in detail. Cellular and whole body imaging using fluorescently labeled molecules have gained popularity compared to procedures using radioactively labeled compounds. The method of fluorescent labeling of peptides and proteins is covered in detail in one chapter. Overall, this volume will serve as a laboratory reference for pharmaceutical chemists, medicinal chemists, and pharmacologists as well as for molecular biologists.

I would like to thank my wife, Latha Nagarajarao, for helping me to edit the chapters. Thanks to Dr. John Walker, chief editor of the series, for his advice and to all the authors who contributed to this series for their valuable time and sharing their detailed knowledge.

Monroe, LA ***Seetharama D. Satyanarayanajois***

Contents

Contributors

PARAYIL KUMARAN AJIKUMAR • *Singapore-Massachusetts Institute of Technology Alliance (SMA), National University of Singapore, Singapore*
Department of Chemical Engineering, Massachusetts Institute of Technology, Cambridge, MA, USA
JENNIFER ARAL • *Peptide Research & Discovery, Amgen, Thousand Oaks, CA, USA*
SATHY V. BALU-IYER • *Department of Pharmaceutical Sciences, SUNY – University, Buffalo, Amherst, NY, USA*
SALEEM BASHA • *James L. Winkle College of Pharmacy, University of Cincinnati, Cincinnati, OH, USA*
HO BOW • *Department of Microbiology, National University of Singapore, Singapore*
VINCENT T.K. CHOW • *Department of Microbiology, National University of Singapore, Singapore*
MAXEY C.M. CHUNG • *Department of Biochemistry, Yong Loo Lin School of Medicine, National University of Singapore, Singapore*
Department of Biological Sciences, Faculty of Science, National University of Singapore, Singapore
CHANNA R. DE SILVA • *Department of Chemistry, University of Arizona, Tucson, AZ, USA*
KHALID A. EL SAYED • *Department of Basic Pharmaceutical Sciences, College of Pharmacy, University of Louisiana at Monroe, Monroe, LA, USA*
PUNEET GAITONDE • *Department of Pharmaceutical Sciences, SUNY – University, Buffalo, Amherst, NY, USA*
PONNAMPALAM GOPALAKRISHNAKONE • *Venom and Toxin Research Program, Department of Anatomy, Yong Loo Lin School of Medicine, National University of Singapore, Singapore*
VINEET GUPTA • *Department of Basic Pharmaceutical Sciences, University of Louisiana at Monroe, Monroe, LA, USA*
VICTOR J. HRUBY • *Department of Chemistry, University of Arizona, Tucson, AZ, USA*
JATINDER S. JOSAN • *Department of Chemistry, University of Arizona, Tucson, AZ, USA*
GLEN E. KELLOGG • *Department of Medicinal Chemistry & Institute for Structural Biology and Drug Discovery, Virginia Commonwealth University, Richmond, VA, USA*
MOHAMMAD KHANFAR • *Department of Basic Pharmaceutical Sciences, College of Pharmacy, University of Louisiana at Monroe, Monroe, LA, USA*
NG JIN KIAT • *Singapore-Massachusetts Institute of Technology Alliance (SMA), National University of Singapore, Singapore*

Teck Kwang Lim • *Department of Biological Sciences, Faculty of Science, National University of Singapore, Singapore*
Qingsong Lin • *Department of Biological Sciences, Faculty of Science, National University of Singapore, Singapore*
Shuo Lin • *Department of Molecular, Cell, and Developmental Biology, University of California, Los Angeles, Los Angeles, CA, USA*
Jining Liu • *Estee Lauder Companies Innovation Institute (China), Shanghai, China*
Yong-Yu Liu • *Department of Basic Pharmaceutical Sciences, University of Louisiana at Monroe, Monroe, LA, USA*
Ronald M. Lynch • *Bio5 Institute, University of Arizona, Tucson, AZ, USA*
Garland R. Marshall • *Center for Computational Biology, School of Medicine, Washington University in St. Louis, St. Louis, MO, USA*
Les P. Miranda • *Peptide Research and Discovery, Amgen, Thousand Oaks, CA, USA*
Justin K. Murray • *Peptide Research & Discovery, Amgen, Thousand Oaks, CA, USA*
Mudit Mudit • *Department of Basic Pharmaceutical Sciences, College of Pharmacy, University of Louisiana at Monroe, Monroe, LA, USA; Department of Pharmaceutical Sciences, D'Youville College, School of Pharmacy, Buffalo, NY, USA*
Giovanni M. Pauletti • *James L. Winkle College of Pharmacy, University of Cincinnati, Cincinnati, OH, USA*
Mark D. Pagel • *Department of Chemistry, University of Arizona, Tucson, AZ, USA*
Too Heng Phon • *Singapore-Massachusetts Institute of Technology Alliance (SMA), National University of Singapore, Singapore*
Delira Robbins • *Department of Pharmacology, Toxicology, & Neuroscience, Louisiana State University Health Sciences Center in Shreveport, Shreveport, LA, USA*
Sharon Ronald • *Department of Basic Pharmaceutical Sciences, College of Pharmacy, University of Louisiana at Monroe, Monroe, LA, USA*
Ramar Perumal Samy • *Venom and Toxin Research Program, Department of Anatomy, Yong Loo Lin School of Medicine, National University of Singapore, Singapore*
Seetharama D. Satyanarayanajois • *Department of Basic Pharmaceutical Sciences, College of Pharmacy, University of Louisiana at Monroe, Monroe, LA, USA*
Girish V. Shah • *Department of Basic Pharmaceutical Sciences, College of Pharmacy, University of Louisiana at Monroe, Monroe, LA, USA*
Fritz Simeon • *Singapore-Massachusetts Institute of Technology Alliance (SMA), National University of Singapore, Singapore*
J. Andrew Surface • *Department of Medicinal Chemistry & Institute for Structural Biology and Drug Discovery, Virginia Commonwealth University, Richmond, VA, USA*
Paul W. Sylvester • *Department of Basic Pharmaceutical Sciences, College of Pharmacy, University of Louisiana at Monroe, Monroe, LA, USA*

HWEE TONG TAN • *Department of Biochemistry, Yong Loo Lin School of Medicine, National University of Singapore, Singapore*
YAT T. TANG • *Center for Computational Biology, School of Medicine, Washington University in St. Louis, St. Louis, MO, USA*
MAUNG MAUNG THWIN • *Venom and Toxin Research Program, Department of Anatomy, Yong Loo Lin School of Medicine, National University of Singapore, Singapore*
ASHUTOSH TRIPATHI • *Department of Medicinal Chemistry & Institute for Structural Biology and Drug Discovery, Virginia Commonwealth University, Richmond, VA, USA*
JOSEF VAGNER • *Bio5 Institute, University of Arizona, Tucson, AZ, USA*
SHRUTHI VAIDHYANATHAN • *James L. Winkle College of Pharmacy, University of Cincinnati, Cincinnati, OH, USA*
BYUNGHEE YOO • *Department of Chemistry, University of Arizona, Tucson, AZ, USA*
QIAN-JIN ZHANG • *Department of Biology, Xavier University of Louisiana, New Orleans, LA, USA*
SHUXING ZHANG • *Department of Experimental Therapeutics, M.D. Anderson Cancer Center, Houston, TX, USA*
YUNFENG ZHAO • *Department of Pharmacology, Toxicology, & Neuroscience, Louisiana State University Health Sciences Center in Shreveport, Shreveport, LA, USA*
HANBING ZHONG • *Laboratory of Chemical Genomics, School of Chemical Biology and Biotechnology, Shenzhen Graduate School of Peking University, Shenzhen University Town Shenzhen, China*

Chapter 1

Virtual Screening for Lead Discovery

Yat T. Tang and Garland R. Marshall

Abstract

The identification of small drug-like compounds that selectively inhibit the function of biological targets has historically been a major focus in the pharmaceutical industry, and in recent years, has generated much interest in academia as well. Drug-like compounds are valuable as chemical genetics tools to probe biological pathways in a reversible, dose- and time-dependent manner for drug target identification. In addition, small molecule compounds can be used to characterize the shape and charge preferences of macromolecular binding sites, for both structure-based and ligand-based drug design. High-throughput screening is the most common experimental method used to identify lead compounds. Because of the cost, time, and resources required for performing high-throughput screening for compound libraries, the use of alternative strategies is necessary for facilitating lead discovery. Virtual screening has been successful in prioritizing large chemical libraries to identify experimentally active compounds, serving as a practical and effective alternative to high-throughput screening. Methodologies used in virtual screening such as molecular docking and scoring have advanced to the point where they can rapidly and accurately identify lead compounds in addition to predicting native binding conformations. This chapter provides instructions on how to perform a virtual screen using freely available tools for structure-based lead discovery.

Key words: Drug discovery, Lead discovery, Molecular docking, Molecular modeling, Structure-based drug design, Virtual screening

1. Introduction

Virtual screening is a computational method for identifying lead compounds from a large and chemically diverse compound library. This computational method is valuable for discovering lead compounds in a faster, more cost-efficient, and less resource-intensive manner compared to experimental methods such as high-throughput screening (1–4). The protocol in this chapter will separate virtual screening into two steps: docking and scoring. AutoDock (5, 6) will perform ligand conformational searches to identify potential bound conformations, and X-Score (7) will

Seetharama D. Satyanarayanajois (ed.), *Drug Design and Discovery: Methods and Protocols*,
Methods in Molecular Biology, vol. 716, DOI 10.1007/978-1-61779-012-6_1,

be used to reevaluate the binding affinity of the predicted structures. AutoDock and X-Score are available for free, widely used and documented, and most importantly, have been successful in identifying novel lead compounds in many studies.

To begin virtual screening, the programs used will be downloaded and installed. The structure files for the compound database and the macromolecule will be downloaded and prepared before screening. The HIV-I protease (8) will be targeted to identify lead compounds from the National Cancer Institute (NCI) Diversity Set (9). For file preparation, ligands in the compound library will have hydrogens added, and will then be converted to a file format compatible with AutoDock. The macromolecule will be prepared by removing the bound ligand and waters from the crystal structure. Hydrogens will be added and partial charges will be calculated. Once the compound library and macromolecule files are prepared, they will be used as input files to begin docking with AutoDock.

After docking is completed, X-Score will be used to rescore the predicted ligand conformations. Binding affinities predicted by X-Score can be used as an alternative scoring method to analyze the results, or it can be used in complement with AutoDock binding energies as a consensus scoring scheme, which has demonstrated to improve discrimination between active and inactive compounds and reduce the number of false positives (10–13). Once the top compound conformations are selected based on the chosen scoring scheme, PyMol will be used to visualize the structures for chemical reasonableness and complementarity.

2. Materials

2.1. AutoDock and AutoGrid (Version 4.2)

1. Download AutoDock and AutoGrid (version 4.2) (6) from the AutoDock webpage (http://autodock.scripps.edu/downloads). Click on "registration form" next to AutoDock 4.2, fill out the information on the registration page, and click on "submit".
2. Select the platform and/or source code, and download the distribution.
3. Follow the installation instructions for your platform to install AutoDock and AutoGrid (http://autodock.scripps.edu/faqs-help/faq/faqsection_view?section=Installing%20AutoDock) (see Note 1).

2.2. AutoDockTools, Autodock and Autogrid (Version 1.5.4, Version 3)

1. Download AutoDockTools (ADT) (version 1.5.4), a preparation and visualization tool for use with AutoDock and AutoGrid, from the Molecular Graphics Lab website (http://mgltools.scripps.edu/downloads). Select the platform and/or source code.

2. Install ADT. For instructions, see http://autodock.scripps.edu/resources/adt.
3. Download a previous version of AutoDock (version 3.0) (5) from the same webpage as AutoDock version 4.2 (http://autodock.scripps.edu/downloads). Click on "instructions".
4. Follow the instructions on obtaining a license and downloading AutoDock.
5. Fill out and sign the Software Distribution Agreement. Once the Agreement has been returned, you will receive an email with instructions on how to download the source code. AutoDock 3.0 contains some scripts that will be useful for file processing.

2.3. AutoDock4 Virtual Screening Tutorial Files

1. Download a set of files from the AutoDock4 virtual screening tutorial (see Note 2) that will be useful for file preparation and analysis with AutoDock4. Go to http://autodock.scripps.edu/faqs-help/tutorial/using-autodock4-for-virtual-screening. Click on the link "VSTutorial files from CVS" to download the file "VSTutorial.tar.gz".
2. After the download is completed make a directory called "VSTutorial", and move the file "VSTutorial.tar.gz" into the new directory with the commands:

   mkdir VSTutorial

   mv VSTutorial.tar.gz VSTutorial
3. Unzip and extract the "VSTutorial.tar.gz" file with the command:

   tar –xvzf VSTutorial.tar.gz.

   This will unzip a number of files used in the virtual screening tutorial from the AutoDock website. Some scripts used in this tutorial will be useful for file formatting.

2.4. X-Score (Version 1.2)

1. Download X-Score (version 1.2) (7) from http://sw16.im.med.umich.edu/software/xtool/. Click on "Click here to get the X-Score v1.2 package now". Read through and accept the license agreement by clicking on "Yes" at the bottom of the page. Fill out the listed information to register, and click on "Submit".
2. Follow the instructions to download and install X-Score.

2.5. OpenBabel (Version 2.2.3)

1. Download OpenBabel, a program for molecular file format conversion, at http://openbabel.org/wiki/Main_Page. Click on "Get OpenBabel".
2. Follow the instructions to download and install OpenBabel for your platform. For more information, see http://openbabel.org/wiki/Guides.

2.6. PyMol

1. Download the PyMol Molecular Viewer at http://pymol.sourceforge.net/. Click on "Download". For education use only, click on "being approved" under "PyMol Starting Points For Potential Project Sponsors". On the next page, click on "registration form", and fill out the information to register.
2. Follow the instructions to download and install PyMol.

2.7. Compound Library (Structure Files)

1. Download a filtered, drug-like version of the NCI Diversity library: Go to http://gfscore.cnrs-mrs.fr/diversity.htm. Click on the link to "Download the 1420 filtered diversity library" to download the file diversity1440.sdf (rename to diversity1420.sdf after download to avoid confusion). This NCI Diversity library contains representative compounds derived from the larger NCI library of 140,000 compounds. These compounds can be ordered for free, making it an attractive library to use for initial screening (see Note 3). For more information, see http://dtp.nci.nih.gov/branches/dscb/diversity_explanation.html.
2. To view structures and details of each compound, visit the Enhanced NCI Database Browser (http://129.43.27.140/ncidb2/).

2.8. Macromolecule

1. The macromolecule target used for this exercise is the HIV-I protease. Search for "1HSG" at the Protein Data Bank (PDB) (http://www.rcsb.org/pdb) (14). This entry contains a high-resolution structure of HIV-I protease with a bound inhibitor. Download the structure in pdb format by clicking on "Download Files" and selecting "PDB File (text)" (see Notes 4 & 5).

3. Methods

The virtual screening workflow can be divided into three steps: file preparation, docking, and scoring. To prepare the receptor, the bound ligand and water molecules will be deleted from the crystal structure. Polar hydrogens will be added, partial charges will be computed, and AutoDock atom types will be assigned for the macromolecule using AutoDockTools. The bound ligand will be prepared for the purpose of setting up the docking grid. To prepare the compound library, the file downloaded from NCI will have hydrogens added to each compound, and subsequently converted from sdf format to mol2 format using OpenBabel. The mol2 file, known as a multi-mol2 file since it contains compounds from the entire NCI Diversity library, will be separated into individual files and renamed. The mol2 files will be converted to the

AutoDock pdbqt format to specify the rotatable bonds for the docking conformational searches.

After the macromolecule is cleaned up, the docking grid will be specified to constrain the search area. Using AutoDockTools, a grid parameter file (gpf) will be generated to state the macromolecule location, size, and atoms types for computing grid maps. AutoGrid takes the parameters from the gpf file and generates grid maps for use with AutoDock.

To run AutoDock, a docking parameter file (dpf) will be generated for each ligand and modified with more exhaustive parameters for the Lamarckian genetic algorithm. After all the files needed for docking have been generated, the virtual screening process can begin. Computing time required for screening will depend on several factors: the size and number of rotatable bonds in the ligand, the size of the docking grid, the genetic algorithm parameters, and the number of runs.

After docking is completed, AutoDock will output the docked structures and binding free energies in the docking log file (dlg). The name of the ligand and pose, structural coordinates, binding free energies, and cluster sizes will be parsed out of the dlg file. The structures will be converted into pdb, and subsequently mol2 formats. X-Score will be used to rescore the docked conformations as an alternative method for scoring and postfiltering. A consensus scoring method can be used by taking into account both the AutoDock binding energies and X-Score binding energies.

Some steps of the virtual screening workflow will be performed with a user interface, while other steps will be performed using terminal commands. In order to automate the preparation and analysis processes, the user will need to have working knowledge on scripting for running commands, parsing files, and editing texts.

3.1. Preparing the Macromolecule in AutoDockTools

1. Start AutoDockTools.
2. Load the macromolecule structure in ADT: Click on File > Read Molecule. This will open up a file browser showing all the files in the directory where ADT was started. Select the file, 1HSG.pdb, and click on Open. The structure of 1HSG will be loaded in the viewer.
3. Color the atoms by atom type: Click on Color > by Atom Type. Select All Geometries, and click on OK. This will set the atom colors according to the atom types. The color scheme is the following: aliphatic carbons (white), aromatic carbons (green), nitrogens (blue), oxygens (red), sulfurs (yellow), hydrogens (cyan).
4. Select the waters to be removed from the structure: Click on Select > Select from String. The Select from String window will appear. Click on the Residue text box, type "HOH*" to

specify all waters, then click on the Atom text box, and type "*" to select all atoms. Click on Add. This will select all atoms in the water molecules. Click on Dismiss to close the Select from String window. At the bottom of the ADT window, you will notice that the Selected window is now in yellow, stating "127 atom(s) have been selected".

5. Remove the selected water molecules: Click on Edit > Delete > Delete AtomSet. A WARNING window will pop-up stating that the deleting cannot be undone. Click on Continue to delete the atom set.
6. Select the bound ligand for removal: Click on Select > Select from String. The Select from String window will appear. Click on the Residue text box, type "MK1*" to specify the ligand, then click on the Atom text window, and type "*". Click on Add. This will select all ligand atoms. Click on Dismiss to close the Select from String window. At the bottom of the ADT window, you will notice that the Selected window has turned yellow, stating "45 atom(s) have been selected".
7. Remove the selected ligand atoms: Click on Edit > Delete > Delete AtomSet. A WARNING window will appear stating that the deleting cannot be undone. Click on CONTINUE to delete the atom set.
8. Add hydrogens to the receptor: Click on Edit > Hydrogens > Add. The Add Hydrogens window will appear. Select Add Hydrogens using Method noBondOrder (for pdb files...). Select yes to renumber atoms to include new hydrogens.
9. Save the receptor file with waters deleted and hydrogens added in the pdb format: Click on File > Save > Write PDB. The Write Options window will appear. In the Filename text box, change the name to 1hsg.pdb. By default the PDB records to be saved are ATOM and HETATM only. Select Sort Nodes under Other write options. Be sure not to write CONECT records. Click on OK to write out 1hsg.pdb.
10. Calculate the partial charges and determine the atom types of the macromolecule: Click on Grid (Fig. 1) > Macromolecule > Choose... A WARNING window will appear stating that it is initializing 1hsg. Click on OK. Initializing the macromolecule includes the following steps: computing Gasteiger partial charges (requires that all hydrogens were added), merging nonpolar hydrogen atoms, and assigning AutoDock atom types. A file browser will appear. Save file as 1hsg.pdbqt and click on Save (Figs. 2 & 3). The pdbqt format includes two additional columns compared to a pdb file: a charge column with Gasteiger partial charges, and an atom type column containing AutoDock atom types. Figure 2a shows a simplified work flow for preparing the macromolecule file.

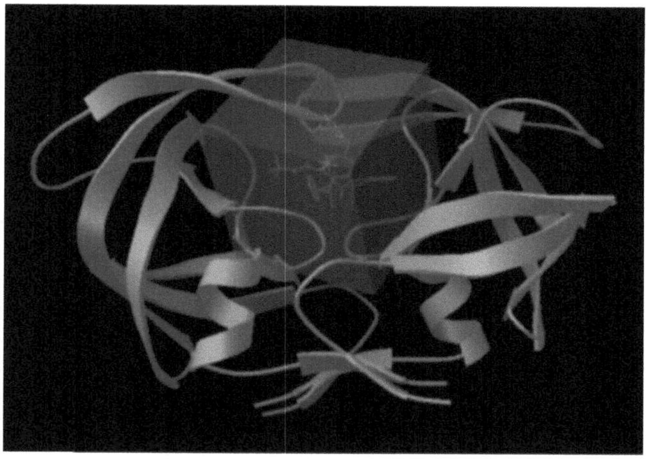

Fig. 1. AutoDockTools is used to set up the docking grid for the macromolecule 1HSG. The macromolecule, HIV-I protease, is shown in *ribbon*, and the bound inhibitor is shown in *sticks*. The grid size used was based on the size of the bound inhibitor from the crystal structure, and the grid spacing is the default value at 0.375 Å.

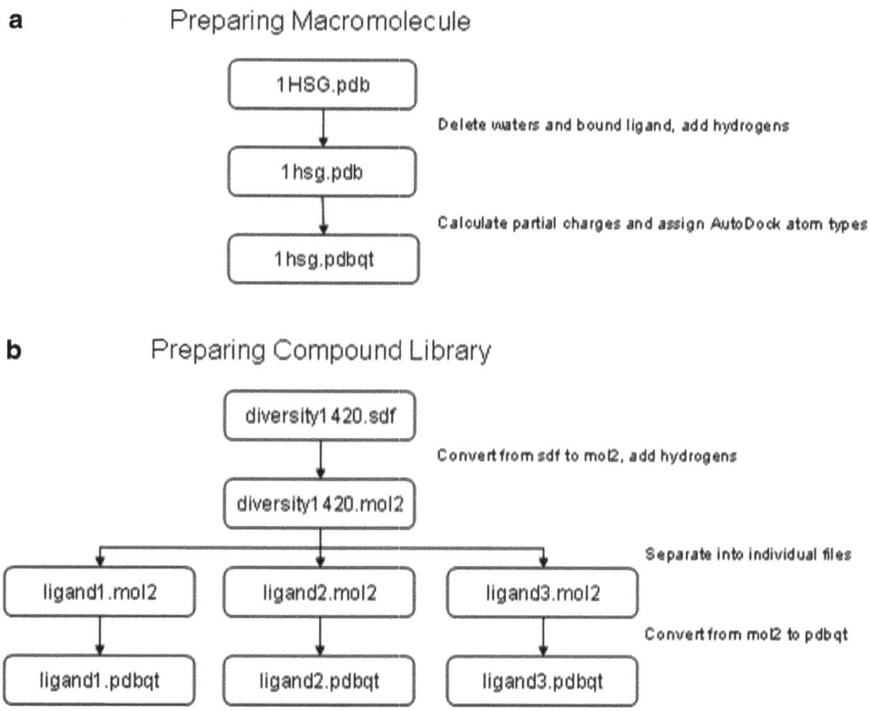

Fig. 2. Workflow chart for processing the compound library and macromolecule files. (**a**) The macromolecular structure file for HIV-I protease (1HSG.pdb) is downloaded from the Protein Data Bank. AutoDockTools will be used to delete all waters and the bound ligand, and also add hydrogens (1hsg.pdb). Next, partial charges and AutoDock atom types will be assigned (1hsg.pdbqt). (**b**) The drug-like filtered version of the compound library, diversity1420.sdf, is downloaded in standard drug format (sdf). OpenBabel is used to convert the sdf format to the SYBYL mol2 format diversity1420.mol2 with all hydrogens added to the compounds. The compound library file will then be separated using the script "split_multi_mol2_file.py" to form individual mol2 files for each compound. Each mol2 file will be converted using the script "prepare_ligand4.py" into AutoDock pdbqt files.

```
REMARK  4 XXXX COMPLIES WITH FORMAT V. 2.0
ATOM      1  N    PRO A   1      29.361  39.686   5.862  1.00 38.10     -0.038 N
ATOM      2  HN1  PRO A   1      28.682  40.038   5.187  1.00  0.00      0.280 HD
ATOM      3  HN2  PRO A   1      29.784  40.592   6.064  1.00  0.00      0.280 HD
ATOM      4  CA   PRO A   1      30.307  38.663   5.319  1.00 40.62      0.259 C
ATOM      5  C    PRO A   1      29.760  38.071   4.022  1.00 42.64      0.259 C
ATOM      6  O    PRO A   1      28.600  38.302   3.676  1.00 43.40     -0.271 OA
ATOM      7  CB   PRO A   1      30.508  37.541   6.342  1.00 37.87      0.042 C
ATOM      8  CG   PRO A   1      29.296  37.591   7.162  1.00 38.40      0.035 C
ATOM      9  CD   PRO A   1      28.778  39.015   7.019  1.00 38.74      0.210 C
ATOM     10  N    GLN A   2      30.607  37.334   3.305  1.00 41.76     -0.338 N
ATOM     11  HN   GLN A   2      31.600  37.358   3.536  1.00  0.00      0.164 HD
ATOM     12  CA   GLN A   2      30.158  36.492   2.199  1.00 41.30      0.160 C
ATOM     13  C    GLN A   2      30.298  35.041   2.643  1.00 41.38      0.251 C
ATOM     14  O    GLN A   2      31.401  34.494   2.763  1.00 43.09     -0.271 OA
ATOM     15  CB   GLN A   2      30.970  36.738   0.926  1.00 40.81      0.042 C
ATOM     16  CG   GLN A   2      30.625  35.783  -0.201  1.00 46.61      0.090 C
ATOM     17  CD   GLN A   2      31.184  36.217  -1.549  1.00 50.36      0.227 C
ATOM     18  OE1  GLN A   2      32.006  35.518  -2.156  1.00 53.89     -0.273 OA
ATOM     19  NE2  GLN A   2      30.684  37.339  -2.061  1.00 51.46     -0.369 N
ATOM     20 1HE2 GLN A   2      31.059  37.630  -2.964  1.00  0.00      0.159 HD
ATOM     21 2HE2 GLN A   2      30.007  37.915  -1.561  1.00  0.00      0.159 HD
ATOM     22  N    ILE A   3      29.160  34.436   2.919  1.00 37.80     -0.338 N
```

Fig. 3. Example of the macromolecule pdbqt file prepared for 1HSG. The pdbqt format is similar to the pdb format, with the exception of two additional columns at the end: the charge column (in this case, Gasteiger charges) and the AutoDock atom type column.

3.2. Preparing the Ligand in AutoDockTools

1. Start AutoDockTools.
2. Load the macromolecule structure in ADT: Click on File > Read Molecule. This will open up a file browser showing all the files in the directory where ADT was started. Select the file, 1HSG.pdb, and click on Open. You will see the structure of 1HSG in the viewer.
3. Select the macromolecule and waters to be removed from the structure: Click on Select > Select from String. The Select from String window will appear. Click on the Residue text box, type "MK1*" to specify the ligand, then click on the Atom text box, and type "*". Click on Add, then click on Invert Selection. This will select all atoms that are not part of the ligand. Click on Dismiss to close the Select from String box. At the bottom of the ADT window, you will notice that the Selected box is now in yellow, stating "1641 atom(s) have been selected".
4. Remove the macromolecule and waters: Click on Edit > Delete > Delete AtomSet. A WARNING box will appear stating that the deleting cannot be undone. Click on CONTINUE to delete the atom set.
5. Add hydrogens to the ligand: Click on Edit > Hydrogens > Add. The Add Hydrogens window will appear. Select Add Hydrogens using Method noBondOrder (for pdb files…). Select yes to renumber atoms to include new hydrogens.

6. Prepare the ligand as pdbqt file: Click on Ligand > Input > Choose. The Choose Molecule for AutoDock4 window will appear. Select 1HSG, and click on Select Molecule for AutoDock4. The window, summary for 1HSG, will appear stating the following setup: added gasteiger charges, merged 42 nonpolar hydrogens, found 17 aromatic carbons, detected 16 rotatable bonds, set TORSDOF to 14. Click on OK.
7. Select the root of the ligand: Click on Ligand > Torsion Tree > Detect Root... ADT will detect the atom to be used as the root, and will be displayed by a green sphere.
8. Choose the torsions in the ligand: Click on Ligand > Torsion Tree > Choose Torsions... The Torsion Count window will appear. This window allows you to select the different types of bonds to be rotatable or nonrotatable. It also states that 14 out of 32 bonds on the ligand are rotatable. The molecular viewer displays rotatable bonds in green, nonrotatable bonds in red, and rotatable but inactive bonds in purple. Click on Done in the Torsion Count window to exit.
9. Save the ligand as a pdbqt file: Click on Ligand > Output > Save as PDBQT... A file browser, Formatted Autotors Molecule File, will appear. Save the file as 1hsg_ligand.pdbqt and click on Save.

3.3. Preparing the Compound Library for AutoDock

1. Convert the compound library from sdf to mol2 format. Use OpenBabel to convert the diversity1420.sdf file to a format that can be used with the AutoDock preparation tools, such as the mol2 format. The OpenBabel command to add hydrogens to the ligands and perform the file format conversion is:

   ```
   babel -isdf diversity1420.sdf -omol2 diversity1420.mol2 -h
   ```

   In the first flag, "-isdf" specifies that the input file is in sdf format. In the second flag, "-omol2" specifies that the output file is in mol2 format. The third flag, "-h", specifies adding hydrogens to the compounds.
2. The mol2 file converted by OpenBabel will need to be separated into individual files. This can be done using the script "split_multi_mol2_file.py" in the VSTutorial directory. Create a new directory, mol2, to keep the individual mol2 files. Copy "split_multi_mol2_file.py" into that directory. The command to use is:

   ```
   ./split_multi_mol2.py -i diversity1420.mol2
   ```

   Be sure to specify the proper directory of diversity1420.mol2. This will now create 1420 individual mol2 files, named according to their NSC number, for each ligand (see Note 6).
3. Convert the mol2 files into the AutoDock pdbqt format. Run the script "prepare_ligand4.py", located in the mgltools

directory (/mgltools_platform_1.5.4/MGLToolsPckgs/AutoDockTools/Utilities24/). The general command for running the script is:

pythonsh prepare_ligand4.py -l ligand.mol2

Before proceeding, there are a few points to consider. First, you will need to do this for all the ligands, so you will need to write a script to run this command for each mol2 file. Also, you need to specify the location of "pythonsh" (/mgltools_platform_1.5.4/bin/), where "platform" is substituted by the platform you are using. The flag, "-l" specifies the name of the ligand file. The output file name will be the same as the input file name, except with the .pdbqt extension (Fig. 4). Figure 2b shows a simplified workflow for preparing the compound library.

```
REMARK  3 active torsions:
REMARK  status: ('A' for Active; 'I' for Inactive)
REMARK    1  A    between atoms: C1_1  and  C2_2
REMARK    2  A    between atoms: C1_1  and  C3_3
REMARK    3  A    between atoms: C2_2  and  C6_6
ROOT
ATOM      1  C2  <1> d           0.000   0.000   0.000  0.00  0.00     0.148 A
ATOM      2  C4  <1> d           0.000   0.000   1.510  0.00  0.00     0.259 A
ATOM      3  N5  <1> d           1.434   0.000  -0.323  0.00  0.00    -0.320 N
ATOM      4  O9  <1> d          -0.983   0.000   2.249  0.00  0.00    -0.270 OA
ATOM      5  N10 <1> d           1.278   0.000   1.879  0.00  0.00    -0.277 N
ATOM      6  C11 <1> d           2.096   0.000   0.830  0.00  0.00     0.324 A
ATOM      7  O16 <1> d           3.343   0.000   0.919  0.00  0.00    -0.247 OA
ATOM      8  H21 <1> d           1.589   0.000   2.840  0.00  0.00     0.173 HD
ATOM      9  H22 <1> d           1.840   0.000  -1.248  0.00  0.00     0.165 HD
ENDROOT
BRANCH   1  10
ATOM     10  C1  <1> d          -0.718  -1.220  -0.575  0.00  0.00     0.085 C
BRANCH  10  11
ATOM     11  C3  <1> d          -2.170  -1.192  -0.159  0.00  0.00    -0.055 A
ATOM     12  C7  <1> d          -3.112  -0.527  -0.953  0.00  0.00     0.007 A
ATOM     13  C14 <1> d          -4.458  -0.501  -0.567  0.00  0.00     0.001 A
ATOM     14  C19 <1> d          -4.861  -1.139   0.612  0.00  0.00     0.000 A
ATOM     15  C15 <1> d          -3.918  -1.803   1.406  0.00  0.00     0.001 A
ATOM     16  C8  <1> d          -2.573  -1.830   1.020  0.00  0.00     0.007 A
ENDBRANCH  10  11
ENDBRANCH   1  10
BRANCH   1  17
ATOM     17  C6  <1> d          -0.710   1.206  -0.568  0.00  0.00    -0.003 A
ATOM     18  C12 <1> d          -0.360   1.707  -1.827  0.00  0.00     0.013 A
ATOM     19  C17 <1> d          -1.038   2.827  -2.325  0.00  0.00     0.020 A
ATOM     20  C20 <1> d          -2.045   3.410  -1.548  0.00  0.00     0.116 A
ATOM     21  N18 <1> d          -2.357   2.907  -0.345  0.00  0.00    -0.272 NA
ATOM     22  C13 <1> d          -1.727   1.837   0.158  0.00  0.00     0.126 A
ENDBRANCH   1  17
TORSDOF 3
```

Fig. 4. Example of a ligand pdbqt file from the NCI Diversity library. The REMARK lines at the beginning of the file state that the ligand has three active torsions that will be considered in the conformational search. The atoms between the ROOT and ENDROOT section will not be moved during the conformational search. The atoms moved by each rotatable bond are stated between the BRANCH and ENDBRANCH section.

3.4. Preparing the Grid Parameter File in AutoDockTools

1. Open the macromolecule file 1hsg.pdbqt in ADT: Click on File > Read Molecule. This will open a file browser in the directory where ADT was started. Select the file, 1hsg.pdbqt, and click on Open.
2. Select 1hsg.pdbqt as the file to use for setting up grids: Click on Grid > Macromolecule > Choose. The Choose Molecule box will appear. Select 1hsg. A window will appear asking to preserve input receptor charges instead of adding Gasteiger charges. Click on Yes to keep the charges. A WARNING box will then pop-up, showing the initialization of the pdbqt file, stating that the autodock_elements and gasteiger charges have already been added. Click on OK.
3. Select the ligand and generate maps: Click on Grid > Set Map Types > Choose Ligand... The Choose Ligand window will appear. Click on 1hsg_ligand and click on Select Ligand (assuming the ligand file is open). By selecting the ligand, the gpf will specify AutoGrid to generate maps for atom types present in the ligand. This line of the gpf file will be edited in a text editor to include additional atom types for virtual screening purposes.
4. Specify the dimensions, spacing, and center of the grid box: Click on Grid > Grid Box. The Grid Options window will appear. Specify the grid box center to be where the ligand is located. In the Grid Options window, click on the Center tab and select Center on ligand. The grid box center is now located at 12.064, 22.47, 5.858 (x center, y center, z center). The size of the grid box, as shown in Fig. 1, is 42×40×40 using a 0.375 Å resolution grid. Click on File and select Close saving current to save the modified grid options parameters (see Note 7).
5. Save the grid parameter file as a 1hsg.gpf: Click on Grid > Output > Save GPF... A file browser will appear. Type in the filename and click on Save.
6. Edit the grid parameter file in a text editor. Two separate gpf files will need to be prepared to calculate all the atom types necessary for virtual screening, since AutoGrid allows only 14 atom types maps to be constructed at a time. Save the gpf files as 1hsg_1.gpf and 1hsg_2.gpf.

   Change line 5 from

   ligand_types A C OA HD N to the following and save as 1hsg_1.gpf

   ligand_types A Br Cl C Fe F HD H HS I and to the following and save as 1hsg_2.gpf

   ligand_types NA N NS OA OS P SA S to include all possible atom types present in the NCI library.

   For each of the addition atom types, add in the corresponding line for creating and naming of the atom type map. For example, v the Br atom type, insert the line "map 1hsg.Br.map"in the section where the lines stating atom-specific affinity maps are located.

Save the modified version of the grid parameter files. See Fig. 5 for examples of the file.

3.5. Running AutoGrid to Create Grid Maps

1. Run AutoGrid to create the grid maps for the macromolecule: Run AutoGrid in the same directory where the ligand, macromolecule, and grid parameter files are located. AutoGrid can be accessed using ADT or by command line. In ADT, click on Run > Run AutoGrid… The Run AutoGrid window will appear. By default, the Macro Name and Host Name will specify your local machine. The Program Pathname specifies where the AutoGrid executable is located. The Parameter Filename specifies the grid parameter file (Fig. 5a, b). The Log Filename specifies the grid log file for the AutoGrid run. By default, the name will be the same as the grid parameter file, except with the extension .glg. The Nice Level specifies the nice level for remote jobs. Cmd specifies the command that will be executed. Click on Launch to start the job. The AutoDock Process Manager window will appear providing status of the job.

   Alternatively, AutoGrid can be run via command line by typing:

   autogrid4 –p 1hsg_1.gpf –l 1hsg_1.glg &

   autogrid4 –p 1hsg_2.gpf –l 1hsg_2.glg &

2. Grid maps will be created for each atom type specified, as well as for the electrostatic potential and desolvation energies. Other files created are the xyz file to specify the grid box size, and the fld file with other information about the grid. The grid log file (glg) will contain a summary from the AutoGrid run.

3.6. Creating the Docking Parameter File in AutoDockTools

1. Because each ligand will require a separate docking parameter file (dpf), scripting will be necessary to automate this procedure. Also, each ligand and its corresponding files that are needed for docking should be placed in separate directories to avoid confusion. For example, in the directory where you are currently working in, create subdirectories for each ligand (e.g., "nsc479" for ligand 479).

2. Run the script prepare_dpf4.py to generate docking parameter files for each ligand. The command for running the script is:

   pythonsh prepare_dpf42.py –l ligand.pdbqt –r 1hsg.pdbqt –o ligand.1hsg.dpf

   Specify the directory where pythonsh (/mgltools_platform_1.5.4/bin/) and prepare_dpf42.py (/mgltools_platform_1.5.4/MGLToolsPckgs/AutoDockTools/Utilities24/) are located, where "platform" will be substituted by the platform you are using. The first flag, -l, a

```
npts 42 40 40                          # num.grid points in xyz
gridfld 1hsg.maps.fld                  # grid_data_file
spacing 0.375                          # spacing(A)
receptor_types A C HD N OA SA          # receptor atom types
ligand_types A Br Cl C Fe F HD H HS I NA # ligand atom types
#ligand_types N NS OA OS P SA S        # ligand atom types
receptor 1hsg.pdbqt                    # macromolecule
gridcenter 12.064 22.47 5.858          # xyz-coordinates or auto
smooth 0.5                             # store minimum energy w/in rad(A)
map 1hsg.A.map                         # atom-specific affinity map
map 1hsg.Br.map                        # atom-specific affinity map
map 1hsg.Cl.map                        # atom-specific affinity map
map 1hsg.C.map                         # atom-specific affinity map
map 1hsg.Fe.map                        # atom-specific affinity map
map 1hsg.F.map                         # atom-specific affinity map
map 1hsg.HD.map                        # atom-specific affinity map
map 1hsg.H.map                         # atom-specific affinity map
map 1hsg.HS.map                        # atom-specific affinity map
map 1hsg.I.map                         # atom-specific affinity map
map 1hsg.NA.map                        # atom-specific affinity map
#map 1hsg.N.map                         # atom-specific affinity map
#map 1hsg.NS.map                        # atom-specific affinity map
#map 1hsg.OA.map                        # atom-specific affinity map
#map 1hsg.OS.map                        # atom-specific affinity map
#map 1hsg.P.map                         # atom-specific affinity map
#map 1hsg.SA.map                        # atom-specific affinity map
#map 1hsg.S.map                         # atom-specific affinity map
elecmap 1hsg.e.map                     # electrostatic potential map
dsolvmap 1hsg.d.map                # desolvation potential map
dielectric -0.1465                     # <0, AD4 distance-dep.diel;>0, constant
```

b

```
npts 42 40 40                          # num.grid points in xyz
gridfld 1hsg.maps.fld                  # grid_data_file
spacing 0.375                          # spacing(A)
receptor_types A C HD N OA SA          # receptor atom types
#ligand_types A Br Cl C Fe F HD H HS I NA # ligand atom types
ligand_types N NS OA OS P SA S        # ligand atom types
receptor 1hsg.pdbqt                    # macromolecule
gridcenter 12.064 22.47 5.858          # xyz-coordinates or auto
smooth 0.5                             # store minimum energy w/in rad(A)
#map 1hsg.A.map                         # atom-specific affinity map
#map 1hsg.Br.map                        # atom-specific affinity map
#map 1hsg.Cl.map                        # atom-specific affinity map
#map 1hsg.C.map                         # atom-specific affinity map
#map 1hsg.Fe.map                        # atom-specific affinity map
#map 1hsg.F.map                         # atom-specific affinity map
#map 1hsg.HD.map                        # atom-specific affinity map
#map 1hsg.H.map                         # atom-specific affinity map
#map 1hsg.HS.map                        # atom-specific affinity map
#map 1hsg.I.map                         # atom-specific affinity map
#map 1hsg.NA.map                        # atom-specific affinity map
map 1hsg.N.map                         # atom-specific affinity map
map 1hsg.NS.map                        # atom-specific affinity map
map 1hsg.OA.map                        # atom-specific affinity map
map 1hsg.OS.map                        # atom-specific affinity map
map 1hsg.P.map                         # atom-specific affinity map
map 1hsg.SA.map                        # atom-specific affinity map
map 1hsg.S.map                         # atom-specific affinity map
elecmap 1hsg.e.map                     # electrostatic potential map
dsolvmap 1hsg.d.map                # desolvation potential map
dielectric -0.1465                     # <0, AD4 distance-dep.diel;>0, constant
```

Fig. 5. The AutoDock grid parameter files (gpf) that are used to generate atom type grid maps for 1HSG. (**a**) This is the first gpf file that will be used to grid maps. Note that the lines commented out, denoted with "#", will be used in the second grid map. (**b**) The second grid map for 1HSG. Using a text editor, the size of the grid (npts), grid spacing (spacing), and gridcenter (gridcenter) can be adjusted to specify the docking search space.

```
autodock_parameter_version 4.2      # used by autodock to validate parameter set
outlev 1
write_all
intelec                             # calculate internal electrostatics
seed pid time                       # seeds for random generator
ligand_types A C HD N NA OA         # atoms types in ligand
fld 1hsg.maps.fld                   # grid_data_file
map 1hsg.A.map                      # atom-specific affinity map
map 1hsg.C.map                      # atom-specific affinity map
map 1hsg.HD.map                     # atom-specific affinity map
map 1hsg.N.map                      # atom-specific affinity map
map 1hsg.NA.map                     # atom-specific affinity map
map 1hsg.OA.map                     # atom-specific affinity map
elecmap 1hsg.e.map                  # electrostatics map
desolvmap 1hsg.d.map                # desolvation map
move nsc479.pdbqt                   # small molecule
about -0.8841 0.2583 0.1357         # small molecule center
tran0 random                        # initial coordinates/A or random
axisangle0 random                   # initial orientation
dihe0 random                        # initial dihedrals (relative) or random
qstep 50.0                          # quaternion step/deg
dstep 50.0                          # torsion step/deg
torsdof 3                           # torsional degrees of freedom
rmstol 2.0                          # cluster_tolerance/A
extnrg 1000.0                       # external grid energy
e0max 0.0 10000                     # max initial energy; max number of retries
ga_pop_size 150                     # number of individuals in population
ga_num_evals 2500000                # maximum number of energy evaluations
ga_num_generations 27000            # maximum number of generations
ga_elitism 1                        # number of top individuals to survive to next generation
ga_mutation_rate 0.02               # rate of gene mutation
ga_crossover_rate 0.8               # rate of crossover
ga_window_size 10                   #
ga_cauchy_alpha 0.0                 # Alpha parameter of Cauchy distribution
ga_cauchy_beta 1.0                  # Beta parameter Cauchy distribution
set_ga                              # set the above parameters for GA or LGA
sw_max_its 300                      # iterations of Solis & Wets local search
sw_max_succ 4                       # consecutive successes before changing rho
sw_max_fail 4                       # consecutive failures before changing rho
sw_rho 1.0                          # size of local search space to sample
sw_lb_rho 0.01                      # lower bound on rho
ls_search_freq 0.06                 # probability of performing local search on individual
set_psw1                            # set the above pseudo-Solis & Wets parameters
unbound_model bound                 # state of unbound ligand
ga_run 10                           # do this many hybrid GA-LS runs
analysis                            # perform a ranked cluster analysis
```

Fig. 6. The AutoDock docking parameter file (dpf) used for docking one of the compounds in the NCI Diversity library. Some of the parameters commonly adjusted for search exhaustiveness are ga_pop_size, ga_num_evals, ga_num_generations, and ga_run. This example contains the default values from AutoDock.

specifies the ligand input file (substitute "ligand" for name of ligand), the second flag, -r, specifies the receptor input file, and the third flag, -o, represents the output docking parameter file. A sample dpf file is shown in Fig. 6.

3. *Optional*: Edit the ligand.1hsg.dpf files using a script to change the following parameters.

   ga_num_evals – from 2,500,000 to 5,000,000

   ga_run – from 10 to 30.

   The parameter, ga_num_evals, specifies the number of times the energy will be evaluated during the docking search. The ga_run parameter is the number of times the docking search is performed, which is also the number of docked ligand conformations generated by AutoDock.

4. Insert the line, “write_all”, after the line, “outlev 1”, to specify the output of docked ligand conformations from each genetic algorithm run (see Note 8).

3.7. Running AutoDock to Perform Virtual Screening

1. Place the ligand and macromolecule pdbqt files, grid map files generated by AutoGrid, and docking parameter file in the same directory for each ligand.
2. Perform docking using AutoDock with the command:

   autodock4 -p ligand.1hsg.dpf -l ligand.1hsg.dlg &

   The first flag, “-p”, specifies the input docking parameter file, and the second flag, “-l”, specifies the docking log file (dlg). After docking is completed, the results will be written to the dlg file.

   A script will be needed to go through each ligand directory and execute AutoDock4. Creating a routine for submitting AutoDock4 virtual screening jobs also varies based on the computer cluster and queuing system that is being used.

3.8. Analyzing AutoDock Docking Results

1. AutoDock results will be written in the docking log file (dlg) as shown if Fig. 7.
2. The tool “get-dockings”, located in the AutoDock3 directory (/AUTODOCK/dist305/share), is used to extract information of the docked conformations in the dlg file and convert it into a pdb file. The get-dockings command is:

   get-dockings ligand.1hsg.dlg

   Specify the directory where “get-dockings” is located. The output file will be named the same, with the pdb extension appended at the end (e.g., ligand.1hsg.dlg.pdb).
3. Modify the atom types in the PDB file. The atom types of chlorine and bromine were incorrectly converted to “l” and “r”, respectively. Use a text editor to edit “l” to “Cl” and “r” to “Br”.
4. Use OpenBabel to add hydrogens and convert the pdb format to mol2 format:

   babel -ipdb protein-ligand.dlg.pdb -omol2 ligand.1hsg.mol2 -h
5. Write a script to parse out the ligand name and run number from the pdb file, and substitute it in as the name of each ligand in the mol2 file. In the pdb file, the ligand name can be found in the line

   “USER DFP”

   and the run number in the line

   “USER Run”

   In the mol2 file, the ligand name and run number (e.g., 479model1) can be overwritten in the second line of the file.

```
DOCKED: MODEL        1
DOCKED: USER    Run = 1
DOCKED: USER    DPF = nsc479.1hsg.dpf
DOCKED: USER
DOCKED: USER    Estimated Free Energy of Binding    =   -6.39 kcal/mol  [=(1)+(2)+(3)-(4)]
DOCKED: USER    Estimated Inhibition Constant, Ki   =   20.84 uM (micromolar)  [Temperature = 29
8.15 K]
DOCKED: USER
DOCKED: USER    (1) Final Intermolecular Energy     =   -7.28 kcal/mol
DOCKED: USER        vdW + Hbond + desolv Energy     =   -7.07 kcal/mol
DOCKED: USER        Electrostatic Energy            =   -0.21 kcal/mol
DOCKED: USER    (2) Final Total Internal Energy     =   -0.58 kcal/mol
DOCKED: USER    (3) Torsional Free Energy           =   +0.89 kcal/mol
DOCKED: USER    (4) Unbound System's Energy  [=(2)] =   -0.58 kcal/mol
DOCKED: USER
DOCKED: USER
DOCKED: USER    NEWDPF move nsc479.pdbqt
DOCKED: USER    NEWDPF about -0.884100 0.258300 0.135700
DOCKED: USER    NEWDPF tran0 8.883953 27.561301 7.319892
DOCKED: USER    NEWDPF quaternion0 -0.061423 0.582569 0.793524 0.164802
DOCKED: USER    NEWDPF axisangle0 -0.062274 0.590645 0.804525 161.028498
DOCKED: USER    NEWDPF quat0 -0.062274 0.590645 0.804525 161.028498 # deprecated
DOCKED: USER    NEWDPF dihe0 -171.26 134.61 148.57
DOCKED: USER
DOCKED: REMARK  3 active torsions:
DOCKED: REMARK  status: ('A' for Active; 'I' for Inactive)
DOCKED: REMARK    1  A    between atoms: C1_1  and  C2_2
DOCKED: REMARK    2  A    between atoms: C1_1  and  C3_3
DOCKED: REMARK    3  A    between atoms: C2_2  and  C6_6
DOCKED: USER                              x       y       z     vdW  Elec       q    Type
DOCKED: USER                           _______ _______ _______ _____ _____   ______ ____
DOCKED: ROOT
DOCKED: ATOM      1  C2  <1> d          8.045  27.213   7.117 -0.27 -0.05    +0.148 A
DOCKED: ATOM      2  C4  <1> d          7.608  28.579   7.591 -0.24 -0.16    +0.259 A
DOCKED: ATOM      3  N5  <1> d          6.793  26.443   7.151 -0.12 +0.09    -0.320 N
DOCKED: ATOM      4  O9  <1> d          8.316  29.574   7.729 -0.44 +0.17    -0.270 OA
DOCKED: ATOM      5  N10 <1> d          6.302  28.487   7.827 -0.20 +0.20    -0.277 N
DOCKED: ATOM      6  C11 <1> d          5.838  27.265   7.575 -0.17 -0.07    +0.324 A
DOCKED: ATOM      7  O16 <1> d          4.643  26.930   7.721 -0.79 -0.03    -0.247 OA
DOCKED: ATOM      8  H21 <1> d          5.732  29.252   8.158 -0.44 -0.23    +0.173 HD
DOCKED: ATOM      9  H22 <1> d          6.680  25.471   6.899 -0.45 -0.10    +0.165 HD
DOCKED: ENDROOT
DOCKED: BRANCH   1  10
DOCKED: ATOM     10  C1  <1> d          8.653  27.258   5.716 -0.34 -0.03    +0.085 C
DOCKED: BRANCH  10  11
DOCKED: ATOM     11  C3  <1> d          8.368  25.958   5.002 -0.21 +0.02    -0.055 A
DOCKED: ATOM     12  C7  <1> d          9.182  24.841   5.230 -0.23 -0.00    +0.007 A
DOCKED: ATOM     13  C14 <1> d          8.918  23.636   4.568 -0.28 -0.00    +0.001 A
```

Fig. 7. The AutoDock docking log file (dlg) contains docking results for one of the compounds in the NCI Diversity library. Shown is the section where the energy and structural coordinates from the first genetic algorithm run are listed. The results are from the first run (denoted in the first two lines as "MODEL 1" and "Run = 1"). The binding free energy (in the line "Estimated Free Energy of Binding") will be used to assess the fitness of the docked poses.

6. To extract the information such as the free energy of the pose and the size of the cluster, write a script to parse out this data from the pdb file. The cluster size is in the line

   "USER Number of conformations in this cluster"

   and the free energy of binding (kcal/mol) in the line

   "USER Estimated Free Energy of Binding".

7. Write a script to append the poses of each ligand from the ligand.1hsg.mol2 files from the separate directories into one

large multi-mol2 file. Name the file dockedresults.mol2. In addition, append together the files stating the binding free energies and cluster sizes of each ligand from separate directories into a single file, so sorting can be performed. Name this file dockedenergies.txt.

8. To assess the best pose from the AutoDock results, the free energy of binding and the cluster size can be considered. In general, conformations with the lowest free energy of binding and the largest cluster size are most likely to be true positive hits. A large cluster size suggests that the search has converged to a particular low energy conformation.
9. Visually inspect the poses with the lowest free energies and also poses with the largest clusters for chemical complementarity (e.g., surface and charge complementarity, possible hydrogen bond donors, and acceptors interacting).
10. The AutoDock free energy of binding can be combined with the X-Score binding affinity in a consensus scoring scheme.

3.9. Rescoring with X-Score

1. Create a new directory called "xscore". Copy the macromolecule pdb file, 1hsg.pdb, to the new directory where rescoring will be performed.
2. Copy the file with all the AutoDock poses, dockedresults.mol2, into the xscore directory.
3. Prepare the receptor pdb file for use with X-Score using the command:

   xscore -fixpdb 1hsg.pdb 1hsg-xscore.pdb
4. Prepare the ligand pose mol2 file for use with X-Score using the command:

   xscore -fixmol2 dockedresults.mol2 dockedresults-xscore.mol2
5. Copy the file, score.input, located in /xscore_v1.2.1/example/trypsin into the directory "xscore". This file will be used as a template for the input file.
6. Edit the score.input file in a text editor: Change the lines "RECEPTOR_PDB_FILE" and "LIGAND_MOL2_FILE" with the names of the receptor file (1hsg-xscore.pdb) and mol2 file of all the docked poses (dockedresults-xscore.mol2). Comment out the line "REFERENCE_MOL2_FILE". Save the changes made to the file score.input as shown in Fig. 8.
7. Run X-Score to compute the binding scores of the ligand poses.

   xscore score.input.

3.10. Analyzing Scoring Results from X-Score

1. The computed scores will be written to the file, xscore.table, as shown in Fig. 9. The file is organized where the scores are sorted from highest to lowest. X-Score uses a combination of

```
###########################################################################
#                                XTOOL/SCORE                              #
###########################################################################
###
FUNCTION        SCORE
###
### specify the input and output files -------------------------------
###
#
RECEPTOR_PDB_FILE    ./1hsg-xscore.pdb
#REFERENCE_MOL2_FILE  ./1ppc_ligand.mol2
#COFACTOR_MOL2_FILE  none
LIGAND_MOL2_FILE     ./dockedresults-xscore.mol2
#
OUTPUT_TABLE_FILE    ./xscore.table
OUTPUT_LOG_FILE      ./xscore.log
###
### how many top hits to extract from the LIGAND_MOL2_FILE?
###
#NUMBER_OF_HITS       100
#HITS_DIRECTORY       ./hits.mdb
###
### want to include atomic binding scores in the resulting Mol2 files?
###
SHOW_ATOM_BIND_SCORE    YES               [YES/NO]
###
### set up scoring functions -----------------------------------------
###
APPLY_HPSCORE           YES               [YES/NO]
        HPSCORE_CVDW  0.004
        HPSCORE_CHB   0.054
        HPSCORE_CHP   0.009
        HPSCORE_CRT  -0.061
        HPSCORE_C0    3.441
APPLY_HMSCORE           YES               [YES/NO]
        HMSCORE_CVDW  0.004
        HMSCORE_CHB   0.101
        HMSCORE_CHM   0.387
        HMSCORE_CRT  -0.097
        HMSCORE_C0    3.567
APPLY_HSSCORE           YES               [YES/NO]
        HSSCORE_CVDW  0.004
        HSSCORE_CHB   0.073
        HSSCORE_CHS   0.004
        HSSCORE_CRT  -0.090
        HSSCORE_C0    3.328
###
### set up chemical rules for pre-screening ligand molecules ---------
###
APPLY_CHEMICAL_RULES    NO           [YES/NO]
        MAXIMAL_MOLECULAR_WEIGHT      600.0
        MINIMAL MOLECULAR WEIGHT      200.0
```

Fig. 8. Input file for use with X-Score. The macromolecule file will need to be specified in the line "RECEPTOR_PDB_FILE", and the docked poses file in the line "LIGAND_MOL2_FILE". X-Score is composed of three separate scoring functions (HPScore, HMScore, HSScore) with adjustable parameters in the input file. A prescreening filter can also be used before the scoring runs.

Rank	Formula	MW	LogP	HPScore	HMScore	HSScore	Average	Name
1	C32H24N6	492.4	7.31	7.97	8.93	7.85	8.25	nsc372046model1
2	C32H24N6	492.4	7.31	7.99	8.84	7.89	8.24	nsc372046model2
3	C32H24N6	492.4	7.31	8.00	8.76	7.94	8.23	nsc372046model9
4	C32H24N6	492.4	7.31	8.00	8.74	7.93	8.23	nsc372046model8
5	C32H24N6	492.4	7.31	8.00	8.73	7.91	8.21	nsc372046model3
6	C32H24N6	492.4	7.31	8.00	8.72	7.91	8.21	nsc372046model4
7	C32H24N6	492.4	7.31	7.95	8.75	7.92	8.21	nsc372046model5
8	C32H24N6	492.4	7.31	7.99	8.72	7.90	8.21	nsc372046model7
9	C32H24N6	492.4	7.31	7.99	8.71	7.89	8.20	nsc372046model10
10	C32H24N6	492.4	7.31	7.91	8.74	7.90	8.18	nsc372046model6
11	C26H24N2O5S	476.4	4.32	7.33	8.65	7.31	7.76	nsc128437model1
12	C27H20O3	392.3	7.12	7.35	8.53	7.28	7.72	nsc13984model4
13	C27H20O3	392.3	7.12	7.33	8.53	7.28	7.71	nsc13984model3
14	C26H24N2O5S	476.4	4.32	7.41	8.05	7.51	7.66	nsc128437model4
15	C28H20N6	440.3	5.97	7.41	8.17	7.37	7.65	nsc371876model3
16	C28H22O6	454.3	6.10	7.24	8.32	7.32	7.63	nsc157307model7
17	C29H20O6	464.3	5.58	7.35	8.09	7.37	7.60	nsc117274model2
18	C26H23N	349.3	8.09	7.16	8.46	7.18	7.60	nsc99543model4
19	C26H23N	349.3	8.09	7.14	8.46	7.17	7.59	nsc99543model9
20	C28H36N2O	416.3	6.67	7.27	8.32	7.18	7.59	nsc39863model9

Fig. 9. Output file from X-Score. The file lists the poses according to their score (AVERAGE), which is the average of the three different scoring functions used in X-Score. The chemical formula (FORMULA), molecular weight (MW), and logP (LogP) are also listed in the output file.

three different scoring functions to compute the binding scores. The column labeled "Average" is the average of the three scores.

2. To apply a consensus scoring method (10) for evaluating the ligand poses, select poses that appear in the top percentage (e.g., top 10%) of both the AutoDock score and X-Score score for experimental testing.

3.11. Visualize Docking Results Using PyMol

1. Open the receptor.pdb file in PyMol.
2. Open a multi-mol2 file of docked poses in PyMol. Be sure not to open the file with all the poses in it, which will be too many structures for viewing.
3. Create a surface representation of the receptor (select "S" for Show on the right menubar next to the name of the receptor file, then select "surface") (see Fig. 10).
4. Select the ligand by clicking on the name of the file on the right menubar.
5. Use the right and left arrows on your keyboard to select through the different poses.

3.12. Ordering Compounds for Experimental Testing

1. Visit the NCI website (15) (http://dtp.nci.nih.gov/branches/dscb/repo_open.html) for details on requesting compounds, shown in Fig. 11. You will need to fill out your information and complete a list for compounds you want to order.

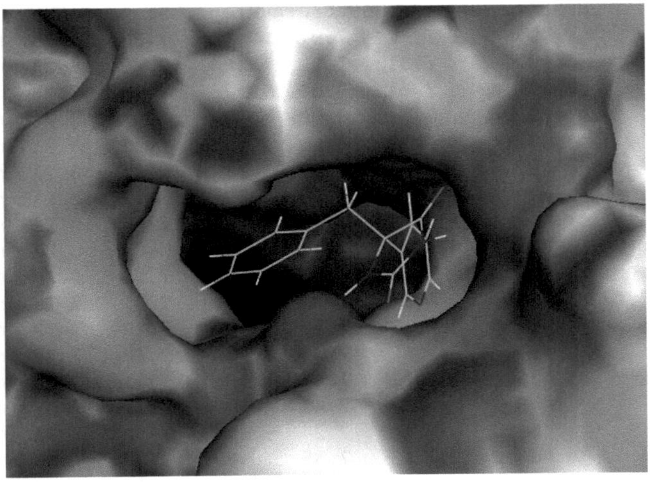

Fig. 10. A docked pose of NSC479 from the NCI Diversity library displayed using PyMol. The compound is displayed in *sticks* and the macromolecule is displayed by *surface.*

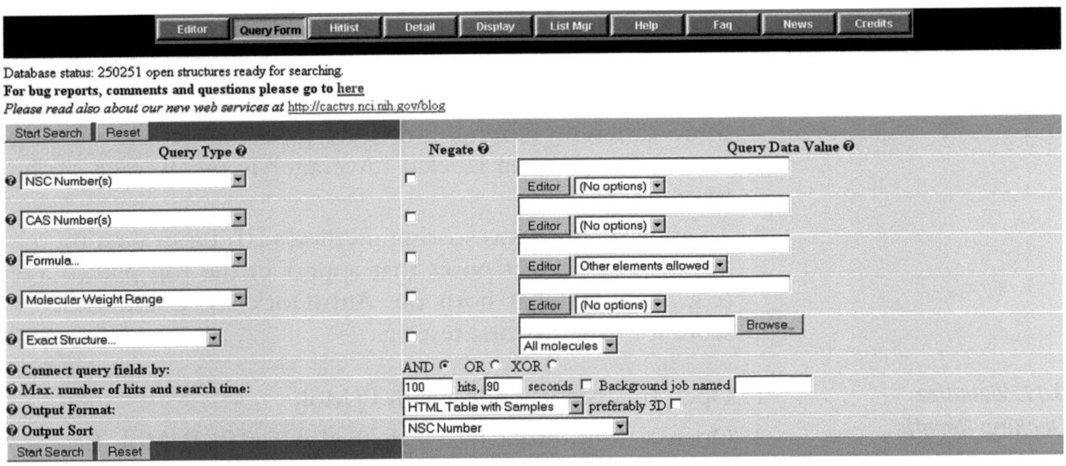

Fig. 11. The query form to find information on the compounds in the NCI Diversity library. The site contains both chemical properties and biological activity data. Similarity searches can also be performed to identify similar compounds in the larger NCI library.

4. Notes

1. Specify the appropriate paths where the downloaded programs are installed.
2. This virtual screening protocol was adapted from the AutoDock4 virtual screening tutorials written by the developers of AutoDock (16). For more information, see http://

autodock.scripps.edu/faqs-help/tutorial/using-autodock4-for-virtual-screening.

3. The NCI Diversity library was chosen in this exercise because compounds can be ordered for free to academics. A larger library to consider screening is ZINC (17) (http://zinc.docking.org). Version 8 of ZINC contains over 13 million purchasable compounds available in ready-to-dock 3-dimensional formats. To filter down the library due to limitations in computational resources, subsets of ZINC can be chosen for screening.
4. Files from the PDB may contain bound ligands, extra subunits, cofactors, and waters, which will need to be removed if they are used as part of the binding site. Files may also contain chain breaks, missing side-chain atoms, or atoms in improper locations that will need to be repaired. AutoDockTools will be used to prepare the macromolecule file. In addition, if more than one high resolution structure is available for your target, docking against the other structures will enhance the sampling of the receptor conformation and possibly increase the probability of identifying hits.
5. If inhibitors are available for the target, they can be added in to your compound database and as a positive control for the screening protocol. For example, if the inhibitors have a high rank, then it suggests that the protocol can identify the true positives.
6. The NCI Database Browser can be used to identify similar compounds, in addition to searching for its chemical properties and biological activities.
7. The grid size can be adjusted by increasing its size to cover more search area of the macromolecule, or decreased to constrain the search area. The resolution can also be adjusted to use a more fine (2.0 Å) or coarse grid. Note that increasing the grid size and using a fine grid will increase the computing time for docking.
8. The AutoDock developers recommend varying some of the genetic algorithm parameters to increase the search exhaustiveness and accuracy. The more important ones are "ga_num_evals", which specifies the number of energy evaluations, and "ga_num_generations", which specifies the number of generations for each genetic algorithm run. The recommended values are 250,000–25,000,000 for "ga_num_evals" for ligands with 1–10 torsions, and 27,000 for "ga_num_generations". To obtain a statistically significant number of binding modes for clustering, 50–100 "ga_runs" should be performed. For more information, see http://autodock.scripps.edu/faqs-help/faq/which-values-of-the-genetic-algorithm-parameters-do-you-normally-use.

Acknowledgments

This work was supported in part by NIH grant GM 68460 (G.R.M.), the Washington University Cancer Biology Pathway (Y.T.T.), and the NIH Vision Sciences Training Grant (Y.T.T.).

References

1. Walters, W. P., Stahl, M. T., and Murcko, M. A. (1998) Virtual screening – an overview. *Drug Discov Today* **3**: 160–178.
2. Shoichet, B. K. (2004) Virtual screening of chemical libraries. *Nature* **432**: 862–865.
3. Kitchen, D. B., Decornez, H., Furr, J. R., and Bajorath, J. (2004) Docking and scoring in virtual screening for drug discovery: Methods and applications. *Nat Rev Drug Discov* **3**: 935–949.
4. Schneider, G., and Bohm, H. J. (2002) Virtual screening and fast automated docking methods. *Drug Discov Today* **7**: 64–70.
5. Morris, G. M., Goodsell, D. S., Halliday, R. S., Huey, R., Hart, W. E., Belew, R. K., and Olson, A. J. (1998) Automated docking using a Lamarckian genetic algorithm and an empirical binding free energy function. *J Comput Chem* **19**: 1639–1662.
6. Huey, R., Morris, G. M., Olson, A. J., and Goodsell, D. S. (2007) A semiempirical free energy force field with charge-based desolvation. *J Comput Chem* **28**: 1145–1152.
7. Wang, R. X., Lai, L. H., and Wang, S. M. (2002) Further development and validation of empirical scoring functions for structure-based binding affinity prediction. *J Comput-Aided Mol Des* **16**: 11–26.
8. Chen, Z. G., Li, Y., Chen, E., Hall, D. L., Darke, P. L., Culberson, C., Shafer, J. A., and Kuo, L. C. (1994) Crystal-Structure at 1.9-Angstrom Resolution of Human-Immunodeficiency-Virus (Hiv)-Ii Protease Complexed with L-735,524, an Orally Bioavailable Inhibitor of the Hiv Proteases. *J Biol Chem.* **269**: 26344–26348.
9. Milne, G. W. A., and Miller, J. A. (1986) The Nci Drug Information-System .1. System Overview. *J Chem Inf Comput Sci* **26**: 154–159.
10. Wang, R. X., Lu, Y. P., and Wang, S. M. (2003) Comparative evaluation of 11 scoring functions for molecular docking. *J Med Chem* **46**: 2287–2303.
11. Charifson, P. S., Corkery, J. J., Murcko, M. A., and Walters, W. P. (1999) Consensus scoring: A method for obtaining improved hit rates from docking databases of three-dimensional structures into proteins. *J Med Chem* **42**: 5100–5109.
12. Wang, R. X., and Wang, S. M. (2001) How does consensus scoring work for virtual library screening? An idealized computer experiment. *J Chem Inf Comput Sci* **41**: 1422–1426.
13. Clark, R. D., Strizhev, A., Leonard, J. M., Blake, J. F., and Matthew, J. B. (2002) Consensus scoring for ligand/protein interactions. *J Mol Graph Model* **20**: 281–295.
14. Berman, H. M., Westbrook, J., Feng, Z., Gilliland, G., Bhat, T. N., Weissig, H., Shindyalov, I. N., and Bourne, P. E. (2000) The Protein Data Bank. *Nucl Acid Res* **28**: 235–242.
15. Ihlenfeldt, W. D., Voigt, J. H., Bienfait, B., Oellien, F., and Nicklaus, M. C. (2002) Enhanced CACTVS browser of the open NCI database. *J Chem Inf Comput Sci* **42**: 46–57.
16. Morris, G. M., Huey, R., and Olson, A. J. (2008) Using AutoDock for ligand-receptor docking. *Curr Protoc Bioinformatics* Chapter 8: Unit 8.14.
17. Irwin, J. J., and Shoichet, B. K. (2005) ZINC – A free database of commercially available compounds for virtual screening. *J Chem Inf Model* **45**: 177–182.

Chapter 2

Computer-Aided Drug Discovery and Development

Shuxing Zhang

Abstract

Computer-aided approaches have been widely used in pharmaceutical research to improve the efficiency of the drug discovery and development pipeline. To identify and design small molecules as clinically effective therapeutics, various computational methods have been evaluated as promising strategies, depending on the purpose and systems of interest. Both ligand and structure-based drug design approaches are powerful technologies, which can be applied to virtual screening for lead identification and optimization. Here, we review the progress in this field and summarize the application of some new technologies we developed. These state-of-the-art tools have been used for the discovery and development of active agents for various diseases, in particular for cancer therapies. The described protocols are appropriate for all drug discovery stages, but expertise is still needed to perform the studies based on the targets of interest.

Key words: Computer-aided drug discovery, High-throughput screening, Ligand-based drug design, Molecular docking, Quantitative structure–activity relationship, Structure-based drug design, Virtual screening

1. Introduction

Drug discovery and development is a time-consuming and expensive process. On average, it takes 10–15 years and US $500–800 million to introduce a drug into the market (1, 2). This is why computer-assisted drug design (CADD) approaches have been widely used in the pharmaceutical industry to accelerate the process (3, 4). CADD helps scientists focus on the most promising compounds so that they can minimize the synthetic and biological testing efforts. In practice, the choice of CADD approaches to be employed is usually determined by the availability of the experimentally determined 3D structures of target proteins. If protein structures are unknown, various methods of ligand-based drug

Seetharama D. Satyanarayanajois (ed.), *Drug Design and Discovery: Methods and Protocols*,
Methods in Molecular Biology, vol. 716, DOI 10.1007/978-1-61779-012-6_2,

design can be employed, such as Quantitative Structure Activity Relationship (QSAR) and pharmacophore analysis. If the target structures are known, structure-based approaches can be used such as molecular docking, which employs the target 3D structures to design novel active compounds with improved potency. As more structures are becoming available, the prediction accuracy will likely to be improved.

1.1. Ligand-Based Drug Design

In the absence of the receptor 3D information, lead identification and optimization depend on available pharmacologically relevant agents and their bioactivities (5–8). The computational approaches include QSAR, pharmacophore modeling, and database mining (8–10). We will use QSAR as an example to illustrate the workflow. QSAR describes mathematical relationships between structural attributes and target properties of a set of chemicals (9, 11, 12). Many different 2D (two-dimensional) and 3D (three-dimensional) QSAR approaches have been developed during the past several decades (13, 14). The major differences of these methods include chemical descriptors and mathematical approaches that are used to establish the correlation between the target properties and the descriptors.

Many 2D QSAR methods have been extensively studied (15, 16) based on graph theoretic indices. Although the physicochemical meaning of these indices is unclear, they certainly represent different aspects of molecular structures. It has been extensively applied to analytical chemistry, toxicity analysis, and other biological activity prediction (17). 3D QSAR approaches have been developed to address the problems of 2D QSAR techniques including their inability to distinguish stereoisomers. These 3D methods include molecular shape analysis (MSA), distance geometry, and Voronoi techniques (18–20). Comparative Molecular Field Analysis (CoMFA) (21) perhaps is the most popular example of 3D QSAR. It has been widely used in medicinal chemistry and toxicity analysis by elegantly combining the power of molecular graphics and partial least square (PLS) technique. QSAR techniques usually assume the linear relationship between a target property and molecular descriptors. However, the explosive growth of structural and biological data has challenged this assumption. To this end, some nonlinear QSAR methods have been proposed and most of them are based on either artificial neural network (ANN) (22–25) or machine learning techniques (26–28). We have concentrated on the development and application of automated algorithms for QSAR studies, including genetic algorithms-partial least squares, k-Nearest Neighbor (29), and support vector machine (30–32).

Machine learning usually is defined as a discipline concerned with the improvement of the performance of computer algorithms based on their previous experiences (33), and these algorithms establish the correlations between the variables and the output of the system (26, 34–37). In engineering field, it is closely related to pattern recognition and has become steadily more successful over the past 20 years. Learning approaches have been widely used in cheminformatics and molecular modeling (38–42). For instance, support vector machine (SVM) was found to yield better results compared to multiple linear regressions (MLR) and radial basis functions (RBF) (31). Various versions of such programs have been applied to the calculation of activities of enzyme inhibitors (43). Lazy learning and kNN approaches were employed in the discovery of anticonvulsant compounds and anticancer agents, respectively (41, 42). Machine learning is also being frequently used to conduct ADMET predictions (44–46). Gaussian kernel SVM was used to successfully classify a set of drugs in terms of their potential to cause an adverse drug reaction TdP (47). Although TdP is involved in multiple mechanisms, the SVM prediction accuracy on an independent set of molecules was 90% more than that with ANN and decision tree methods.

1.2. Structure-Based Drug Design

Structure-based design has played an important role in drug discovery and development (48–50). This approach requires the understanding of receptor–ligand interactions. If the target 3D structure is known, it can be used for the design of new ligands (49–51). The structural information is either from X-ray crystallography, NMR, or from homology modeling. SBDD approaches are responsible for evaluating the complementarities and predicting the possible binding modes and affinities between small molecules and their macromolecular receptors. The success of SBDD is well documented (52, 53) and the computational approaches vary widely in methodology, performance, and speed. Some are capable of providing accurate binding modes, while others are more suitable for fast searching of large databases (50, 54–61). Herein we will focus on the most commonly used strategies: molecular docking and scoring.

Molecular docking is used for computational schemes that attempt to find the best matches between a receptor and a ligand. It involves the prediction of ligand conformations and orientation (or posing) within a binding site and attempts to place the ligand into the binding site in configurations and conformations appropriate for interacting with the receptor (62). Docking methods can be divided into matching and simulation methods. The former approaches create a binding site model, typically including the favorable hydrogen binding and steric interactions, and then attempt to dock a ligand into this model by geometrical matching (63). Although early attempts of matching methods only considered the translational and orientational degrees of freedom of the ligand, most of recently developed programs take into account the conformational flexibility of ligands and the limited flexibility of the receptor (63, 64). The examples of this class include DOCK (65, 66), FlexX (67, 68), etc. Simulation methods put a molecule into a binding site by exploring the translations, orientations, and conformations until an ideal binding mode is found. Autodock is the most representative example of this class (69).

One of the major challenges is the scoring function problem, i.e., the problem of fast and accurate evaluation of binding affinities. Several approaches to address this problem have been proposed and developed. Force field scoring is based on the classical molecular force fields, such as AMBER (70), CHARMM (71), MMFF94 (72), etc., to compute nonbonded interaction terms between the receptor and ligand atoms. Additional empirical terms taking into account the solvation and entropy effects have been also considered (73). The second family of methods is the empirical scoring functions, which include LUDI (74–76)and VALIDATE (77). They have been introduced several years ago and are based on the concept that the receptor–ligand interaction energy can be approximated by a multivariate regression of different parameters such as the number of hydrogen bonds, lipophilicity, ionic interactions, entropy penalties, etc. Recently, a third family of methods, knowledge-based scoring functions (DrugScore (78) SmoG (79), PMF (80), BLEEP (81), etc.) has been introduced. These methods employ the statistical analysis of known receptor–ligand complexes to define pairwise interatomic potentials of protein–ligand interactions. After the calibration on the training set of complexes, these scoring functions are validated by predicting binding affinities for the complexes of the test sets.

Recently advances in networking, high-end computers, large data stores, and middleware capabilities are ushering in a new era of high-performance parallel and distributed simulations (82). Based on these technologies, novel high-throughput docking approaches have been developed to enable efficient and inexpensive drug discovery. For instance, we developed an automated DOcking-based VIrtual Screening (DOVIS) system (59), which makes sophisticated docking strategies to be carried out on HPC clusters to screen millions of compounds more efficiently. In this chapter, we will discuss the methods using our recent implementation HiPCDock (61).

2. Materials (Hardware and Software)

2.1. Ligand-Based Design Approaches

1. Computer workstations with Linux operating systems.
2. ChemDraw or other molecular structure drawing programs.
3. Descriptor generators such as DRAGON, MolConnZ, and OEChem.
4. Text editors such as UltraEdit, vi, and EMACS.
5. Descriptors normalization programs.
6. Data splitting program such as SE8.
7. Databases such as ZINC, PubChem, and ChemDiv.
8. ALL-QSAR Program.
9. Activity testing facility.

2.2. Structure-Based Design Approaches

1. High-performance computing (HPC) clusters with Linux operating systems.
2. LSF queuing systems for the HPC clusters.
3. Java environment.
4. Perl and Python modules.
5. HiPCDock program.
6. AutoDock3 program.
7. AutoDockTools package.
8. Matlab package.
9. OpenBabel program.

3. Methods

3.1. Ligand-Based Design Approaches

Different programs have different protocols to perform the task. Here we use ALL-QSAR as an example to demonstrate the procedures (Fig. 1). For special notes, please refer Section 4.

1. Prepare molecular structures of interest. Most of programs accept sdf, mol2, or some other formats. The structures can be 2D or 3D, depending on the studies. If 3D QSAR (Fig. 2) is conducted, then 3D structures of the molecules are required.
2. Calculate descriptors for the molecules using the molecular file created above. Most descriptor generation programs just need the molecular file as input. Depending on the study, some options may need to be specified. For instance, with MOE descriptors, you can specify 1D, 2D, or 3D descriptors, or all of them. Other commonly used descriptors include DRAGON descriptors, MolConnZ descriptors, OEChem shape descriptors, etc. During this step, some molecules may be skipped due to the inability to calculate the descriptors by the programs. This can be due to the limitations of the programs or the inaccuracy of the molecule structures.
3. Prepare the molecular activity file. Usually two columns are required: the first column is the molecular name and the second

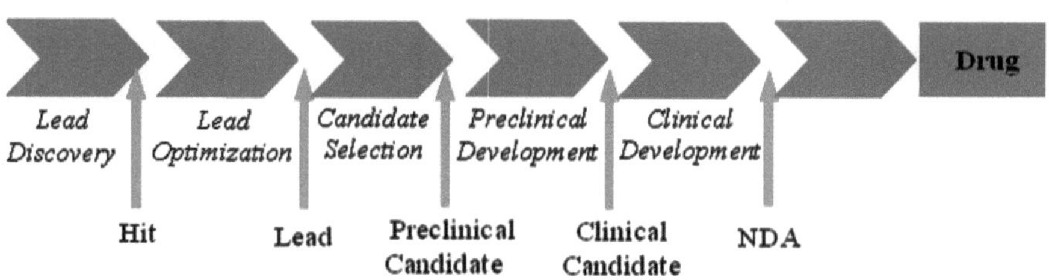

Fig. 1. Drug discovery and development pipeline. The process is very time consuming and expensive. It mainly includes lead discovery and optimization, preclinical and clinical trial, and final NDA and marketing.

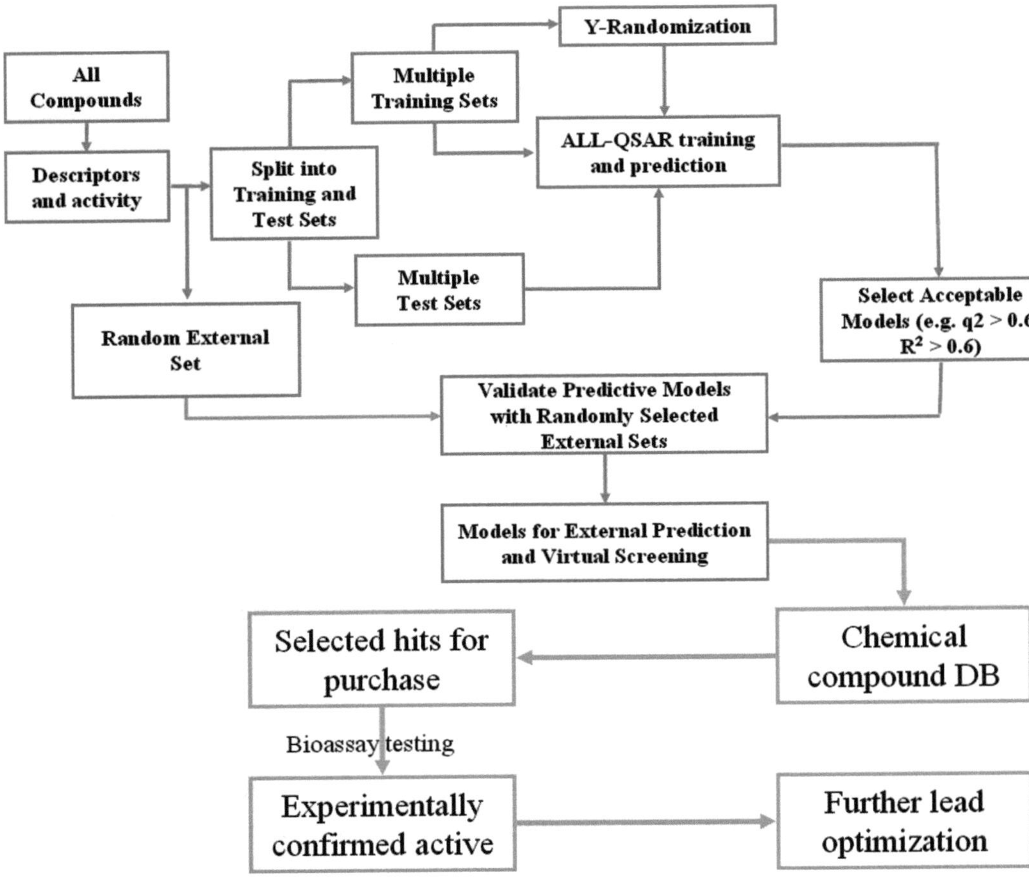

Fig. 2. QSAR and virtual screening workflow. Starting from molecular structures and their bioactivities, QSAR models can be built to perform external predictions and virtual screening. The identified hits are experimentally tested, and the active compounds will be further optimized and the new data can be further fed back to the process.

is the activity values. The order of the molecules in the activity file should be corresponding to the order in the descriptor file.

4. Descriptor normalization. Usually the values of the descriptors are quite different as many of them represent completely different properties with different scale. For instance, the molecular weight is in hundreds but the LogP is usually below 10. To exclude the disproportional influence by the descriptor values, normalization is recommended. The way to do this is to find the maximum and minimum values for all molecules for each descriptor and normalize each values with $(X_i - X_{min})/(X_{max} - X_{min})$. There are many other ways to do the normalization.
5. Once the descriptors are normalized, the dataset will be split into multiple training and test sets for model building. This can be achieved with SE8 (Sphere Exclusion version 8) algorithm (83).

6. The procedures of SE8 start with the calculation of the distance matrix **D** between representative points in the descriptor space. Let D_{min} and D_{max} be the minimum and maximum elements of **D**, respectively. N probe sphere radii are defined by the following formulas $R_{min} = R_1 = D_{min}$, $R_{max} = R_N = D_{max}/4$, $R_i = R_1 + (i-1) \times (R_N - R_1)/(N-1)$, where $i = 2,\ldots,N-1$.
7. Each probe sphere radius corresponds to one division into the training and test set. In our studies it consisted of the following steps. (i) Select randomly a compound. (ii) Include it in the training set. (iii) Construct a probe sphere around this compound. (iv) Select compounds from this sphere and include them alternatively into test and training sets. (v) Exclude all compounds from within this sphere for further consideration. (vi) If no more compounds left, stop. Otherwise let *m* be the number of probe spheres constructed and *n* be the number of remaining compounds. Let d_{ij} ($i = 1,\ldots,m$; $j = 1,\ldots,n$) be the distances between the remaining compounds and probe sphere centers. Select a compound corresponding to the lowest d_{ij} value and go to step (ii).
8. Once the dataset is split into training and test sets, our ALL-QSAR will load the training set descriptors and activities space into memory and assign a lowest predefined value to the kernel width *K*.
9. Take a query compound from the test set and calculate the Euclidean distances between it and all compounds of the training set. If the distance from the test set compound to its nearest neighbor is higher than D_{max}, this compound is out of the applicability domain. Since the activity prediction for it is believed to be not accurate, it will not be predicted. In this case return to step 9 and process the next compound of the test set, or, if there are no more compounds in the test set, go to step 16. If the compound of the test set is within the applicability domain, go to step 10. The applicability domain is calculated as the following: $APD = \hat{y} + Z\sigma$, where $\hat{y}$ is the average of weighted Euclidean distance for the training set. Z is an empirical cutoff value to control the significance (or confidence) level with the default value as 0.5. σ is the standard deviation of all pairwise Euclidean distance in the training set.
10. The weight of every compound in the training set is calculated for the query compound.
11. Calculate coefficients β.
12. Using the values of β, weights and descriptors to predict the target property of the query compound.
13. Repeat step 9 for the next compound. If the procedure was repeated for all compounds, go to step 14.

14. Calculate the correlation coefficient between the predicted and experimental activity values of the test set compounds.
15. If kernel width is lower than the predefined value, add a predefined step to it and repeat the process starting from step 9 for *N* times until the prediction is converged.
16. Sort models by the R^2 starting from the highest value, and RMSD between predicted and actual target property values and select the top 10 best models.
17. The models can be used for predictions of new molecules or virtual screening.
18. In virtual screening, top hits based on predicted activity (e.g., top 100) are selected for investigation.
19. The selected hits will be inspected for their scaffold, potential toxicity, and other properties by both modelers and synthetic chemists.
20. Only those accepted by both modelers and chemists are submitted to experimental testing.
21. Experimentally confirmed hits will be used to perform lead optimization and new molecule design.
22. The newly designed molecule will be predicted for their activity, starting from step 1, and the measured activities are fed back to our model building process.

3.2. Structure-Based Design Approaches

Here by splitting it into multiple steps including preprocessing of molecules, parallel docking, and postprocessing of result analysis, the overall workflow in Fig. 3 demonstrates how our new HiPCDock (61) works as high-throughput molecular docking protocols for drug discovery and development. For special notes, please refer Section 4.

3.2.1. Preprocessing of Receptors

1. The protein structure is directly downloaded from PDB (pdb format). Hydrogens are added to the structures and appropriate charges are assigned by executing a Python script, which uses the related functions from AutoDockTool (Fig. 4).
2. The structure is converted from pdb format to pdbq format by adding an extra column of charges. If users prefer adding hydrogens and assigning charges with other software, such as SYBYL, it can be done and the saved mol2 file can be used as input into our pipeline.
3. Once our program loads the structure, it uses AutoDock utility program *mol2fftopdbq* to convert the mol2 file to pdbq format.
4. After the pdbq file is obtained, the solvation process is performed using *addsol* module from AutoDock to convert the pdbq file to pdbqs format. The current acceptable input file formats include pdb, pdbq, and mol2.

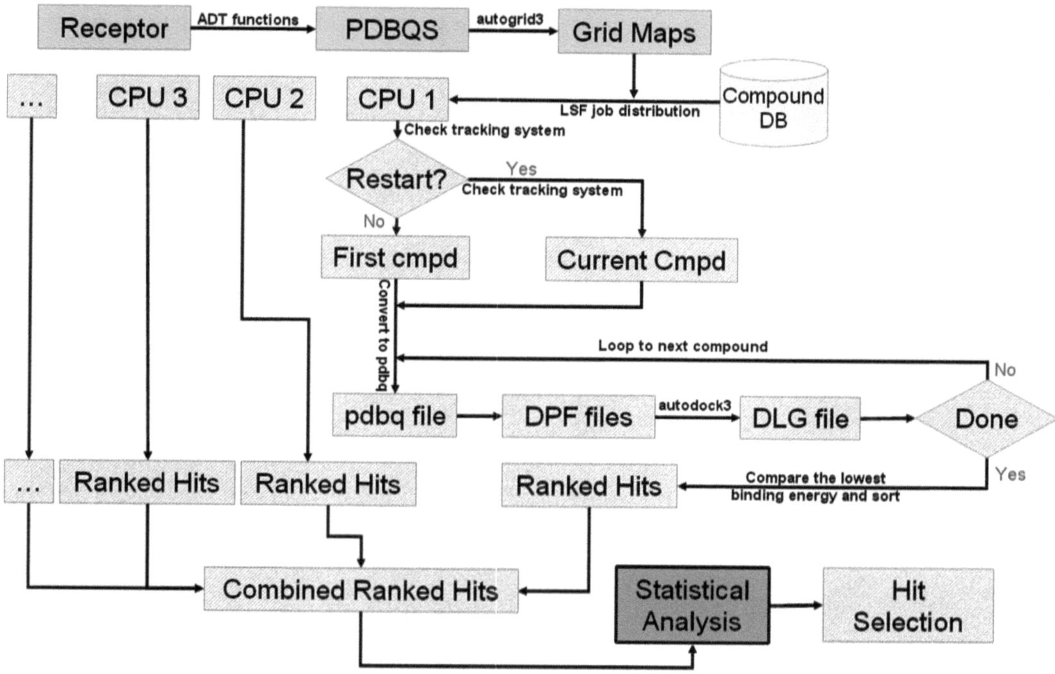

Fig. 3. Overall workflow of HiPCDock. The whole process includes target and ligand preparation, distribution of parallel docking onto multiple CPUs, and final analysis of the results to select promising hits. This is involved in a statistical analysis (77) of docking scores as indicated in the *black box*.

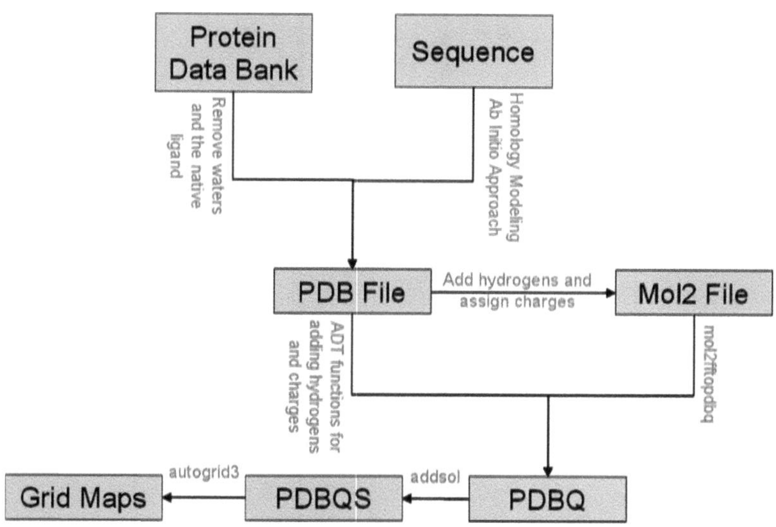

Fig. 4. Workflow for protein preparation. Target preparation starts from the 3D structure of the proteins. Hydrogens and charges are automatically added and grid maps are created using autogrid3, and the pdbqs file is generated for docking process.

5. After the solvation, the created pdbqs is used to generate a grid parameter file (GPF). Currently, ten atom types are used for proteins, including carbon (C), nitrogen (N), oxygen (O), sulfur (S), hydrogen (H), metal (M), phosphorus (P), Zinc (Z), Calcium (L), and X for unknown type.
6. The 3D grids of interaction energy for all possible atom types are calculated at one time. These uniquely defined atom types include nonaromatic carbon (C), aromatic carbon (A), nitrogen (N), oxygen (O), sulfur (S), phosphorus (P), hydrogen (H), metal (M), fluorine (F), chlorine (c), bromine (b), iodine (I), zinc (Z), calcium (L), iron (f), and unknown type (X). They basically cover most of the possible ligand atom types included in databases.
7. The center of the common grids can be either the center of mass coordinates of the ligand that had been removed from the binding site of the target protein under consideration or the geometrical center of a series of key residues provided by users.
8. A modified script (from *gpfgen*) is used to generate the GPF file with our customized atom types and the parameter values provided by users.
9. Based on the GPF file, *autogrid3* is executed to create 16 atom type maps, plus an additional electron density map.

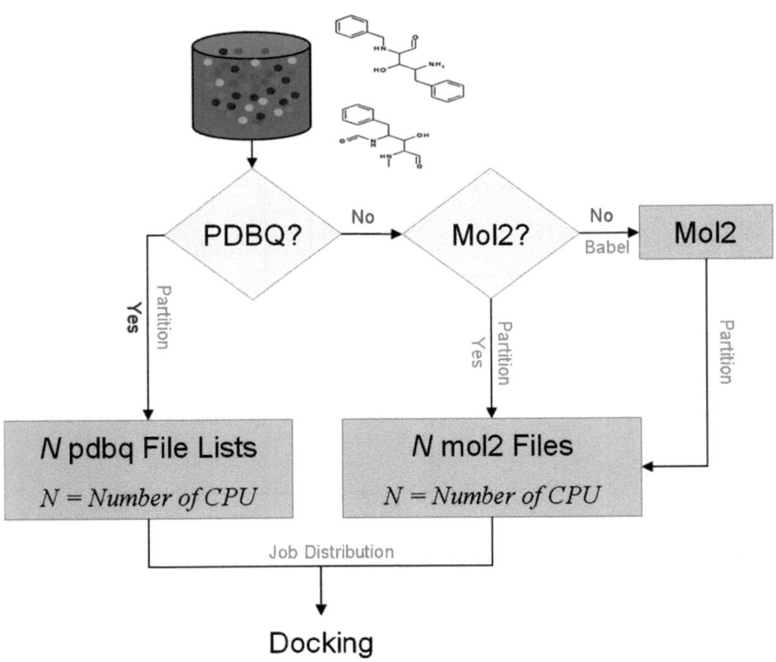

Fig. 5. Workflow for chemical compound preparation. Chemical compound preparation is also performed on multiple CPUs to speed up the process as the chemical database can include millions of compounds. The process will result in ligand pdbq files, which can be repeatedly used in docking.

3.2.2. Preprocessing of Ligand Compounds

The chemical compounds also need to be preprocessed for our program as demonstrated in Fig. 5. The current acceptable ligand input file formats are SMILE strings (smi), sdf/sd, mol, mol2, and pdbq. Files in the first four formats may have single or multiple molecule(s). Each pdbq file can comprise one molecule. The input of chemical compounds is a directory, so it can include multiple files. The pipeline requires that the directory contains either pdbq or acceptable non-pdbq files. The protocol is as follows:

1. HiPCDock converts each non-mol2 file using OpenBabel to mol2 format, which possesses Gasteiger charges.
2. Then each mol2 file is partitioned into multiple pieces of roughly equal size. The number of pieces is determined by the number of CPU requested by users.
3. If the directory has pdbq files, HiPCDock generates multiple (equals to the number of CPU) file lists. Each list includes approximately equal number of compounds.

3.2.3. Parallel Docking on HPC Clusters

Once the grid maps are generated and the chemical compounds are partitioned into the right format, parallel docking can be performed using high-performance computing clusters for virtual screening. Here are the procedures:

1. Each partition is submitted to a CPU and the docking process is performed automatically. The current implementation is using Load Sharing Facility (LSF) queuing system.
2. The LSF job array function is used for the job distribution and scheduling. Once a CPU is available, HiPCDock distributes a job on that CPU and starts docking. Otherwise, it is pending in the queue.
3. The workflow on each CPU is illustrated in Fig. 4. If the chemical database is in mol2 format, *autotors* is executed for each molecule (by looping through all of the molecules in the partition) to define the torsions of the compound and then convert it to pdbq format.
4. The new pdbq file will be saved in a directory so that it can be re-used directly in future runs.
5. If the input is already in pdbq format or the built-in database is used, the above process is skipped and the docking starts to run by executing *autodock3* module.
6. The docking parameter file (DPF) is automatically generated by HiPCDock based on the input from users.
7. After docking each molecule, the result in its docking log file (DLG) is analyzed and the lowest estimated free energy of binding is recorded. This is used for the comparison with other molecules to determine whether this molecule is a strong enough binder to be a hit. If yes, its DLG is kept, otherwise its related files will be deleted in order to save disk space.

8. Since this is the most time-consuming part with a big loop (e.g., tens of thousands of compounds on each CPU if we dock millions of compounds on hundreds of CPUs), a restart function is implemented to improve the robustness of the program. Basically, each successfully processed molecule is recorded in a tracking file. Every time HiPCDock runs, it first checks the tracking file and starts from the molecule where the last run was stopped.

3.2.4. Postprocess of Docked Results

Once the jobs on all CPUs are done, the HiPCDock postprocess module starts to analyze the results.

1. It collects all of the individual hit lists together and generates an overall list.
2. The list is sorted according to their free energy of binding, and the top ranked compounds, as requested by users (e.g., 10% of all database compounds), are selected as the final hits.
3. These hits can be further refined by chemists' knowledge as well as by molecular visualization provided by HiPCDock.
4. For each final hit, all of docked conformations are extracted from the DLG and are converted to sdf files so that the users can visualize their interactions with the receptor.
5. OpenBabel function is utilized to calculate some molecular properties for each hit.

4. Notes

1. The molecular descriptors should be normalized to exclude the influence of those disproportional descriptor values.
2. The descriptors used in training, testing, or new datasets should be consistent.
3. Usually descriptor correlation analysis should be conducted to keep only independent descriptors, also for the reduction of descriptor dimensions.
4. Parameter tuning is usually necessary to obtain best models for predictions, and therefore, it might be a good idea to run the model building multiple times by changing the parameters.
5. Y randomization should be performed to exclude chance correlation between the descriptors and target properties.
6. Databases for virtual screening should be cleaned and their descriptors should be normalized based on training set normalization parameters.

7. Receptors structures should be cleaned by removing its water molecules and by fixing the wrong or missing residues for docking.
8. Different charge types can be tried during docking.
9. The starting conformations of ligands (or chemical databases) should be minimized by using the lowest energy conformations.
10. If the docking process is disrupted, it can be restarted and the docking will continue until finished.
11. The hit selection is based on the conformation with the lowest predicted binding free energies but not necessarily the best binding poses due to the approximation and imperfection of scoring functions.
12. Multiple scoring functions can be applied to conduct consensus docking/scoring to obtain the best predictions.

Acknowledgments

We are grateful to John Morrow for proofreading this chapter, and this work was supported in part by MD Anderson faculty startup fund.

References

1. Workman, P. (2003). How much gets there and what does it do?: The need for better pharmacokinetic and pharmacodynamic endpoints in contemporary drug discovery and development. *Curr Pharm Des.* **9:** 891–902.
2. Brown, D. & Superti-Furga, G. (2003). Rediscovering the sweet spot in drug discovery. *Drug Discov Today.* **8:** 1067–1077.
3. Gomeni, R., Bani, M., D'Angeli, C., Corsi, M. & Bye, A. (2001). Computer-assisted drug development (CADD): an emerging technology for designing first-time-in-man and proof-of-concept studies from preclinical experiments. *Eur J Pharm Sci.* **13:** 261–270.
4. Veselovsky, A. V. & Ivanov, A. S. (2003). Strategy of computer-aided drug design. *Curr Drug Targets Infect Disord.* **3:** 33–40.
5. Stahura, F. L. & Bajorath, J. (2004). Virtual screening methods that complement HTS. *Comb Chem High Throughput Screen.* **7:** 259–269.
6. Guner, O., Clement, O. & Kurogi, Y. (2004). Pharmacophore modeling and three dimensional database searching for drug design using catalyst: Recent advances. *Curr Med Chem.* **11:** 2991–3005.
7. Hansch, C., Leo, A., Mekapati, S. B. & Kurup, A. (2004). Qsar and Adme. *Bioorg Med Chem.* **12:** 3391–3400.
8. Parvu, L. (2003). QSAR – a piece of drug design. *J Cell Mol Med.* **7:** 333–335.
9. Langer, T. & Wolber, G. (2004). Virtual combinatorial chemistry and in silico screening: Efficient tools for lead structure discovery? *Pure App Chem.* **76:** 991–996.
10. Dror, O., Shulman-Peleg, A., Nussinov, R. & Wolfson, H. J. (2004). Predicting molecular interactions in silico: I. A guide to pharmacophore identification and its applications to drug design. *Curr Med Chem.* **11:** 71–90.
11. Perkins, R., Fang, H., Tong, W. D. & Welsh, W. J. (2003). Quantitative structure-activity relationship methods: Perspectives on drug discovery and toxicology. *Environ Toxicol Chem.* **22:** 1666–1679.
12. Tropsha, A. & Zhang, W. F. (2001). Identification of the descriptor pharmacophores using variable selection QSAR: Applications to database mining. *Curr Pharm Design.* **7:** 599–612.
13. Leo, A. J. & Hansch, C. (1999). Role of hydrophobic effects in mechanistic QSAR. *Perspect Drug Discov Design.* **17:** 1–25.

14. Garg, R., Kurup, A., Mekapati, S. B. & Hansch, C. (2003). Searching for allosteric effects via QSAR. Part II. *Bioorg Med Chem.* **11:** 621–628.

15. Kier, L. B. & Hall, L. H. (1993). The generation of molecular-structures from a graph-based Qsar equation. *Quant Struct Act Relat.* **12:** 383–388.

16. Hall, L. H. & Kier, L. B. (2001). Issues in representation of molecular structure – The development of molecular connectivity. *J Mol Graph Model.* **20:** 4–18.

17. Anker, L. S., Jurs, P. C. & Edwards, P. A. (1990). Quantitative structure retention relationship studies of odor-active aliphatic-compounds with oxygen-containing functional-groups. *Anal Chem.* **62:** 2676–2684.

18. Crippen, G. M. (1982). Distance geometry analysis of the benzodiazepine binding-site. *Mol Pharmacol.* **22:** 11–19.

19. Hopfinger, A. J. (1980). A Qsar Investigation of dihydrofolate-reductase inhibition by baker triazines based upon molecular shape-analysis. *J Am Chem Soc.* **102:** 7196–7206.

20. Boulu, L. G. & Crippen, G. M. (1989). Voronoi binding-site models – calculation of binding modes and influence of drug-binding data accuracy. *J Comb Chem.* **10:** 673–682.

21. Cramer, R. D., III, Patterson, D. E. & Bunce, J. D. (1988). Comparative molecular field analysis (CoMFA). 1. Effect of shape on binding of steroids to carrier proteins. *J Am Chem Soc.* **110:** 5959–5967.

22. So, S. S. & Richards, W. G. (1992). Application of neural networks – quantitative structure-activity-relationships of the derivatives of 2,4-diamino-5-(substituted-benzyl)pyrimidines as Dhfr inhibitors. *J Med Chem.* **35:** 3201–3207.

23. Tetko, I. V., Tanchuk, V. Y., Chentsova, N. P., Antonenko, S. V., Poda, G. I., Kukhar, V. P. & Luik, A. I. (1994). Hiv-1 reverse-transcriptase inhibitor design using artificial neural networks. *J Med Chem.* **37:** 2520–2526.

24. Ajay, A. & Murcko, M. A. (1995). Computational methods to predict binding free energy in ligand-receptor complexes. *J Med Chem.* **38:** 4953–4967.

25. Andrea, T. A. & Kalayeh, H. (1991). Applications of neural networks in quantitative structure-activity-relationships of dihydrofolate-reductase inhibitors. *J Med Chem.* **34:** 2824–2836.

26. Bolis, G., Dipace, L. & Fabrocini, F. (1991). A machine learning approach to computer-aided molecular design. *J Comput Aided Mol Des.* **5:** 617–628.

27. King, R. D., Muggleton, S., Lewis, R. A. & Sternberg, M. J. E. (1992). Drug design by machine learning – the use of inductive logic programming to model the structure-activity-relationships of trimethoprim analogs binding to dihydrofolate-reductase. *Proc Natl Acad Sci U S A.* **89:** 11322–11326.

28. Jain, A. N., Dietterich, T. G., Lathrop, R. H., Chapman, D., Critchlow, R. E., Bauer, B. E., Webster, T. A. & Lozanoperez, T. (1994). Compass – a shape-based machine learning tool for drug design. *J Comput Aided Mol Des.* **8:** 635–652.

29. Zheng, W. F. & Tropsha, A. (2000). Novel variable selection quantitative structure-property relationship approach based on the k-nearest-neighbor principle. *J Chem Inf Comput Sci.* **40:** 185–194.

30. Xue, C. X., Zhang, R. S., Liu, H. X., Yao, X. J., Liu, M. C., Hu, Z. D. & Fan, B. T. (2004). An accurate QSPR study of O-H bond dissociation energy in substituted phenols based on support vector machines. *J Chem Inf Comput Sci.* **44:** 669–677.

31. Yao, X. J., Panaye, A., Doucet, J. P., Zhang, R. S., Chen, H. F., Liu, M. C., Hu, Z. D. & Fan, B. T. (2004). Comparative study of QSAR/QSPR correlations using support vector machines, radial basis function neural networks, and multiple linear regression. *J Chem Inf Comput Sci.* **44:** 1257–1266.

32. Kovatcheva, A., Golbraikh, A., Oloff, S., Xiao, Y. D., Zheng, W. F., Wolschann, P., Buchbauer, G. & Tropsha, A. (2004). Combinatorial QSAR of ambergris fragrance compounds. *J Chem Inf Comput Sci.* **44:** 582–595.

33. Mjolsness, E. & DeCoste, D. (2001). Machine learning for science: State of the art and future prospects. *Science* **293:** 2051–2055.

34. Herbrich, R. & Williamson, R. C. (2003). Algorithmic luckiness. *J Mac Learn Res.* **3:** 175–212.

35. Schneider, G. & Downs, G. (2003). Machine learning methods in QSAR modelling. *QSAR Comb Sci.* **22:** 485–486.

36. Sebastiani, P., Kohane, I. S. & Ramoni, M. F. (2003). Machine learning in the Genomics era – Editorial: Methods in functional genomics. *Machine Learning* **52:** 5–9.

37. Smith, M. G. & Bull, L. (2003). Feature construction and selection using Genetic Programming and a Genetic Algorithm. *Genetic Programming, Proceedings* **2610,** 229–237.

38. Armengol, E. & Plaza, E. (2003). Discovery of toxicological patterns with lazy learning. *Knowledge-Based Intellignet Information and Engineering Systems, Pt 2, Proceedings* **2774,** 919–926.

39. Oloff, S., Zhang, S., Sukumar, N., Breneman, C. & Tropsha, A. (2006). Chemometric analysis of ligand receptor complementarity: identifying complementary ligands based on receptor information (CoLiBRI). *J Chem Inf Model.* **46:** 844–851.
40. Zhang, S., Golbraikh, A. & Tropsha, A. (2006). Development of quantitative structure-binding affinity relationship models based on novel geometrical chemical descriptors of the protein-ligand interfaces. *J Med Chem.* **49:** 2713–2724.
41. Zhang, S., Golbraikh, A., Oloff, S., Kohn, H. & Tropsha, A. (2006). A novel automated lazy learning QSAR (ALL-QSAR) approach: method development, applications, and virtual screening of chemical databases using validated ALL-QSAR models. *J Chem Inf Model* **46:** 1984–1995.
42. Zhang, S., Wei, L., Bastow, K., Zheng, W., Brossi, A., Lee, K. H. & Tropsha, A. (2007). Antitumor agents 252. Application of validated QSAR models to database mining: discovery of novel tylophorine derivatives as potential anticancer agents. *J Comput Aided Mol Des.* **21:** 97–112.
43. Duch, W., Swaminathan, K. & Meller, J. (2007). Artificial intelligence approaches for rational drug design and discovery. *Curr Pharm Des.* **13:** 1497–1508.
44. Clark, D. E. & Grootenhuis, P. D. (2002). Progress in computational methods for the prediction of ADMET properties. *Curr Opin Drug Discov Dev.* **5:** 382–390.
45. Davis, A. M. & Riley, R. J. (2004). Predictive ADMET studies, the challenges and the opportunities. *Curr Opin Chem Biol.* **8:** 378–386.
46. Li, H., Yap, C. W., Ung, C. Y., Xue, Y., Li, Z. R., Han, L. Y., Lin, H. H. & Chen, Y. Z. (2007). Machine learning approaches for predicting compounds that interact with therapeutic and ADMET related proteins. *J Pharm Sci.* **96:** 2838–2860.
47. Yap, C. W., Cai, C. Z., Xue, Y. & Chen, Y. Z. (2004). Prediction of torsade-causing potential of drugs by support vector machine approach. *Toxicol Sci.* **79:** 170–177.
48. Kubinyi, H. (2003). Drug research: myths, hype and reality. *Nat Rev Drug Discov.* **2:** 665–668.
49. Reddy, M. R. & Erion, M. D. (1998). Structure-based drug design approaches for predicting binding affinities of HIV1 protease inhibitors. *J Enzyme Inhib.* **14:** 1–14.
50. Taylor, R. D., Jewsbury, P. J. & Essex, J. W. (2002). A review of protein-small molecule docking methods. *J Comput Aided Mol Des.* **16:** 151–166.
51. Kuntz, I. D., Meng, E. C. & Shoichet, B. K. (1994). Structure-based molecular design. *Acc Chem Res.* **27:** 117–123.
52. Hardy, L. W. & Malikayil, A. (2003). The impact of structure-guided drug design on clinical agents. *Curr Drug Discov.* **3:** 15–20.
53. Maryanoff, B. E. (2004). Inhibitors of serine proteases as potential therapeutic agents: The road from thrombin to tryptase to cathepsin G. *J Med Chem.* **47:** 769–787.
54. Chen, L. S., Nowak, B. J., Ayres, M. L., Krett, N. L., Rosen, S. T., Zhang, S. & Gandhi, V. (2009). Inhibition of ATP synthase by chlorinated adenosine analogue. *Biochem Pharmacol.* **78**: 583–591.
55. Du-Cuny, L., Song, Z., Moses, S., Powis, G., Mash, E. A., Meuillet, E. J. & Zhang, S. (2009). Computational modeling of novel inhibitors targeting the Akt pleckstrin homology domain. *Bioorg Med Chem.* **17:** 6983–6992.
56. Mahadevan, D., Powis, G., Mash, E. A., et al. (2008). Discovery of a novel class of AKT pleckstrin homology domain inhibitors. *Mol Cancer Ther.* **7:** 2621–2632.
57. Moses, S. A., Ali, M. A., Zuohe, S., Du-Cuny, L., Zhou, L. L., Lemos, R., Ihle, N., Skillman, A. G., Zhang, S., Mash, E. A., Powis, G., Meuillet, E. J. (2009). In vitro and in vivo activity of novel small-molecule inhibitors targeting the pleckstrin homology domain of protein kinase B/AKT. *Cancer Res.* **69**: 5073–5081.
58. Zhang, S., Ying, W. S., Siahaan, T. J. & Jois, S. D. S. (2003). Solution structure of a peptide derived from the beta subunit of LFA-1. *Peptides.* **24:** 827–835.
59. Zhang, S., Kumar, K., Jiang, X., Wallqvist, A. & Reifman, J. (2008). DOVIS: an implementation for high-throughput virtual screening using AutoDock. *BMC Bioinformatics* **9:** 126.
60. Zhang, S., Kaplan, A. H. & Tropsha, A. (2008). HIV-1 protease function and structure studies with the simplicial neighborhood analysis of protein packing method. *Proteins.* **73:** 742–753.
61. Zhang, S. & Du-Cuny, L. (2009). Development and evaluation of a new statistical model for structure-based high-throughput virtual screening. *Int J Bioinform Res Appl.* **5:** 269–279.
62. Kitchen, D. B., Decornez, H., Furr, J. R. & Bajorath, J. (2004). Docking and scoring in virtual screening for drug discovery: Methods and applications. *Nat Rev Drug Discov.* **3:** 935–949.
63. Morris, G. M., Goodsell, D. S., Halliday, R. S., Huey, R., Hart, W. E., Belew, R. K. & Olson, A. J. (1999). Automated docking using a

Lamarckian genetic algorithm and an empirical binding free energy function. *J Comput Chem.* **19:** 1639–1662.

64. Halperin, I., Ma, B., Wolfson, H. & Nussinov, R. (2002). Principles of docking: An overview of search algorithms and a guide to scoring functions. *Proteins* **47:** 409–443.
65. Makino, S. & Kuntz, I. D. (1997). Automated flexible ligand docking method and its application for database search. *J Comb Chem.* **18:** 1812–1825.
66. Shoichet, B. K. & Kuntz, I. D. (1991). Protein docking and complementarity. *J Mol Biol.* **221:** 327–346.
67. Kramer, B., Metz, G., Rarey, M. & Lengauer, T. (1999). Ligand docking and screening with FlexX. *Med Chem Res.* **9:** 463–478.
68. Rarey, M., Kramer, B., Lengauer, T. & Klebe, G. (1996). A fast flexible docking method using an incremental construction algorithm. *J Mol Biol.* **261:** 470–489.
69. Goodsell, D. S., Morris, G. M. & Olson, A. J. (1996). Automated docking of flexible ligands: applications of AutoDock. *J Mol Recognit.* **9:** 1–5.
70. Cornell, W. D., Cieplak, P., Bayly, C. I., et al. (1996). A second generation force field for the simulation of proteins, nucleic acids and organic molecules. *J Am Chem Soc.* **117:** 5179–5197.
71. MacKerell, A. D., Jr., Banavali, N. & Foloppe, N. (2000). Development and current status of the CHARMM force field for nucleic acids. *Biopolymers.* **56:** 257–265.
72. Halgren, T. A. (1996). Merck molecular force field: 1. Basis, form, scope, parameterization, and performance of MMFF94. *J Comput Chem.* **17:** 490–519.
73. Shoichet, B. K., Leach, A. R. & Kuntz, I. D. (1999). Ligand solvation in molecular docking. *Proteins.* **34:** 4–16.
74. Bohm, H. J. (1992). Ludi – rule-based automatic design of new substituents for enzyme-inhibitor leads. *J Comput Aided Mol Des.* **6:** 593–606.
75. Bohm, H. J. (1992). The computer-program Ludi – a new method for the denovo design of enzyme-inhibitors. *J Comput Aided Mol Des.* **6:** 61–78.
76. Bohm, H. J. (1998). Prediction of binding constants of protein ligands: a fast method for the prioritization of hits obtained from de novo design or 3D database search programs. *J Comput Aided Mol Des.* **12:** 309–323.
77. Head, R. D., Smythe, M. L., Oprea, T. I., Waller, C. L., Green, S. M. & Marshall, G. R. (1996). VALIDATE: a new method for the receptor-based prediction of binding affinities of novel ligands. *J Am Chem Soc.* **118:** 3959–3969.
78. Gohlke, H., Hendlich, M. & Klebe, G. (2000). Knowledge-based scoring function to predict protein-ligand interactions. *J Mol Biol.* **295:** 337–356.
79. DeWitte, R. S. & Shakhnovich, E. I. (1996). SMoG: de novo design method based on simple, fast, and accurate free energy estimates. 1. Methodology and supporting evidence. *J Am Chem Soc.* **118:** 11733–11744.
80. Muegge, I. & Martin, Y. C. (1999). A general and fast scoring function for protein-ligand interactions: a simplified potential approach. *J Med Chem.* **42:** 791–804.
81. Mitchell, J. B. O., Laskowski, R. A., Alex, A. & Thornton, J. M. (1999). BLEEP-potential of mean force describing protein-ligand interactions: I. Generating potential. *J Comput Chem.* **20:** 1165–1176.
82. Johnston, W. E., Jacobson, V. L., Loken, S. C., Robertson, D. W. & Tierney, B. L. (1992). High-performance computing, high-speed networks, and configurable computing environments: progress toward fully distributed computing. *Crit Rev Biomed Eng.* **20:** 315–354.
83. Golbraikh, A., Shen, M., Xiao, Z. Y., Xiao, Y. D., Lee, K. H. & Tropsha, A. (2003). Rational selection of training and test sets for the development of validated QSAR models. *J Comput Aided Mol Des.* **17:** 241–253.

Chapter 3

Using Active Site Mapping and Receptor-Based Pharmacophore Tools: Prelude to Docking and De Novo/Fragment-Based Ligand Design

Ashutosh Tripathi, J. Andrew Surface, and Glen E. Kellogg

Abstract

Understanding the three-dimensional aspects of drug-receptor interactions and their specificity at the molecular level has become a focal point in modern drug discovery. Herein, we describe a set of methods by which the binding site on a protein can be located and mapped and the protein–ligand intermolecular interactions can be studied in the context of drug discovery. The methodology we describe is based on the empirical Hydropathic INTeraction (HINT) force field. Applications of the novel cavity detection algorithm, VICE, are demonstrated in delineating the binding pockets. The binding site environment is mapped using hydropathic "complementary map." The two binding sites are compared by calculating their 3D differences and the intermolecular interactions between a bound ligand and protein was further studied by HINT intermolecular maps. We illustrate the applications of these different types of HINT maps through an example from the development of selective COX-2 inhibitors.

Key words: Cavity detection, Cavity mapping, Computer-aided drug design, De novo drug design, Docking, HINT, Pharmacophore

1. Introduction

Structural and physicochemical characterization of an active site associated with a protein of health interest has become a major goal in drug discovery, i.e., understanding the chemistry behind molecular recognition is a central issue in drug design. For many years computational medicinal chemists have attempted to develop computer tools that can evaluate protein structure and aid in the design of drugs with higher affinity and selectivity (1, 2). It is perhaps an overworn analogy, but ligand "drug" molecules can be labeled as "keys," and protein receptors labeled as "locks," and

Seetharama D. Satyanarayanajois (ed.), *Drug Design and Discovery: Methods and Protocols*, Methods in Molecular Biology, vol. 716, DOI 10.1007/978-1-61779-012-6_3,

the idea is to find the perfect key to fit a particular lock. With advances in the experimental techniques of X-ray crystallography and NMR, the elucidation of binding features on a protein structure has certainly become more convenient in the last decade or two (3). Concomitantly, technology that enables the computational "mapping" of binding sites to generate pharmacophore models directly from a protein crystal structure has also advanced (4). This combination of experimental structure and computational analysis can reveal key elements in protein–ligand binding. Such knowledge is indispensable for rational drug design because in the majority of cases, receptor–drug interaction is very specific in nature. Correctly mapping the binding site is an important step in structure-based drug design and can be used as the starting point for finding new lead compounds or drug candidates.

While a wide variety of methods of searching for and discovering new drug candidates have been developed in recent years (5, 6), interest has continued to grow in docking, virtual screening of large libraries, and de novo ligand design approaches (7–11). The success of placing, constructing, and validating molecules in a specific target site is ultimately dependent on the accuracy of how well the active site is characterized. After locating and determining the extents of a binding site, the first crucial step involves locating its interaction points or "hot spots." This step more or less unequivocally identifies and delineates the binding site for docking. It is a critical step as it defines and sets the constraints for positioning the ligand in the defined binding region, even though the actual fitting or docking is a geometrical optimization process that can be solved by generating thousands of poses within the given constraints on active site. The next important step is energetically assessing the docked position of ligand, either with a scoring protocol or by a ranking metric for the protein–ligand complex. It is crucial to understand the intermolecular interactions between a protein and a ligand to effectively predict the correct binding mode of a candidate and thus design more potent drugs.

Although many force fields and scoring functions accurately describe most of the expected intermolecular interactions (12, 13), these force fields and scoring functions are mathematical expressions that often tend to overemphasize certain aspects of the physics of the interactions rather than the physicochemical description of binding process. Also, most Newtonian force fields estimate the enthalpic components of binding much more accurately than the entropic. The primary goal of any drug design endeavor is to understand the binding environment in a manner that can help in the design of more selective and potent drugs. As force fields provide energy information regarding the system it would be more useful and meaningful if the physicochemical properties and/or interaction can be represented as fields that can be mapped and visualized, interactively, in three dimensions. Using a map, the spatial distributions of properties such as charge, hydrophobicity, etc. can easily be qualitatively analyzed. Points of interaction between the ligand and active site might be understood and also qualitatively and even semiquantitatively assessed.

1.1. Three-Dimensional Mapping of Protein Properties and Interactions

We have recently described a computational method for determining the location, shape, and size of cavities and pockets on proteins (14). Our method is unique in its particular algorithm, and produces many more metrics describing the cavities it identifies than others, but this type of technology is commonly available from a number of sources, including some on public web servers, e.g., Q-SiteFinder (15), PocketFinder (16), Ligsite^{csc} (17).

A number of computational approaches have been developed to locate and map binding pockets in proteins (1, 2, 4). A pioneering and novel 3D grid-based approach was conceived by Peter Goodford in his GRID program (18). In GRID, a binding region on a protein is mapped by calculating interaction energies between (functional) probe groups placed at each grid point and the atoms of the protein. In a similar approach (MCSS), about 1,000–5,000 small functional groups (probes) are interacted with the protein surface simultaneously and energy minima are calculated to define favorable interaction sites (19). In the above approaches, interaction energy for the probe is calculated and retained as the field value for a contour map of that region. The resultant generated functional maps of the binding site indicate the most favorable regions for placing ligand groups with properties similar to the probes. This map can be contoured at specific energy levels and by visual inspection one can determine the energetically likely locations where that fragment or molecule may be found. This provides the skeleton for positioning a ligand or creating ligands de novo based on the mapped properties of their target. This process intuitively makes sense as rational drug design is fundamentally based on the structure of its receptor (20, 21).

In cases where the structure of the receptor is not known, the putative environment of the active site can be deciphered and mapped from the property fields of a diverse set of ligands that are presumed to bind at that site. The prototype approach, CoMFA (Comparative Molecular Field Analysis), explores the electrostatic and steric interaction field around a set of ligands superimposed on each other (22). Steric and electrostatic fields are calculated for each molecule by interaction with a probe atom at a series of grid points surrounding the aligned 3D structures. These property field energies can be correlated with biological activity data to generate predictive models that guide the optimization of a lead compound. The property field energy can be contoured to generate hypothetical complementary binding features of the active site where a ligand shows optimal electrostatic and steric interactions. CoMSIA, a similar approach, maps hydrogen bond donors, hydrogen bond acceptors, and hydrophobic fields in addition to steric and electrostatic features (23). In short, these methods attempt to model the receptor environment from the perspective of the ligands' structures and properties.

In a variation of the GRID/MCSS approaches and the property fields generated in CoMFA/CoMSIA, where interaction energies are calculated between a probe and a protein atom on a grid, the properties of existing molecules (and atoms) can be *projected* into unoccupied space to propose the properties of a "complement." In other words, it is assumed that the nature of unknown species is complementary in its properties to, or will make ideal interactions with, the defining atom(s) and that the optimum distance between a complementary atom and the defining atom is the sum of their van der Waals radii.

A third paradigm for map creation is one where the interactions between species, e.g., between the protein and its ligand, are encoded and displayed. In this map, the quality of interactions whether favorable or unfavorable for binding, are visualized and putative molecular modifications that would change those interactions can be intuitively examined.

All three dimensional maps are normally and most simply displayed as isopotential contour maps that display solid surfaces of constant value, similar to, two dimensional topographical contour maps of landscape features on Earth.

1.2. The HINT Interaction Model

HINT (Hydropathic INTeractions) is a computational medicinal chemistry research tool that provides map visualization output as was described above. The HINT force field is based on empirically-derived Log $P_{o/w}$ values that intuitively estimate free energy of binding, ΔG (24–26). Log $P_{o/w}$ is a thermodynamic quantity that encodes both enthalpic and entropic contributions and is related to the free energy of solvent transfer between water and 1-octanol for a small molecule. Terms for hydrogen-bonding, acid–base interactions, Coulombic attractions as well as hydrophobic interactions are evaluated. HINT was created specifically to calculate all noncovalent interactions. The HINT model describes specific atom–atom interactions between two molecules, using the equation:

$$H_{\mathrm{TOT}} = \sum\sum b_{ij} = \sum\sum (a_i S_i a_j S_j R_{ij} T_{ij} + r_{ij}) \qquad (1)$$

where a is the hydrophobic atom constant for a single atom (derived from log $P_{o/w}$), S is the solvent accessible surface area, T is a function that differentiates polar – polar interactions (acid–acid, acid–base or base–base), and R and r are functions of the distance between atoms i and j. Usually, R is given by a simple exponential of the distance between the interacting atoms and r is a 6–12 Lennard-Jones potential. The interaction score b_{ij} describes the specific atom–atom interaction between atoms i and j, and H_{TOT} represents the total HINT interaction score. The HINT model is based on the assumption that each b_{ij} approximates a partial δg value for a specific atom–atom interaction, thus the total HINT score, $\Sigma\Sigma\, b_{ij}$, which is the cumulative sum of all the atom–atom interactions, correlates with $\Delta G_{interaction}$, i.e., $\Delta G = \Sigma(\delta G)$.

Depending on the character of the interacting atoms (i.e., $a < 0$ or $a > 0$), the type of an interaction can be quantified, i.e., hydrophobic, polar, etc. Among the possible polar interactions of (Lewis) acid–acid, acid–base or base–base, only acid–base is scored favorably. Hydrophobic–hydrophobic interactions are scored favorably whereas, hydrophobic–polar interactions are categorized as unfavorable. Taking a clue from the nature of these atom constants, the general microenvironment of the binding site can also be characterized and more intuitively, complementary binding points within the binding pocket can also be derived. Analogously, molecular and complementary property maps, with hydrophobicity and polarity scales, can be generated with HINT, using much the same methodology as electrostatic grid mapping programs such as GRID and other mapping algorithms (27): a three-dimensional "grid" is superposed over the molecule or region of interest. At each grid point is a test atom that has hydrophobic atom constant (a_t) and solvent accessible surface area (S_t) both equal to one. The field value of each grid point is then given by $A_t = \Sigma\, a_i\, S_i\, R_{it}$, where R_{it} is a function of the distance between each atom in the system (i) and the grid point (t), which is usually a simple exponential. In complement maps a custom R_{it} function that has its maximum value at twice the van der Waals radius for the projecting atom is used. In addition, the acid/base characters of the projecting atoms are inverted in complement space.

Interaction HINT maps can be envisioned as a calculation where the test (grid) points are acting as observers to the interactions at their locations. Each test point measures the effects from atoms i on one interacting molecule and atoms j on the other interacting molecule with

$$C_t = \sum\sum a_i S_i R_{it} a_j S_j R_{jt}, \quad (2)$$

where C_t is the interaction grid point value.

Herein, we illustrate through several examples the application of various kinds of HINT 3D maps in rational drug design. Taking a case study from the design and development of COX-1 and COX-2 inhibitors, we illustrate how HINT can effectively be used to rationally analyze a protein–ligand complex and optimize a lead molecule. COX-1 and COX-2 are two isoforms of cyclooxygenase enzyme with high structural similarity (28, 29). While COX-1 is expressed in most cells and is believed to be responsible for producing the prostaglandins that provide gastrointestinal tolerability, COX-2 is an inducible form that is expressed in inflammatory tissue. Understanding the architecture and environment of active site is important in designing more potent and selective drugs. Thus, in this method we analyze the active site of COX-1 and COX-2 by utilizing HINT maps and revisit the design and optimization process of a series of analogs, with an illustrative retrospective HINT structure–activity relationships (SAR) analysis.

Recently, second generation NSAIDs have been developed that selectively inhibit the COX-2 isozyme (30). While DuP-697 was one of the first leads reported in 1990 by DuPont Company to be a selective COX-2 inhibitor, Searle Monsanto (now Pfizer) developed an extensive series of compounds that lead to the identification and development of Celecoxib (traded as Celebrex), a potent and selective COX-2 inhibitor (31) (see Fig. 1). Compound SC558, a celecoxib prototype, was developed by substituting the methyl-sulfonyl group with a sulfonamide moiety; it was cocrystallized and reported (29) as the culmination of much research, development, and evaluation. One lead compound developed from DuP-697 was SC58125 with a pyrazole scaffold. Another such compound, SC57666, with a cyclopentene scaffold showed that the function of the heterocyclic ring is to provide the necessary spatial geometry to the 1,2-diaryl rings and that a heterocycle ring is not necessary for activity. A number of selective COX-2 analogs were developed by substitution on the two phenyl rings and the heterocyclic ring (31).

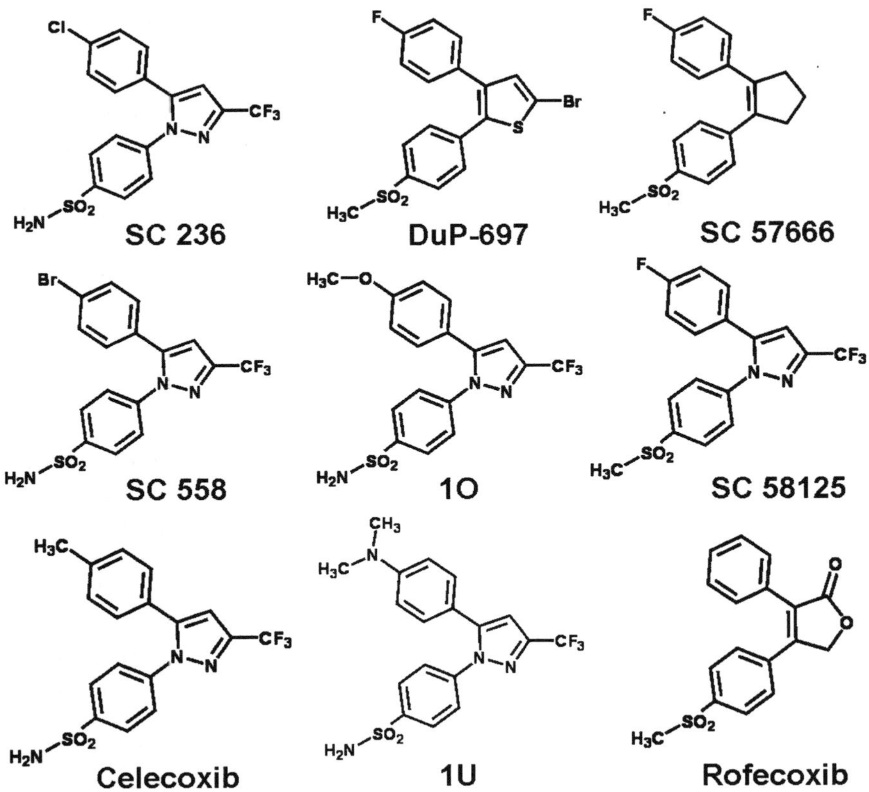

Fig. 1. Structures of selective COX-2 inhibitors. Development of second generation NSAIDs began with improvements on a series of compounds starting with the lead *DuP-697*.

2. Materials

2.1. Model Building

The dataset in this study consists of X-ray crystal structures of COX-1 and COX-2 enzyme cocrystallized with different marketed drugs and known inhibitors. These crystal structures were selected from the literature. The X-ray crystal structure coordinates of COX-1 complexed with Flurbiprofen (PDB code: 1EQH) (32) and COX-2 complexed with SC558 (PDB code: 6COX) (29) and flurbiprofen (PDB code: 3PGH) (29), in PDB format, were retrieved from the RCSB (Brookhaven) Protein Data Bank (3). Molecular modeling was performed using the Sybyl 7.3 program suite (www.tripos.com) on Linux workstations. The HINT module with its associated computational tools is available as a Sybyl add-on or as a programmable toolkit from eduSoft LC (www.edusoft-lc.com).

3. Methods

3.1. Preparation of Protein Models

There are a number of experimental factors and uncertainties, as well as flaws in the commonly used file formats, which require some "preparation" of protein molecular models before they can be effectively used in computational studies. The following steps illustrate a minimal set of steps that may be applied to "clean up" a structure. More extensive preparation such as unrestrained energy minimization may be necessary if there are errors in the experimental structure data, e.g., nonhydrogen atoms that are too close to one another, etc.

1. The protein and protein–ligand structures were prepared for this study by removing all the water molecules and ions associated with the structure. The ligands were extracted and their bond orders and atom types (hybridization and environment) were checked against the published chemical structures. Hydrogen atoms were added to complete valences as necessary. The ligand structures, thus modified, were remerged with the protein models. Hydrogen atoms were next added to the protein structures using the tool within the Sybyl Biopolymer module and the positions of all hydrogens in the system were optimized to an energy gradient of 0.005 kcal Å mol^{-1} with the Tripos force field (in Sybyl 7.3) while keeping heavy atom positions fixed (i.e., heavy atoms were treated as an immobile aggregate). The models for the ligand analogs were then reextracted from the crystal structures (see Note 1).
2. To compare and analyze COX-1 and COX-2 active sites, the two structures were overlaid on the basis of their sequence

similarity using the "Align Structures by Homology" feature under Sybyl's Biopolymer module, taking COX-2 as the reference structure.

3. LogP, also referred to as the ***hydrophobicity***, is a key factor in drug design, and is the first step in all HINT calculations as it provides the primary atom-based metric for analyses (*vide supra*). Thus, all proteins and ligands need to be "Partitioned" before running any other HINT calculations on them.
4. For proteins and small molecules, the "Partition Method" should be set to "Dictionary" and "Calculate," respectively. The latter option uses the molecules' Sybyl atom types and bond connections as input data to the HINT partition algorithm.
5. To somewhat simplify calculations, some atoms are not explicitly used. For the protein and ligand, only "Essential" hydrogens are treated explicitly. Essential hydrogens are bonded to polar atoms and may potentially become involved in hydrogen bonds. All other hydrogen atoms are treated implicitly, e.g., a methyl is treated as a methyl "atom" rather than an sp^3 carbon plus three distinct hydrogen atoms. The "Solvent Condition" was set to "Inferred," which sets the protonation state for each protein amino acid monomer based on the number and connectivity of the hydrogens present.

3.2. Cavity Map Detection

The Cavity search module of HINT invokes the new VICE algorithm (14) to locate and delineate the binding site on a protein. The module generates cavity maps that can be visualized graphically along with sets of descriptive data metrics providing both qualitative and quantitative information about the (putative) protein active sites.

1. The first step of cavity detection is to define parameters for creating and calculating a grid box around the entire protein or just the region of interest. In either case, a 3D Cartesian grid box is created and its extents and grid-spacing are defined. The 3D grid points typically have a spacing of 1.0 Å, but the resolution can be varied depending upon the computational requirements. To define a region of interest, either an atom centered- or a coordinate centered-box can be used, or when the cavity location is well-defined by the presence of a ligand in the binding site, that ligand's extents can be used. In the COX-1 and COX-2 cases, the ligands present in the binding sites defined the regions of interest, and their extents enhanced by a 5-Å margin and a grid resolution of 1 Å were used as grid boxes.
2. The "Maximum Unrestrained Pathlength (MUP)" is set to 10 Å; this is the vector length limit for scanning grid points

within the defined grid box. The algorithm detects cavities by determining the fraction of vectors emanating from each grid point that encounter atoms rather than the box edge. The MUP limits false positives due to other molecules or curved cavity entrances. The "Cavity Definition," which is the fraction of vectors encountering atoms, is set to 0.50, and this value is contoured in creating the cavity map. This cavity definition can be adjusted to tailor the profile of the cavity entrance, whether flat, concave, or convex.

3. The calculated raw cavity, thus calculated, can further be refined with a "Shaping Factor" parameter that smoothes the cavity by eliminating vague tendrils, etc. that project from the cavity. This works by requiring each grid point within the cavity to have a defined fraction of its neighbors to also be within the cavity. The default value is set to 0.5, but the user can interactively smooth out the cavity by varying this value, through visual inspection, and/or iterative applications.
4. Further, small clusters of unoccupied spaces are eliminated based on the value of minimum volume for retention. The default value is set to 100 Å^3. If there is ambiguity or multiple cavities of interest, the user can interactively change parameters and/or region definition and focus on just one of the pockets and investigate it in detail.
5. Once the cavity of interest is isolated and defined with a map, the surface of the pocket can be contoured and displayed with translucent, solid surface, line, or dot rendering. The user can also generate a set of cavity analysis metrics with detailed information about the volume and surface area (including an estimate of the opening size), as well as lists of atoms, residues, and/or chains lining the binding pocket.

Figures 2a–c illustrates the cavity maps for COX-1 (a, in orange translucent surface) and COX-2 (b, in yellow translucent surface). The proteins are aligned on the same coordinate system (*vide infra*) for convenience. On inspecting the two cavities, there are clearly slightly different shapes of the two cavities with COX-2 cavity slightly larger in size with a much more well-defined subpocket in the lower right quadrant (Fig. 2b) than the likely to be inaccessible subpocket in this region of COX-1 (Fig. 2a). This is echoed in the quantitative data that estimates the volume of the COX-1 active site pocket to be ~690 Å^3 and that of COX-2 to be ~790 Å^3. Figure 2c illustrates these two pockets superimposed and thus indicates the regions, of particularly COX-2, that can be exploited for the design of selective inhibitors.

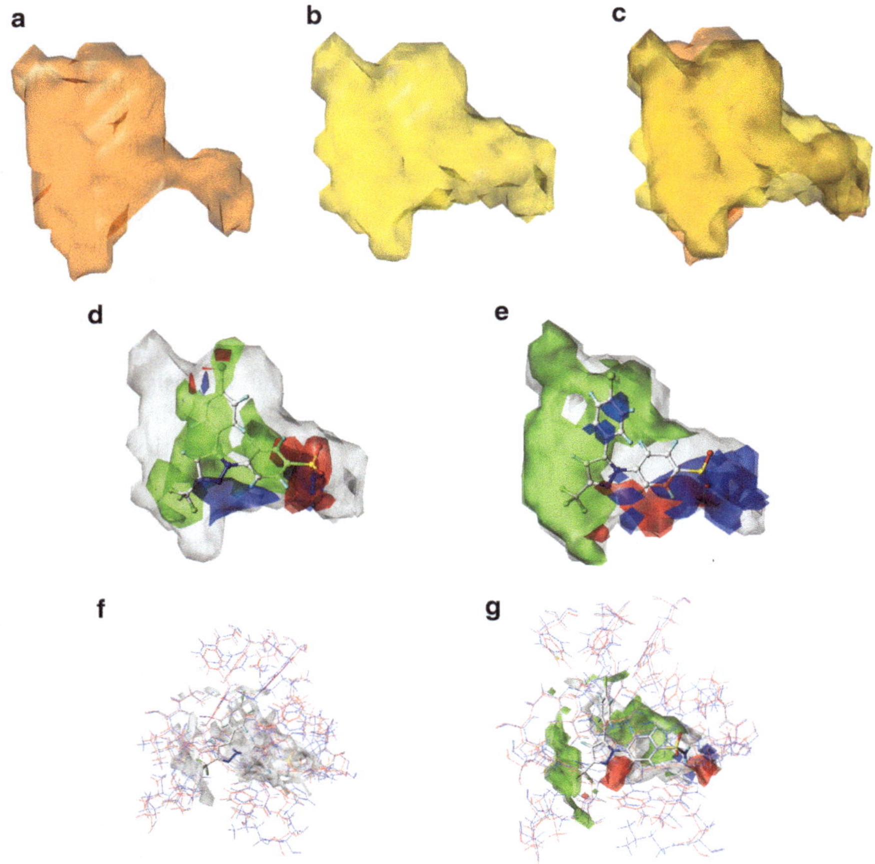

Fig. 2. Contoured displays of various maps calculated in this report. *Cavity Volumes and extents*. (**a**) COX-1; (**b**) COX-2; (**c**) COX-1 and COX-2 superimposed. The orientation of the COX-1 molecular model was transformed to match that of the COX-2 molecular model. (**d**) *Intermolecular HINT interaction map between COX-2 and SC558. Green contours* show favorable hydrophobic interactions, *blue contours* show favorable polar interactions and *red contour* shows unfavorable polar interactions. (**e**) *Complement map of the COX-2 active site*. (**f**) *Difference map*. Figure illustrates difference map between COX-1 and COX-2. The white shaded mapped region shows the exclusive regions COX-2 cavity. (**g**) *Difference map*. Figure shows exclusive complementary site present in COX-2 but absent in COX-1 active site. *Green regions* are hydrophobic regions, *red* and *blue* are acid and basic complementary regions present in COX-2 but absent in COX-1.

3.3. Intermolecular Interaction Table and Map

Once the active site is defined, the next step in any drug design project is to thoroughly characterize the binding site. In cases where the target protein is cocrystallized with a small molecule inhibitor/modulator, it is very instructive to study and analyze intermolecular interaction between the protein and this bound ligand. HINT 3D intermolecular and complement maps can provide crucial information about the intermolecular interaction and nature of the active site. In the following step, we investigate the binding of the SC558 (inhibitor/lead) to COX-2, quantitatively via HINT Table analysis and graphically via HINT Maps.

1. The Intermolecular Table module tabulates all the interaction between a protein and a ligand and data is written to HINT Table files (.tab) (Fig. 3). All interactions, within a cutoff radius of typically 8 Å, are recorded and summed. The .tab file reports, however, a subset of these interactions defined by the table "Extents," which excludes interactions outside a range of (usually) 6 Å, and table "Value," which excludes interactions with absolute value of HINT score (*bij* in (1)) below a threshold of (usually) 10. The total HINT interaction score (H_{TOT}) is an indicator of the binding efficiency between the inhibitor and COX-2. The correlation of these HINT interaction scores with experimental binding data for a set of several compounds may lead to a QSAR-like model that can be used to predict binding for new, untested molecular inhibitors. Figure 3 is an example HINT interaction (.tab) file for SC558 bound to COX-2.
2. Intermolecular interactions can be visualized using 3D intermolecular maps. Maps for hydrophobic and polar interactions are calculated separately so that polar binding interactions

Monomer Type	Monomer Name	Atom Name	Atom Type	Hydrophobic Atom Const.	SASA	Atom Name	Atom Type	Hydrophobic Atom Const.	SASA	Distance Angstroms	Distance VDW	Interaction Score	Interaction Type
HIS	HIS90	CE1	C.2:1	-0.652	60.00	N3	N.am	-1.540	101.26	3.698	113.80	137	Acid/Base
HIS	HIS90	CE1	C.2:1	-0.652	60.00	01	0.2	-1.915	40.05	3.023	94.46	108	Acid/Base
HIS	HIS90	CE1	C.2:1	-0.652	60.00	S1	S.o2	1.980	25.89	3.935	112.43	-32	Hydroph./Polar
ARG	ARG120	NH1	N.pl3	-1.540	49.00	C3	C.co	1.165	24.36	3.588	110.40	-41	Hydroph./Polar
ARG	ARG120	NH1	N.pl3	-1.540	49.00	C4	C.3	-0.940	18.08	3.577	110.06	34	Hydroph./Polar
ARG	ARG120	NH1	N.pl3	-1.540	49.00	N2	N.2	-1.871	32.29	3.966	127.95	50	Acid/Base
SER	SER353	O	0.2	-1.915	26.00	N3	N.am	-1.540	101.26	2.785	91.32	70	Hydrogen Bond
SER	SER353	O	0.2	-1.915	26.00	01	0.2	-1.915	40.05	4.598	153.28	-13	Base/Base
SER	SER353	O	0.2	-1.915	26.00	S1	S.o2	1.980	25.89	4.132	125.22	-23	Base/Base
TYR	TYR355	OH	0.3	-0.440	40.00	C6	C.ar:1	0.355	40.88	3.468	108.38	32	Hydrogen Bond
TYR	TYR355	OH	0.3	-0.440	40.00	C7	C.ar:1	0.355	40.87	4.015	125.47	20	Acid/Base
TYR	TYR355	OH	0.3	-0.440	40.00	N2	N.2	-1.871	32.29	4.010	131.48	34	Acid/Base
LEU	LEU359	CD2	C.3:3	0.820	65.00	C4	C.3	-0.940	18.08	4.227	124.32	15	Hydrophobic
LEU	LEU359	CD2	C.3:3	0.820	65.00	F2	F.cf3	0.243	41.23	3.238	101.20	18	Hydrophobic
LEU	LEU384	CD1	C.3:3	0.820	66.00	BR1	Br	1.030	54.18	3.739	106.83	54	Hydrophobic
ARG	ARG513	NH1	N.pl3	-1.540	49.00	01	0.2	-1.915	40.05	3.336	109.39	125	Hydrogen Bond
ARG	ARG513	NH1	N.pl3	-1.540	49.00	02	0.2	-1.915	40.05	5.511	180.68	12	Acid/Base
ARG	ARG513	NH1	N.pl3	-1.540	49.00	S1	S.o2	1.980	25.89	4.496	134.21	34	Acid/Base
VAL	VAL523	CG2	C.3:3	0.818	61.50	02	0.2	-1.915	40.05	3.650	114.06	-64	Hydroph./Polar
VAL	VAL523	CG2	C.3:3	0.818	61.50	S1	S.o2	1.980	25.89	3.607	103.06	69	Hydrophobic

```
Total Interaction Constant        1.333215e+03

 Contributions:
        5.271311e+02 Hydrogen Bond
        1.336454e+03 Acid/Base
        1.406055e+03 Hydrophobic
       -1.856216e+02 Acid/Acid
       -6.445333e+02 Base/Base
       -1.106271e+03 Hydroph./Polar
```

Fig. 3. An example of a HINT interaction (.tab) file for SC558 bound to COX-2. The first two columns show the name and type of protein residue involved in the interaction. Atom Name and Atom Type columns describe Sybyl atom name and atom type, respectively (for example C.2:1 describes an sp^2 hybridized carbon with one hydrogen attached to it). Hydrophobic Atom Const. and SASA are empirically derived atom constant and Solvent Accessible Surface Area for that particular atom (see (1)). The next four columns give the same type of information about the interacting ligand/molecule. The Distance column gives information about the distance between the two interacting atom in Angstroms, while VDW is the percentage of the sum of van der Waals of two interacting atom (i.e., 100 would be perfect van der Waals distance between them). The last column gives the HINT interaction score (as calculated by (1)) and type of interaction between the two interacting atom. At end of the file, Total HINT interaction score is given with breakdown of all the contributing interaction types.

can be more accurately classified. In the hydrophobic map, grid points with positive values arise from hydrophobic–hydrophobic interactions and grid points with negative values arise from hydrophobic–polar nonbinding interactions. The latter interaction class can be considered as representing, to a large extent, the cost of desolvation. There are four interaction classes represented in a polar map: hydrogen bond, acid–base, acid–acid and base–base. Polar interactions are all those that do not involve hydrophobic atoms. Hydrogen bonding interactions are special cases of (favorable) acid–base interactions where the interacting atoms and interatomic distances are consistent with hydrogen bonds being formed. Both acid–acid and base–base interactions are unfavorable interactions and contribute negative-valued grid points and are thus unfavorable (see Note 2).

3. The dimensional extents of the map region are usually defined using the molecular extents of the inhibitor with a margin of 4 Å. The "Distance Function" is the definition of the R_{ij} and r_{ij} terms in (1). While there are a lot of adjustable parameters in the distance function, for this exercise we kept the default parameters, i.e., $R_{ij} = e^{-r}$, a simple exponential of the distance between interacting atoms.
4. Both the hydrophobic and polar (acid/base) interaction density maps were calculated using identical map regions and distance functions. These maps can be visualized by contouring the corresponding map for display. Loading a map produces a histogram of the contour data with a range of values from maximum (positive) to minimum (negative). Generally, one plots maps at the +20% and –20% levels as a first look. The color convention that we recommend is green for favorable (+) hydrophobic/hydrophobic interactions that promote the binding, blue for favorable (+) polar/polar interactions such as acid/base and hydrogen bonding that promote the binding and red regions for unfavorable (–) polar/polar interactions that appear to hinder the binding. While the unfavorable (–) hydrophobic/polar interactions may also be plotted, they often make the maps too busy and complicated.

Figure 2d illustrates the intermolecular HINT interaction map between COX-2 cocrystallized with its inhibitor SC558. The three contours represent the significant interactions between COX-2 and SC558; the color conventions are as described above. Close examination of these maps, particularly in the red regions, suggests that either there is an ionization state mismatch like two (negatively charged) carboxylates in close proximity that should be corrected by protonation of one in the molecular model, or, more interestingly, that careful design might produce a new ligand better-suited for the active site. Also, it is often instructive to examine the interaction table in concert with the intermolecular map.

3.4. Complement Map

When the structure of a receptor is known, it is useful to qualitatively identify the hydropathic structural features of the binding site or to generate a structure/receptor-based pharmacophore. In generating a complement map of the binding site, it may be possible to identify pharmacophoric features that should be present in the "ideal" substrate for that receptor site. The pharmacophoric features can then be compared to the bound molecules that can subsequently be optimized for better interactions.

1. To generate complementary maps, it is desirable to partition the molecule with "Directionality Vectors" *on* in order to focus the hydropathic map density along physically meaningful vectors associated with the molecule structure. The "Directionality Vector Types" are set to "Hybridized Pi/Lone Pairs," an option that emphasizes polar density in π clouds and lone pairs. The vector focus represents how tightly the polar hydropathic density will adhere to the vector directions; hydrophobic density is treated as nondirectional (spherical). With no directionality, hydropathic density in complement maps is uniformly spherical.
2. As with all maps, complement maps need to be generated within the active site region. In this example, the region of interest can be defined using the molecular (dimensional) extents of the inhibitor. The hydrophobic/polar and acid/base complement maps are calculated and saved separately for later visualization. Generally, all parameters are set as they were in intermolecular interaction map calculations. New, however, is the option to use a cavity map to "focus" the complement map within the cavity. The idea of cavity focusing is simply implemented: if the cavity map is represented as a TRUE (1)/FALSE (0) map where TRUE represents grid points inside the cavity and FALSE represents grid points outside, then multiplying that map by the complement map will restrict the complement map to grid points within the boundaries of the cavity.
3. The hydrophobic/polar and acid/base complement maps are calculated and then focused as above. The focused complement maps can be visualized by contouring them. Generally, contour values are chosen such that their values are around 50% of the maximum (or minimum) field value (see Note 3).

The hydrophobic/polar complement map produces a map where positive field values represent hydrophobic regions of space, and negative field values represent polar (hydrophilic) regions. The acid/base complement map produces a map where the acidic polar and basic polar regions of space are coded with positive and negative field values, respectively. Figure 2e illustrates the complement map of the COX-2 active site. The net display of contoured maps shows regions of the active site most hospitable to hydrophobic groups (green contour) and differentiates between the two types of polar regions (acid-like in red and base-like in blue) based on the Lewis definition of acids and bases.

3.5. Difference Maps

The active site of COX-1 and COX-2 is highly conserved with a sequence identity of ~87%. Understanding the *differences* between the active sites of two isoforms is critical in designing more selective inhibitors with lower toxicity. Comparative analysis of the COX-1 and COX-2 active sites can be performed by calculating difference maps between the two active sites.

1. Contour files (**.cnt*) of COX-1 and COX-2 cavity maps are given as input. Subtracting the COX-1 cavity map from COX-2 cavity map will highlight the difference in the shape of the two cavities.
2. More to the point, we can find the features exclusively present in one cavity by finding the difference between the complement maps of one active site and the other. Using the previously calculated hydrophobic/polar and acid/base complement maps for both the COX-1 and COX-2 active site aligned on the same Cartesian coordinate system, difference maps can be calculated by subtracting the hydrophobic/polar complement map of COX-1 from the hydrophobic/polar complement map of COX-2. Similarly, the acid/base complement map of COX-1 is subtracted from that of COX-2. Once both difference maps are generated, they can be visually inspected. Figure 2f illustrates the difference map between the cavity maps of COX-1 and COX-2: the gray-colored contours delineate the portion of cavity that is present in COX-2 but absent in COX-1. Figure 2g illustrates the complementary map regions exclusive to COX-2.

It becomes clearer on analyzing the cavity maps and their difference maps that COX-2 pocket extends into a subpocket that is somewhat restricted in COX-1. This additional subpocket is relatively polar in nature and is responsible for selectivity of second generation COX-2 inhibitor. Figure 2f shows difference in complement map between COX-1 and COX-2. Difference between the two sites can be seen in the extended subpocket region where sulfonamide group snugly fits in the pocket of COX-2. Sulfonamide group is important for activity as conversion of sulfonamide to methylsulfone leads to loss-in-activity as observed in the cases of cmpd39/SC58125, DuP607, SC57666, and Rofecoxib. On the other side is a hydrophobic region that is lined by residues Phe381, Leu384, Tyr385, Trp387, Phe513 where catalysis occurs. Extensive SAR studies have been performed at this site. Substitution on 5-aryl ring with methyl (1i/Celecoxib), methoxy (1o), and N,N-dimethyl group (1u) resulted in superior COX-2 activity.

Structure–activity relationship analysis showed substitution on 4-position that leads to increase in activity (31). HINT Intermolecular interaction analysis and Complementary map analysis further validated this result and was observed from the map analysis.

4. Notes

1. During the preparation of protein, water molecules, ions, or cofactors should only be retained if they are structurally conserved and contribute in protein–ligand interaction. It is important to save the modified protein in the mol2 file format because the traditional PDB format does not save all hybridization and bond order information.
2. The presence of negative interactions is an inescapable consequence of biological interactions, and it may be tempting to extract too much significance from them.
3. The Contour Value is the numerical value for the contouring operation. It represents the isopotential to be enclosed by the contour surfaces. Generally, choose a Contour Value that is around 50% of the maximum (or minimum) field value. Ultimately, however, maps are meant to be visually pleasing and informative, so avoid choosing Contour Values that are misleading, e.g., implying a greater contribution of hydrophobic interaction than is present, etc.

References

1. Sotriffer, C., Klebe, G. (2002) Identification and mapping of small-molecule binding sites in proteins: computational tools for structure-based drug design. *Il Farmaco.* **57**: 243–251.
2. Campbell, S. J., Gold, N. D., Jackson, R. M., Westhead, D. R. (2003) Ligand binding: functional site location, similarity and docking. *Curr Opin Struct Biol* **13**: 389–395.
3. Berman, H. M., Westbrook, J., Feng, Z., Gilliland, G., Bhat, T. N., Weissig, H., Shindyalov, I. N., Bourne, P. E. (2000) The protein data bank. *Nucleic Acid Res.* **28**: 235–242.
4. Pazos, F., Sternberg, M. J. E. (2004) Automated prediction of protein function and detection of functional sites from structure. *Proc Natl Acad Sci.* **101**: 14754–14759.
5. Bleicher, K. H., Böhm, H., Müller, K., Alanine, A. I. (2003) Hit and lead generation: beyond high-throughput screening. *Nat Rev Drug Discov.* **2:** 369–378.
6. Walters, W. P., Murcko, A., Murcko, M. A. (1999) Recognizing molecules with drug-like properties. *Curr Opin Chem Bio.* **3:** 384–387.
7. Walters, W. P., Stahl, M. T., Murcko, M. A. (1998) Virtual screening – an overview. *Drug Discov Today.* **3:** 160–178.
8. Smith, A. (2002) Screening for drug discovery: the leading question. *Nature.* **418**: 483–459.
9. Schneider, G., Böhm, H. (2002) Virtual screening and fast automated docking methods. *Drug Discov Today.* **7:** 64–70.
10. Erlanson, D. A., McDowell, R. S., O'Brien, T. (2004) Fragment-based drug discovery. *J Med Chem.* **47:** 3463–3482.
11. Martin, Y. C. (1992) 3D database searching in drug design. *J Med Chem.* **35:** 2145–2154.
12. Ferrara, P., Gohlke, H., Price, D. J., Klebe, G., Brooks III, C. L. (2004) Assessing scoring functions for protein-ligand interactions. *J Med Chem.* **47:** 3032–3047.

13. Gohlke, H., Klebe, G. (2002) Approaches to the description and prediction of the binding affinity of small-molecule ligands to macromolecular receptors. *Angew Chem Int Ed.* **41**: 2644–2676.
14. Tripathi, A., Kellogg, G. E. (2010) A novel and efficient tool for locating and characterizing protein cavities and binding sites. *Protein Struct Funct Bioinf.* **78**: 825–842.
15. Laurie, A. T. R., Jackson, R. M. (2005) Q-SiteFinder: an energy-based method for the prediction of protein-ligand binding sites. *Bioinformatics.* **21**: 1908–1916.
16. An, J., Totrov, M., Abagyan, R. (2005) Pocketome via comprehensive identification and classification of ligand binding envelopes. *Mol Cell Proteomics.* **4**: 752–761.
17. Huang, B., Schroeder, M. (2006) LIGSITE^{csc}: predecting ligand binding sites using the Connolly surface and degree of conservation. *BMC Struct Biol.* **6**: 19.
18. Goodford, P.J. (1985) A computational procedure for determining energetically favorable binding sites on biologically important macromolecules. *J Med Chem.* **28**: 849–857.
19. Miranker, A., Karplus, M. (1991) Functionality maps of binding sites: a multiple copy simultaneous search method. *Proteins Struct Funct Genet.* **11**: 29–34.
20. Joseph-McCarthy, D. (1999) Computational approaches to structure-based ligand design. *Pharmacol Ther.* **84**: 179–191.
21. Anderson, A.C. (2003) The process of structure-based drug design. *Chem Biol.* **10**: 787–797.
22. Cramer III, R. D., Patterson D. E., Bunce, J. D. (1988) Comparative molecular field analysis (CoMFA). 1. Effect of shape on binding of steroids to carrier proteins. *J Am Chem Soc.* **110**: 5959–5967.
23. Klebe, G., Abraham, U., Mietzner, T. (1994) Molecular similarity indices in a comparative analysis (CoMSIA) of drug molecules to correlate and predict their biological activity. *J Med Chem.* **37**: 4130–4146.
24. Kellogg, G. E., Abraham, D. J. (2000) Hydrophobicity: is LogP(o/w) more than the sum of its parts? *Eur J Med Chem.* **35**: 651–661.
25. Cozzini, P., Fornabaio, M., Marabotti, A., Abraham, D. J., Kellogg, G. E., Mozzarelli, A. (2002) Simple, intuitive calculations of free energy of binding for protein-ligand complexes. 1. Models without explicit constrained water. *J Med Chem.* **45**: 2469–2483.
26. Spyrakis, F., Amadasi, A., Fornabaio, M., Abraham, D. J., Mozzarelli, A., Kellogg, G. E., Cozzini, P. (2007) The consequences of scoring docked ligand conformations using free energy correlations. *Eur J Med Chem.* **42**: 921–933.
27. Kellogg, G. E., Abraham, D. J. (1992) KEY, LOCK, and LOCKSMITH: Complementary hydropathic map predictions of drug structure from a known receptor-receptor structure from known drugs. *J Mol Graphics.* **10:** 212–217.
28. Filizola, M., Perez, J. J., Palomer, A., Mauleo´n, D. (1997) Comparative molecular modeling study of the three-dimensional structures of prostaglandin endoperoxide H2 synthase 1 and 2 (COX-1 and COX-2). *J Mol Graph Mod.* **15**: 290–300.
29. Kurumbail, R.G., Stevens, A. M., Gierse, J. K., McDonald, J. J., Stegeman, R. A., Pak, J. Y., Gildehaus, D., Miyashiro, J. M., Penning, T. D., Seibert, K., Isakson, P. C., Stallings, W. C. (1996) Structural basis for selective inhibition of cyclooxygenase-2 by anti-inflammatory agents. *Nature.* **384**: 644–648.
30. Flower, R. J. (2003) The development of COX-2 inhibitor. *Nat Rev Drug Discov.* **2**: 179–191.
31. Penning, T. D., Talley, J. J., Bertenshaw, S. R., Carter, J. S., Collins, P. W., Docter, S., Graneto, M. J., Lee, L. F., Malecha, J. W., Miyashiro, J. M., Rogers, R. S., Rogier, D. J., Yu, S. S., Anderson, G. D., Burton, E. G., Cogburn, J. N., Gregory, S. A., Koboldt, C. M., Perkins, W. E., Seibert, K., Veenhuizen, A. W., Zhang, Y. Y., Isakson, P. C. (1997) Synthesis and biological evaluation of the 1,5-Diarylpyrazole class of cyclooxygenase-2 inhibitors: identification of 4-(5-(4-Methylphenyl)-3-(trifluoromethyl)-1H-pyrazol-1-yl) benzenesulfonamide (SC-48635, Celecoxib). *J Med Chem.* **40**: 1347–1365.
32. Selinsky, B. S., Gupta, K., Sharkey, C. T., Loll, P. J. (2001) Structural analysis of NSAID binding by prostaglandin H2 synthase: Time-dependent and time-independent inhibitors elicit identical enzyme conformations. *Biochemistry.* **40**: 5172–5180.

Chapter 4

Methods for Evaluation of Structural and Biological Properties of Antiinvasive Natural Products

Mudit Mudit, Mohammad Khanfar, Girish V. Shah, and Khalid A. El Sayed

Abstract

Prostate cancer is considered the most common cancer form among males in Western countries. Very limited options are available for the treatment of advanced metastatic prostate cancer. More than 50% of today's anticancer drugs are natural products or derived from a natural origin. To discover new entities with potential to treat prostate cancer at androgen-refractory stages, 36 structurally diverse natural products were screened using functional-based assays. The tested compounds were selected broadly from major secondary metabolites of plants, marine invertebrates, and fungi. These diverse entities were prescreened for their antiinvasive ability against prostate cancer cells, PC-3M, using spheroid disaggregation assay. Active representatives including three selected structural classes, a macrolide, a β-carboline alkaloid, and a phenylmethylene hydantoin (PMH), were then tested for their ability to stabilize junctional complexes and enhance cell–cell adhesion of androgen independent prostate cancer cells. Transepithelial resistance (TER) and paracellular permeability assays were used to elicit the aforementioned properties. These studies led to the emergence of PMHs as a small molecule class from the marine sponge *Hemimycale arabica* with a unique potential to attenuate CT-stimulated prostate cancer growth, metastasis, paracellular permeability, and enhance TER and cell–cell adhesion of prostate cancer cells. The unique activities of PMHs were validated using several in vitro assays followed by in vivo testing in two mice models. A 3D QSAR was established using SYBYL 8.1-Comparative Molecular Field Analysis (CoMFA) model. This chapter includes the methodology for evaluation of structural and biological properties of new antiinvasive molecules with an exceptional potential to stabilize junctional complexes from diverse natural product sources.

Key words: Antimetastatic, Cell–cell adhesion, CoMFA, Junctional complexes, LPB-Tag mice, Natural products, Nude mice, Phenylmethylene hydantoin, Prostate cancer, Red Sea sponge *Hemimycale arabica*, Spheroid disaggregation assay

1. Introduction

Prostate cancer is the second leading cause of cancer-related death in men in the United States (1). Surgery, radiation therapy, and watchful waiting constitute the current available treatment options

Seetharama D. Satyanarayanajois (ed.), *Drug Design and Discovery: Methods and Protocols*, Methods in Molecular Biology, vol. 716, DOI 10.1007/978-1-61779-012-6_4,

for localized and early-stage prostate cancer (2). However, disease relapsing is common in patients with advanced metastatic disease (2). The disease when treated with androgen ablation therapy eventually becomes androgen-independent in nature and the tumor becomes metastatic, chemoresistant, and life threatening (3–5). It is believed that a key mechanism associated with calcitonin (CT)-stimulated prostate cancer progression and metastasis is the disruption of cell–cell adhesion (6, 7). The poor clinical outcome with chemotherapeutic agents such as doxorubicin, mitoxantrone, and docetaxel in patients with hormone refractory prostate cancer urges the critical need for the discovery and development of effective therapeutic agents for the treatment of the disease.

For the discovery and development of new drugs, natural products proved to be an unparalleled source of molecular diversity. Drugs from the natural origin can be classified as "original natural products," "semi-synthetically-derived natural products," and "synthetic products based on natural product models" (8). For the discovery of new natural products class that can enhance cell–cell adhesion and attenuate prostate tumor growth and metastasis, in-house library of various isolated natural products was screened (Fig. 1). These compounds were isolated from a wide-range of sources like plants, fungi, and marine invertebrates (Fig. 2). The isolated compounds with diverse molecular skeleton were selected for the prescreening in support of antigrowth and antiinvasive properties against the highly metastatic PC-3M cells in MTT assay, Matrigel™-invasion assay, spheroid disaggregation assay, and other function-based assays. MTT assay was used to measure the viable (living) cell count, and hence to demonstrate any cytotoxic effect of the tested compounds. In addition, the effect of the abovementioned compounds on PC-3M cell proliferation was also evaluated in the presence and absence of CT (CT causes modest but significant increase in PC-3M proliferation). The objective was to identify those compounds which can inhibit CT-induced cell proliferation in prostate cancer cells. For the development of metastasis, tumor invasion of basement membrane is considered one of the crucial steps in the complex multistep event. Matrigel-invasion assay was used to measure the degree of metastasis, which latter was replaced by spheroid disaggregation assay. Spheroid disaggregation assay is considered a better mimic of in situ tumor metastasis compared to the linear invasion assays, because tumor cells are generally released in clumps, attach to the preferred extracellular matrix (ECM), and then radially migrate in all directions (9–12).

Interestingly, three compounds with diverse molecular skeleton were identified with the ability to suffice the above postulated aim. Latrunculin A (a macrolide), manzamine A (a β-carboline alkaloid), and phenylmethylene hydantoin (PMH) (a cyclic imide, hydantoin)

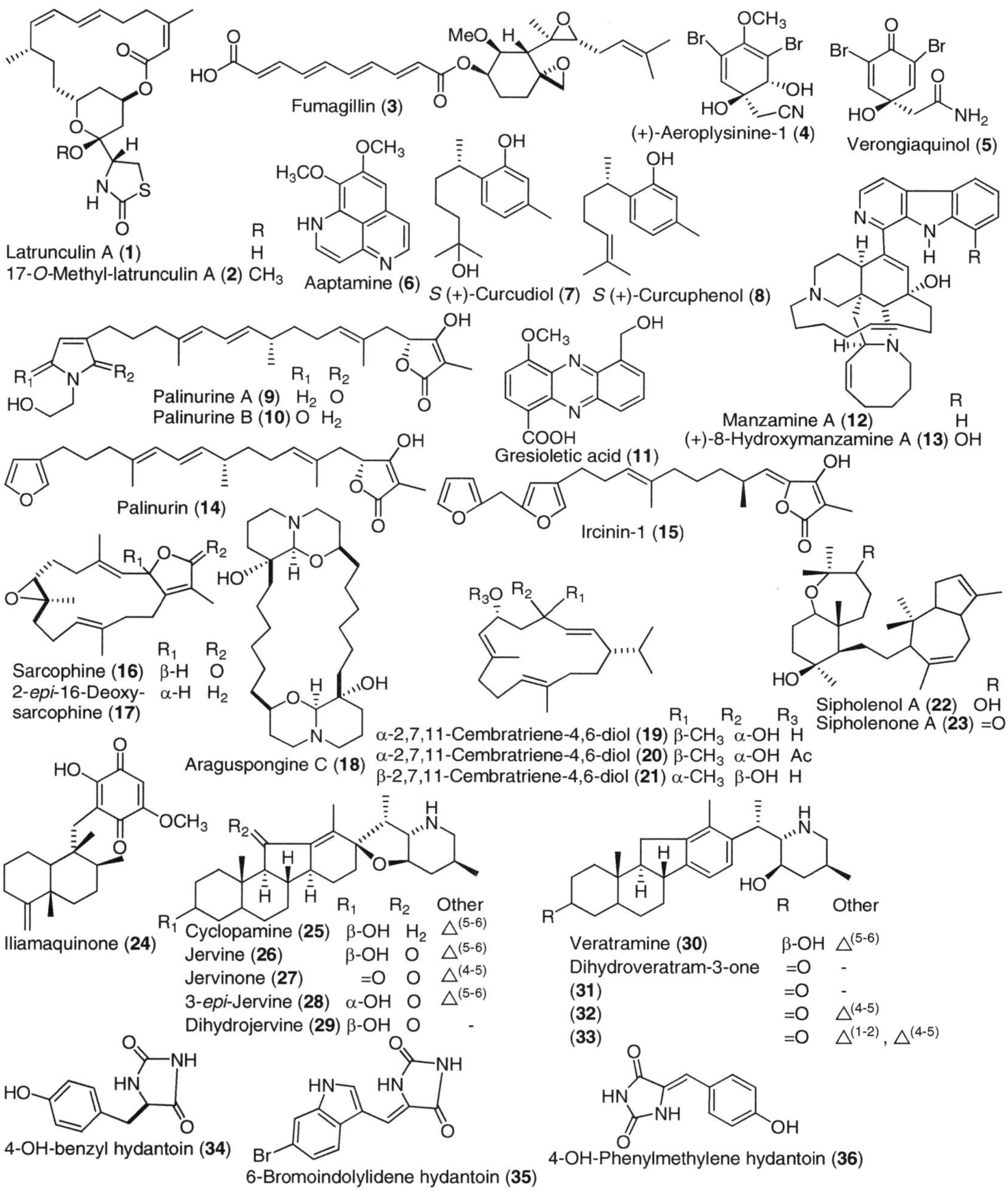

Fig. 1. In-house library of isolated natural products from plants, fungi, and marine invertebrates.

with their respective structurally diverse class showed significant antiinvasive properties. These marine-derived compounds were isolated from the diverse Red Sea sponges and soft corals. Sponges are well known for their high biodiversity, widespread distribution, and unique biology, which make them an incredibly attractive research target (13). These antiinvasive compounds acted as

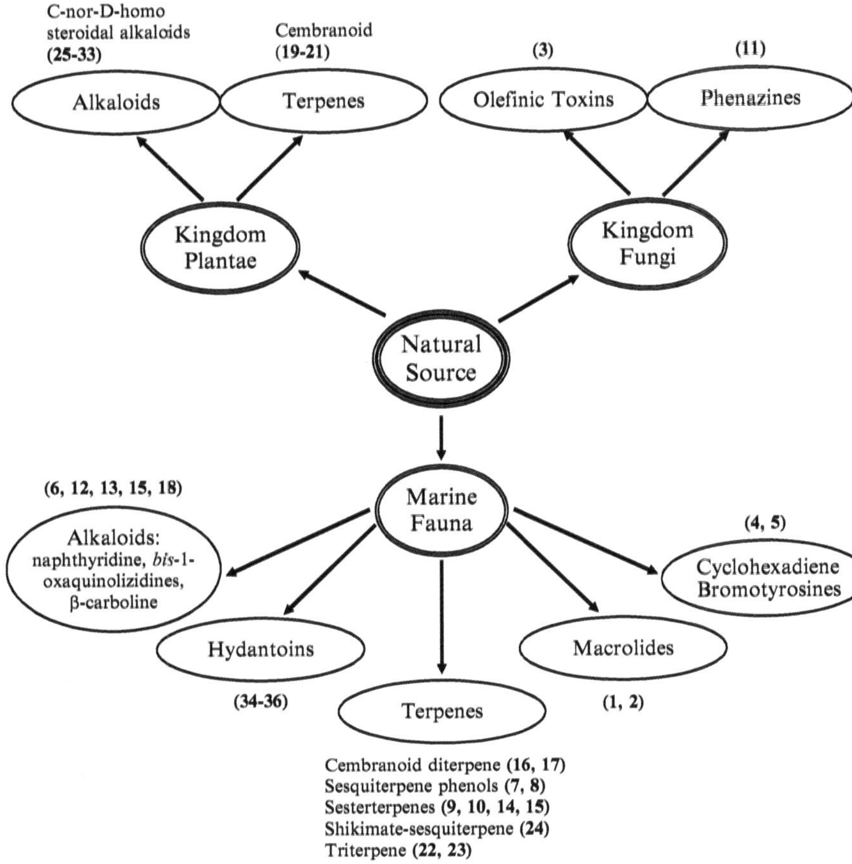

Fig. 2. Schematic diagram of various isolated natural product classes with their respective examples (**1–36**).

an impetus for the beginning of the second screening, which screened the most promisingly active class in terms of their junctional complexes stabililization properties in addition to their ability to attenuate CT-stimulated tumor growth and metastasis of prostate cancer cells. Transepithelial resistance (TER) assay was used to observe the effect of selected compounds on the junctional complexes, confluence of the cellular monolayer, in the presence and absence of CT. This assay was applied in the present study to see the beneficial effect of these compounds on tight junctions. Additionally, TJs barrier function can be quantified by the ability of TMR-dextran to penetrate through the PC-3M cell layer, therefore, paracellular permeability assay was used to see individual compound effect on diluent- and CT-treated PC-3M cell layers. PMH was discovered as a lead small molecule class from the marine sponge *Hemimycale arabica* that attenuates CT-stimulated prostate cancer growth and metastasis in conjunction with its ability to stabilize cell–cell adhesion complexes of prostate cancer cells (14, 15).

This "inspirational molecular structure class" served as a scaffold for further optimization as a potential therapeutic lead. Limited sustainable supply of most bioactive natural products is the main obstacle that may hinder their further development as drug leads (16–18). Feasible, regioselective, and cost effective synthesis of the pharmacologically active marine natural product, 4-hydroxyphenylmethylene hydantoin 36, was then achieved. Complete synthesis of this small molecule not only secured adequate supply for in vitro and animal studies, but it also permitted the synthesis of a number of related analogs for the structure–activity relationship study (14). Forty diversely substituted PMH analogs were then synthesized by selecting a wide array of substituted aldehydes possessing electron-withdrawing (+σ), lipophilic (+π), electron-donating (−σ), and less lipophilic (−π) substituents, in order to increase their antimetastatic potential (Table 1). Spheroid disaggregation assay was selected to access this activity (9–12). Most known PMHs including **36** and **45–73** showed no significant cytotoxic effects in the CNS or other organs when tested in animals at doses >100 μM (19). Moreover, PMH 36 did not display any noticeable toxic effects on prostate cancer cells (PC-3M) at doses up to 200 μM in spheroid disaggregation assays (no observed dead cells) or up to 50 μM in MTT assays. These PMHs were then tested for their antiinvasive effects at 200 μM in spheroid disaggregation assays. If a PMH was not active at this particular dose, it was deemed inactive. PMHs **36** and **37** inhibited PC-3M-CT+ spheroid disaggregation and cell migration in a dose-dependent manner with EC_{50} values of 150 and 30 μM, respectively. These results showed that the migration of cells as indicated by the spheroidal disaggregation was inhibited in the presence of PMH derivatives in a dose-dependent manner. This was not associated with cytotoxicity since PMH **36** did not affect cell viability in MTT assay.

Nude mice model with orthotopic xenograft of PC-3M cells was then selected to assess the antimetastatic activity of PMH 36 and 37 in vivo (15). PMHs **36** and **37** decreased the orthotopic tumor growth and inhibited the formation of tumor micrometastases in distant organs without apparent cytotoxic effects at the tested doses (15). PMH **37**, being the most active one, was tested in LPB-Tag transgenic mice model (15). It decreased the morbidity and extended the survival of the LPB-Tag mice with remarkable reduction of the growth of primary tumors and their metastasis in reproductive organs (15). Therefore, PMHs **36** and **37** were suggested as potent lead attenuators of the disassembly of junctional complexes which are key events in the progression of a localized prostate tumor to its metastatic form (15).

Based on the abovementioned results, PMHs are considered potential leads for the control and prevention of metastatic prostate cancer (14). To establish the structure–activity relationship of

Table 1
Synthesized phenylmethylene hydantoin analogs (reproduced from ref. (14) with permission from Elsevier Science.)

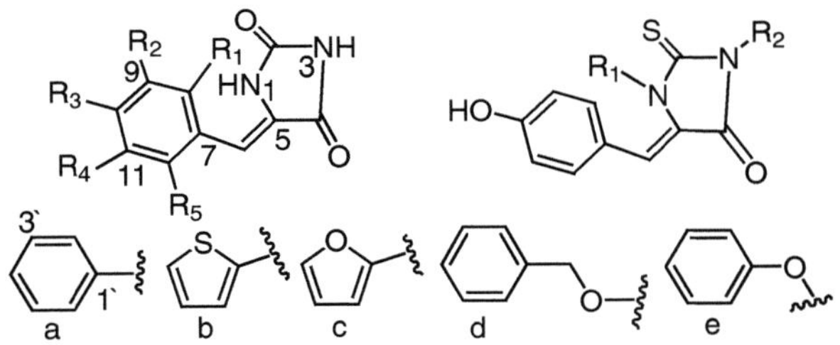

	R_1	R_2	R_3	R_4	R_5		R_1	R_2
36	H	H	OH	H	H	74	Me	Me
37	H	H	S-Et	H	H	75	H	H
38	F	F	Me	H	H			
39	a	H	H	H	H			
40	H	a	H	H	H			
41	b	H	H	H	H			
42	H	H	b	H	H			
43	c	H	H	H	H			
44	H	CN	H	H	H			
45	H	H	Cl	H	H			
46	Cl	H	H	H	Cl			
47	Br	H	H	H	H			
48	H	H	Br	H	H			
49	F	H	H	H	H			
50	H	H	F	H	H			
51	H	F	F	H	H			
52	CF_3	H	H	H	H			
53	H	CF_3	H	H	H			
54	H	H	CF_3	H	H			
55	H	OMe	H	H	H			
56	H	H	OMe	H	H			
57	OMe	H	OMe	H	H			
58	OEt	H	H	H	H			

(continued)

Table 1 (continued)

	R_1	R_2	R_3	R_4	R_5	R_1	R_2
59	H	H	OEt	H	H		
60	H	H	OBu	H	H		
61	H	OH	H	H	H		
62	H	H	N-Et_2	H	H		
63	d	H	H	H	H		
64	H	e	H	H	H		
65	H	NO_2	H	H	H		
66	H	H	NO_2	H	H		
67	H	H	H	H	H		
68	Me	H	Me	Me	H		
69	H	H	a	H	H		
70	H	H	*t*-But	H	H		
71	H	H	*n*-But	H	H		
72	Cl	H	H	H	H		
73	H	Cl	H	H	H		

this class and to justify this prominent activity, molecular modeling studies were done using comparative molecular field analysis (CoMFA) (14). To illustrate the activity of most potent compound, CoMFA steric and electrostatic fields from PLS analysis were plotted. The most active PMH 37 is displayed in the contour maps of QSAR model (Fig. 3) (14). The regions of high and low steric tolerance are shown in green and yellow polyhedra, respectively (Fig. 3a). Areas of high steric bulk tolerance (80% contribution) were observed near the *p*-position of the benzylidene group in 37. The enhanced activity of PMHs 37, 42, and 62 may also be attributed to the presence of bulky groups in *p*-position, which is surrounded by green contours in steric field plot. The sterically unfavored yellow regions were observed near the *o*-position of benzylidine group at the opposite direction of *N*-1 of hydantoin moiety. CoMFA electrostatic fields are shown as blue (more positive charge) and red (more negative charge) polyhedra in (Fig. 3b) phenyl ring of 37 (14). Therefore, compounds possessing electronegative groups near these regions (high electron density) may show more activity. The distal part of the benzylidene group have an electronegative group with prominent red contour, which is consistent with the observation that the three most active PMHs with migration values less than

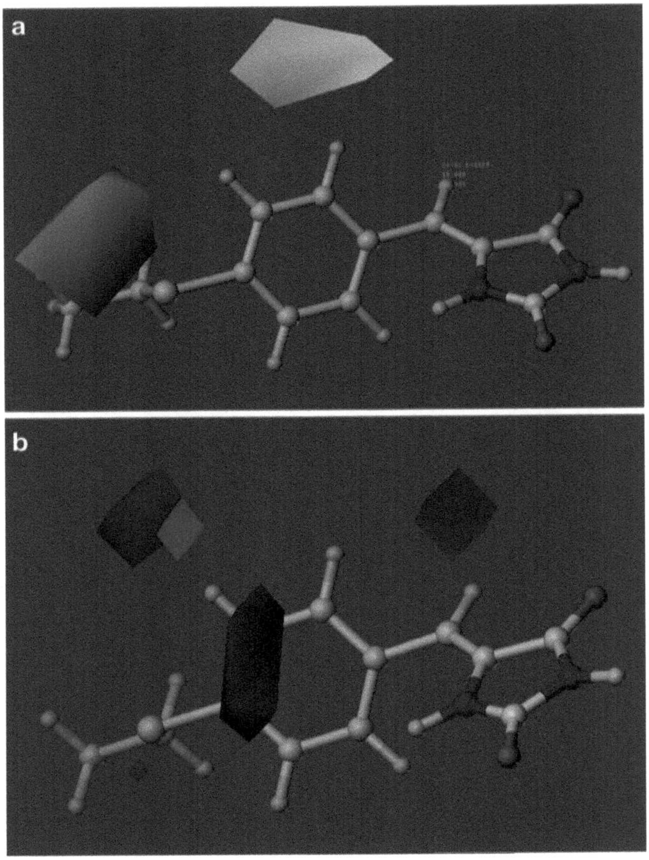

Fig. 3. Graphical representation of CoMFA STDEV*COEFF analysis based field fit alignment. (**a**) Steric contour plots: sterically favored (80% contribution level) are represented by green polyhedra predicted to increase activity. Sterically disfavored (10% contribution level) are represented by yellow polyhedra predicted to decrease activity. (**b**) Electrostatic contour plots: negative charge-favored areas (80% contribution level) are represented by red polyhedra. Negative charge-disfavored areas (20% contribution level) are represented by blue polyhedra. (Reproduced from ref. (14) with permission).

30 μm (55, 62 and 37) posses oxygen, nitrogen, and sulfur atoms, respectively in the *p*-position (14). These compounds have H-accepting properties that could contribute to hydrogen bonding interaction near this position. Blue contours reside around the upper right-hand and upper left-hand corners of 37, which brace the hydrogen atoms of the aromatic and ethylene moieties, indicating that electropositive groups near this area are predicted to increase the activity (14). This could also be a possible indication that H bond donor groups in this position could be favored. The red contours near the *p*-position of the benzylidene group coincide with the sterically favorable green contours. Therefore, substituents at these positions should be electron-donating but with high steric bulk for better activity. Blue contour at the *o*-position

of benzylidene group was observed. Therefore, a low electron density in this area will have a positive effect on the antimetastatic activity. Due to the low substitution variability in the training set around the hydantoin ring, no contours were observed in this area (14).

In conclusion, PMH is a novel antimetastatic lead class that was discovered based on functional-based assays. It can be easily, regioselectively, and cost-effectively synthesized. These advantages entail the emergence of future PMHs as potential therapeutics for the control and prevention of metatstatic prostate cancer.

2. Materials

2.1. Extraction and Isolation

1. Sponge *Hemimycale Arabica*: obtained from Red Sea, stored at −80°C (see Note 1).
2. Waring commercial blender (blended at room temperature).
3. Ethanol, chloroform, methanol.
4. Si gel 60 (particle size 63–200 μm), C-18 Si gel (Bakerbond, Octadecyl, 40 μm), Sephadex LH-20.
5. For $CHCl_3$–MeOH gradient elution, several solutions with increasing percentages of MeOH were made, starting with 0.5% MeOH in $CHCl_3$ up to 100% of MeOH at which the most polar compound is eluted. Almost 5 mL of elute was collected in each 10 mL – culture tube (13 × 100 mm) (see Note 2).
6. For H_2O–MeOH gradient elution, fractionation started at 0.5% MeOH in H_2O and reached up to 50% MeOH in H_2O, or till the elution of the most nonpolar compound.
7. Final purification was achieved by using high performance liquid chromatography (HPLC), Dionex HPLC system, semipreparative Phenomenex column; Ultracarb 5 μ ODS (250 × 10 mm), pump flow rate 3.3 mL/min using 40% MeOH in H_2O (see Note 3).

2.2. Tools for Early and Concluding Characterization

1. Thin layer chromatography (TLC): precoated silica gel 60 F_{254} 500 μm TLC plates, using MeOH–$CHCl_3$ (1:9) as a developing solvent.
2. TLC developing chamber (see Note 4).
3. NMR sample preparation; 5 mm, 8″ L NMR sample tubes (see Note 5).
4. NMR spectrometer (see Note 6).
5. FT-IR spectrophotometer.
6. Micromass LCT spectrometer.

2.3. Semisynthetic Method of Preparation of PMH

1. Two-necked round bottom flask, 25 mL.
2. Oil bath with temperature regulator.
3. Alkacid test ribbon (pH range 2–10) (Fisher scientific company).
4. Saturated solution of $NaHCO_3$.
5. Ethanolamine.
6. 4-hydroxybenzaldehyde (Sigma).

2.4. Spheroid Disaggregation Assay

1. 96-well, flat bottom, ultralow-attachment tissue culture plates.
2. ECM-coated 24-well microplate.
3. Gyrotory shaker, (see Note 7).
4. CO_2 incubator.
5. Diff-Quik stain set, (Dade-Behring, Newark, DE).
6. Calcitonin peptide (human), >99% pure(Bachem Americas, Inc. Torrance, CA).

2.5. Junctional Complex Stabilization Studies

1. 12-well transwell filters (0.4-μm pore size).
2. EVOM V-ohm meter.
3. Tetramethyl rhodamine – labeled dextran (TMR-dextran, 4 kDa).
4. Bio-Tek ELISA plate reader (Ex 530 nm/Em 590 nm).

2.6. In Vivo Assays

1. Male BALB/c nu/nu mice (6–8 week old) (Harlan Laboratories).
2. LPB-Tag transgenic mice (12T-7fast) (14, 15). Positive adult mice is used in the present study.
3. PMHs 100× concentration in 10% DMSO and diluted to 1× with normal saline.
4. Molecular Imaging Software version 6.05f7 (Kodak).
5. Retiga 2000 RT digital camera connected to a microscope (Nikon Optiphot 2) and a computer.
6. IPLab Image Analysis Software (BD Biosciences).

2.7. 3D QSAR Model

1. Molecular modeling software (CoMFA, SYBYL 8.0 suit of programs, Tripos Discovery Informatics, St. Louis, Missouri) installed on a DELL desktop workstation equipped with a 1.0-GHz Intel® Xeon® processor running the Red Hat Enterprise Linux (version 4) operating system.
2. The chemical structures of hydantoin derivatives were sketched in SYBYL 8.0 and assigned Gasteiger partial charges and energy minimized using Energy Force Field to a final root-mean-square gradient of 0.01 kcal/mol.

3. Methods

3.1. Extraction and Isolation

1. About 1 Kg frozen sponge was blended with EtOH and filtered. The blended sponge material was extracted with EtOH at room temperature (4 × 2 L). Ethanolic extracts were pooled and then evaporated under vacuum.
2. The dried extract (~32.0 g) was then subjected to Si gel 60 medium pressure liquid chromatography (MPLC) using $CHCl_3$-MeOH gradient elution to afford several fractions containing PMHs. Pooled fractions were further chromatographed on Si gel 60 using $CHCl_3$–MeOH gradient elution.
3. Further purification was achieved on C-18 Si gel with H_2O–MeOH gradient elution or Sephadex LH-20 using $CHCl_3$-MeOH gradient elution (see Note 8).
4. HPLC was used for the final purification. Semipure mixture was injected carefully in the injector valve, 2,000 μL, of the HPLC and fractions containing PMH were collected (retention time = 11.6 min) (see Note 9).

3.2. Tools for Early and Final Characterization

1. TLC (Thin layer chromatography) is a chromatographic technique, which involves two phases, a solid (stationary phase) and a liquid (mobile phase). TLC was used to support the identity of isolated and synthetic PMH, and also to monitor the progress of reactions (R_f value = distance traveled by the compound/distance traveled by the solvent front). Briefly, the diluted reaction mixture was applied (spotted) at the start line, 0.5 cm above the bottom of the TLC plate (5 × 10 cm) with the use of a thin capillary tube. Appropriate mobile phase was selected, usually MeOH–$CHCl_3$ (1:9), to develop the plate in presaturated TLC chamber with the desired solvent system.
2. NMR spectroscopy was used to determine the structural identity of PMHs. It is a very selective technique to distinguish proton and carbon atoms within a molecule. In brief, the olefinic proton singlet at δ 6.35 correlated with the methine carbon at δ 110.4, in HMQC spectrum, was assigned H-6. Proton H-6 showed ^3J-HMBC correlations with the downfield hydantoin ring amide carbonyl carbon C-4, δ_C 166.7, and the aromatic methine carbons C-8/C-12 at δ 132.3, which confirmed the presence of an intact PMH moiety. The symmetric aromatic proton doublets H-8/H-12 showed COSY correlations with protons H-9/H-11. Protons H-8/H-12 showed ^3J-HMBC correlations with the quaternary carbon C-10 (δ_C 126.4) (see Note 10).
3. Infra Red (IR) spectroscopy was used in conjunction with NMR to gather information about compound's distinctive

functional groups. Briefly, the compound was dissolved in $CHCl_3$ and was placed in IR cell. IR υ_{max} ($CHCl_3$), for characteristic keto functionality was confirmed at 1,708, 1,749 cm^{-1}, and hydroxyl functional group was present at 3,344 cm^{-1}.

4. For the final confirmation of molecular mass of PMH, Micromass LCT spectrometer was used. HREIMS spectra confirmed the presence of intact PMH.

3.3. Synthetic Method of Preparation of PMH

1. Two-necked round bottom flask was used to dissolve (1.0 g) hydantoin in 10 mL water (19). It was heated at 70°C in an oil bath with continuous stirring. Saturated solution of $NaHCO_3$ was used to maintain the pH at 7.0. Ethanolamine (0.9 mL) was then added and temperature was increased to 90°C (19) (see Note 11).
2. To this, an equimolar quantity of 4-hydroxybenzaldehyde solution in 10 mL of ethanol was added, dropwise. The reaction was kept under reflux for 10 h. The endpoint of the reaction was visualized by the formation of yellow precipitate.
3. The reaction mixture was then cooled at 4°C and the precipitate was filtered. Precipitate was washed using EtOH–H_2O (1:5) and then recrystallized with EtOH (see Note 12).

3.4. Spheroid Disaggregation Assay

1. In brief, a 100-μL suspension of 5×10^4/mL PC-3M cells in RPMI 1640 serum-free medium was placed on 96-well low-attachment tissue culture plates (14, 15).
2. The plates were rocked on gyrotory shaker in a CO_2 incubator at 37°C for 2 days, at the end of which the spheroids measuring 150–300 μm diameter (4×10^4 cells per spheroid) were formed.
3. A single spheroid was then placed in the center of each well of ECM-coated 24-well microplate in 200 μL of serum-free medium, was allowed to attach to the ECM for 1 h, and digitally photographed ($t = 0$) (14, 15) (see Note 13).
4. The spheroids were then cultured at 37°C for 48 h, fixed, stained with Diff-Quik (Dade-Behring), and rephotographed. The diameter of the area covered with cells was measured in a microscope calibrated with a stage and ocular micrometer. The results are presented as μm migration ± SE, where migration = (diameter of the area covering migrated cells − diameter of the spheroid)/two from three separate experiments, totaling five to ten spheroids. (14, 15).

3.5. Junctional Complex Stabilization Studies

3.5.1. Transepithelial Resistance

1. Approximately 1×10^5 cells were plated and grown to confluency on 12-well transwell filters (0.4-μm pore size) in complete medium for the first 12 h and then in serum-free medium (15).
2. Electrodes were placed at the upper and lower chambers and TER was measured in triplicate wells at multiple time points after CT/PMH addition with EVOM V-ohm meter (15).
3. The TER values were normalized to the area of the monolayer filter and calculated by subtracting the blank values derived from the filters containing only bathing medium. The integrity and cell density of monolayers was carefully monitored during TER measurement studies (15).

3.5.2. Paracellular Permeability

1. This assay was used to measure the diffusion of tetramethyl rhodamine-labeled dextran across a cell layer grown on a membrane of transwell insert (paracellular permeability) (15).
2. PC-3M cells were seeded (1×10^5 per insert) and cultured to form a monolayer for 5 days. The culture medium was then replaced with HBSS a few minutes before the addition of TMR-dextran (1 mg/mL in HBSS) (15).
3. TMR-dextran was added to the upper chamber and 100 μL of the samples were removed from the lower chamber after 1 h. Fluorescence was measured on an ELISA plate reader (Ex 530 nm/Em 590 nm) (15).
4. The diffusion of TMR-dextran across the insert without cells was also measured to ascertain the integrity of cell monolayers. Each data point was in quadruplicates.

3.6. In Vivo Assays

1. Orthotopic xenograft model was used to test the effect of PMH-36/37 on tumor growth/metastasis of PC-3MCT+ cells in nude mice. Because 37 displayed potent antimetastatic effects in orthotopic xenograft model, this molecule was tested in LPB-Tag mice. The detailed description of both models is mentioned in reference (15).

3.7. 3D QSAR Model

3.7.1. Design of 3D QSAR Model

1. A data set of 35 PMH derivatives was used for this study (14).
2. The antimetastatic activity for these compounds was determined using PC-3M spheroid disaggregation assay. The activity was expressed as migration distance in μm. The ($-\log EC_{50}$) which is the concentration required to decrease migration distance by 50% was used in CoMFA.
3. To evaluate the predictability of the generated 3D QSAR model, PMHs were divided into training set and test set.

Each set possessed PMH analogs with a similar range of antimetastatic activity. Thus, the test set is the true representative of the training set. This was achieved by arbitrarily setting aside six compounds as a test set with a regularly distributed antimetastatic activity. The mean (standard deviation) of the activity of the training and test set was 96.32 (40.04) and 87.67 (57.18), respectively (14).

4. The predicted activities of training and test set values were obtained by multiplying the values of each descriptor for a particular row generated by CoMFA by its corresponding coefficient from the PLS equation in the model (20).

3.7.2. Alignment Rule

1. The SYBYL QSAR rigid body field fit command was used for this alignment (see Note 14).
2. Compound 37, one of the most active PMHs, was used as a reference, on which other molecules were aligned. Values of the steric and electrostatic fields were truncated at 30 kcal/mol.

3.7.3. Partial Least Square (PLS) Analysis

1. The partial least squares algorithm was used in conjugation with the cross-validation (leave-one-out) option to obtain the optimum number of components which were used to generate the final CoMFA model without cross validation (20, 21).
2. The result from a cross-validated analysis was expressed as q^2, which is defined as $q^2 = 1 - \text{PRESS}/\Sigma(Y - Y_{mean})^2$ where $\text{PRESS} = \Sigma(Y - Y_{Pred})^2$. The q^2 can take up values in the range from 1, suggesting a perfect model, to less than 0, where the errors of prediction are greater than the error from assigning each compound mean activity of the model (14).
3. Cross-validated PLS analysis using the leave-one-out procedure employed six components, in which each compound is systematically excluded from the set and its activity was predicted by a model derived from the rest of the compounds.
4. The optimum number of components was defined as that which yielded the highest q^2 value, which normally had the smallest RMS error of prediction (SEP). Equal weights were assigned to the steric and electrostatic descriptors using the CoMFA_STD scaling option (14).
5. The final PLS analysis was then performed using the optimum number of components with no cross-validation. The final PLS analysis was then performed using the optimum number of components with no cross-validation (14).
6. To obtain the statistical confidence limits on the analysis, PLS analysis using 100 bootstrap (bs) groups with the optimum number of components was performed (20, 21).

3.7.4. Predictive r^2 Values

1. The predictive ability was determined from a set of six compounds that were not included in the training set. These

compounds were aligned, and their activities were predicted by PLS analysis (14).

4. Notes

1. Exposure to extreme temperatures should be avoided, optimal temperature −20 to −80°C. For the experiments described in this chapter, sponge *Hemimycale arabica* was collected at a depth of 10 m, and 12.4 miles of Hurghda at the Egyptian Red Sea coast.
2. In normal phase chromatography, the polarity of the solvent should be gradually increased. A ratio of 1:100, mixture to be fractionated/stationary phase was used.
3. The selection of semipreparative column varies from one compound class to another. Extreme caution must be taken for solvent system selection and pump flow rate, both may directly affect the base line and consequently the purity of compound.
4. Very diluted sample should be applied on the TLC. To avoid tailing of the band, the TLC chamber must be completely presaturated with the solvent system of interest, 60 min before development. A blank filter paper may be kept vertically inside the jar and attached to the inner jar wall to improve the pre-saturation process.
5. Use of DMSO should be avoided, if possible, as sample recovery usually requires chromatographic purification. Main advantage of DMSO use is its ability to dissolve both polar and nonpolar compounds.
6. Samples should always be kept at 0°C to avoid any possible chemical degradation.
7. The shaker speed must be optimally selected to avoid any deformation of the spheroids.
8. This step should be completed as early as possible to avoid any compound degradation on the column.
9. Diluted mixture of compounds should be injected to avoid saturation of the HPLC detector.
10. Appropriate mass of the compound should be used to acquire good NMR spectra. Although it depends on the molecular size, usually 5–20 mg should be sufficient.
11. Aldehyde solution in water is usually acidic, saturated 10% $NaHCO_3$ solution should be added slowly to avoid extreme basic solution.

12. To increase the reaction yield, it is advisable to keep the reaction mixture at 4°C for 1–2 h after completion of the reaction.
13. Extreme care should be taken in transferring the formed spheroid from 96-well plates to 24-well plates to avoid disturbing and dismantling the delicate spheroid aggregates. Complete spheroid should be placed at the center of 24-well plates.
14. Alignment is the most important parameter; all the molecules should be properly aligned (field fit alignment) to have consistency in the model results.

References

1. Jemal, A., Siegel, R., Ward, E., Hao, Y., Xu, J., Thun, M.J. (2009) Cancer statistics. *CA Cancer J Clin.* **59**: 225–249.
2. American Cancer Society. http://www.cancer.org. Accessed 03/15/2009.
3. Jongsma, J., Oomen, M.H., Noordzij, M.A., Van Weerden, W.M., Martens, G.J., van der Kwast, T.H., Schröder, F.H., van Steenbrugge, G.J. (2002) Different profiles of neuroendocrine cell differentiation evolve in the PC-310 human prostate cancer model during long-term androgen deprivation. *Prostate.* **50**: 203–215.
4. Furuya, Y., Akakura, K., Akimoto, S., Inomiya, H., Ito, H. (1999) Pattern of progression and survival in hormonally treated metastatic prostate cancer. *Int J Urol.* **6**: 240–244.
5. Segawa, N., Mori, I., Utsunomiya, H., Nakamura, M., Nakamura, Y., Shan, L., Kakudo, K., Katsuoka, Y. (2001) Prognostic significance of neuroendocrine differentiation, proliferation activity, and androgen receptor expression in prostate cancer. *Pathol Int.* **51**: 452–459.
6. Shah, G.V., Shibu, T., Anbalagan, M., Liu, Y., Hermonat, P.L., Williams, J., Chaudhary, J. (2008) Calcitonin promotes in vivo metastasis of prostate cancer cells by altering cell signaling, adhesion, and inflammatory pathways. *Endocr Relat Cancer.* **15**: 953–964.
7. Shah, G.V., Anbalagan, M., Gokulgandhi, M., Soan, K., Thomas, S. (2009) Cadherin Switching and activation of beta-catenin signaling underlie proinvasive actions of calcitonin-calcitonin receptor axis in prostate cancer. *J Biol Chem.* **284**: 1018–1030.
8. Newman, D.J, Cragg, G.M. (2008) Anticancer drug discovery and development from natural products. In: Colegate SM, Molyneux RJ (eds) Bioactive Natural Products, 2nd edn. CRC Press: Boca Raton. pp 323–370.
9. Thomas, S., Chigurupati, S., Anbalagan, M., Shah, G. (2006) Calcitonin increases tumorigenicity of prostate cancer cells: evidence for the role of protein kinase A and urokinase-type plasminogen receptor. *Mol Endocrinol.* **20**: 1894–1911.
10. Thomas, S., Chiriva-Internati, M., Shah, G.V. (2007) Calcitonin receptor-stimulated migration of prostate cancer cells is mediated by urokinase receptor-integrin signaling. *Clin Exp Metastasis.* **24**: 363–377.
11. Heuser, M., Ringert, R.H., Zoeller, G., Hemmerlein, B. (2003) Dynamic assessment of angiogenesis in renal cell carcinoma spheroids by intravital microscopy. *J Urol.* **169**: 1267–1270.
12. Hoevel, T., Macek, R., Swisshelm, K., Kubbies, M. (2004) Reexpression of the TJ protein CLDN1 induces apoptosis in breast tumor spheroids. *Int J Cancer.* **108**: 374–383.
13. Sashidhara, K.V., White, K.N., Crews, P. (2009) A selective account of effective paradigms and significant outcomes in the discovery of inspirational marine natural products. *J Nat Prod.* **72**: 588–603.
14. Mudit, M., Khanfar, M., Muralidharan, A., Thomas, S., Shah, G.V., van Soest, R.W., El Sayed, K.A. (2009) Discovery, design, and synthesis of anti-metastatic lead phenylmethylene hydantoins inspired by marine natural products. *Bioorg Med Chem.* **17**: 1731–1738.

15. Shah, G.V., Muralidharan, A., Thomas, S., Gokulgandhi, M., Mudit, M., Khanfar, M., El Sayed, K.A. (2009) Identification of a small molecule class to enhance cell-cell adhesion and attenuate prostate tumor growth and metastasis. *Mol Cancer Ther.* **8**: 509–520.
16. Newman, D.J., Cragg, G.M. (2007) Natural products as sources of new drugs over the last 25 years. *J Nat Prod.* **70**: 461–477.
17. Molinski, T.F., Dalisay, D.S., Lievens, S.L., Saludes, J.P. (2009) Drug development from marine natural products. *Nat Rev Drug Discov.* **8**: 69–95.
18. McChesney, J.D., Venkataraman, S.K., Henri, J.T. (2007) Plant natural products: back to the future or into extinction? *Phytochemistry.* **68**: 2015–2022.
19. Thenmozhiyal, J.C., Wong, P.T., Chui, W.K. (2004) Anticonvulsant activity of phenylmethylenehydantoins: a structure-activity relationship study. *J Med Chem.* **47**: 1527–1535.
20. Cramer III, R.D., Patterson, D.E., Bunce, J.D. (1988) Comparative molecular field analysis (CoMFA). Effect of shape on binding of steroids to carrier proteins. *J Am Chem Soc.* **110**: 5959–5967.
21. Böhm, M., St rzebecher, J., Klebe, G. (1999) Three-dimensional quantitative structure-activity relationship analyses using comparative molecular field analysis and comparative molecular similarity indices analysis to elucidate selectivity differences of inhibitors binding to trypsin, thrombin, and factor Xa. *J Med Chem.* **42**: 458–477.

Chapter 5

Solid-Phase Peptide Synthesis Using Microwave Irradiation

Justin K. Murray, Jennifer Aral, and Les P. Miranda

Abstract

Since the advent of solid-phase peptide synthesis (SPPS) in the late 1950s, numerous advancements in the underlying chemistry (i.e., orthogonal protection strategy, coupling reagents, and solid support matrices) have greatly improved the efficiency of the technique. More recently, application of microwave radiation to SPPS has been found to reduce reaction time and/or increase the initial purity of synthetic peptide products. In this protocol, conditions are described to accomplish rapid peptide coupling and 9-fluorenylmethoxycarbonyl (Fmoc) removal reactions under temperature-controlled conditions in either a manual or automated synthesis format using a microwave reactor. These microwave-assisted peptide synthesis procedures have been used to rapidly prepare a "difficult" peptide sequence from the acyl carrier protein, ACP(65-74), in less than 3 h and the reduced, linear precursor to human hepcidin, in high initial purity.

Key words: Hepcidin, MAOS, Microwave irradiation, Solid-phase peptide synthesis

1. Introduction

Solid-phase peptide synthesis (SPPS) was first conceptualized and demonstrated by Bruce Merrifield in the late 1950s and early 1960s (1). Five decades later, the fundamental concept of stepwise C- to N-terminal assembly of a polypeptide chain immobilized on a solid support matrix is still the most widely adopted strategy; however, the practical application of the technique has been greatly improved through chemical innovation (2). SPPS (Fig. 1) is accomplished by: (a) coupling the activated ester of an N^{α}-protected amino acid residue with the free N^{α}-amine of a resin-bound amino acid at the N-terminus of a growing oligopeptide chain; (b) removing the base-labile N^{α}-9-fluorenylmethoxycarbonyl (Fmoc) group from the newly incorporated amino acid residue by treatment with piperidine

Seetharama D. Satyanarayanajois (ed.), *Drug Design and Discovery: Methods and Protocols*, Methods in Molecular Biology, vol. 716, DOI 10.1007/978-1-61779-012-6_5,

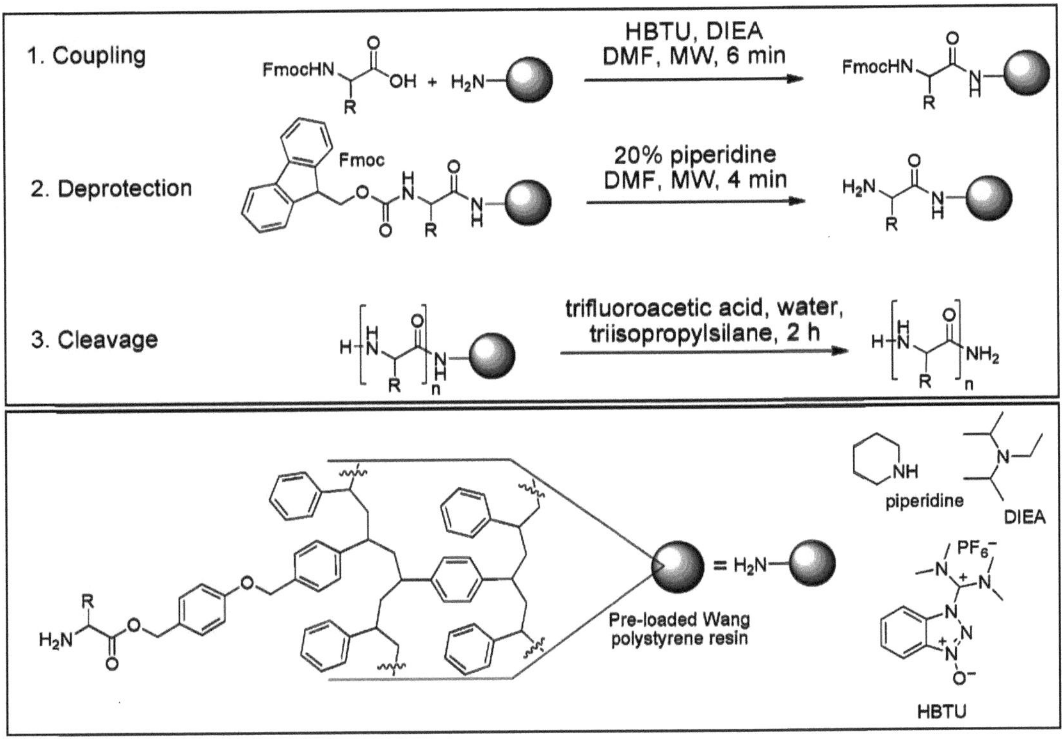

Fig. 1. Solid-phase peptide synthesis (SPPS) reaction scheme (*MW* microwave irradiation). Steps 1 and 2 are repeated to extend the polypeptide chain before performing step 3.

(chain elongation proceeds as steps 1 and 2 are repeated until the desired oligomer length is achieved); (c) cleavage of the peptide from the solid support with simultaneous global side chain deprotection by treatment with trifluoroacetic acid (TFA). As described, the Fmoc/*tert*-butyl amino acid protection strategy has largely supplanted the original *tert*-butyloxycarbonyl (Boc)/benzyl approach, replacing the hazardous final cleavage reagent hydrofluoric acid with TFA (3). Aminium/uronium salts, such as *N*-[(1H-benzotriazol-1-yl)(dimethylamino)methylene]*N*-methylmethanaminium hexafluorophosphate *N*-oxide (HBTU) in the presence of a tertiary amine base, are both convenient and effective, replacing earlier carbodiimde-based coupling reagents as the primary form of activation chemistry (4, 5). Cross-linked polystyrene resins have been superseded by hydrophilic polymers and copolymers that improve solvation of the growing peptide chain (6). Chemical advancements made to improve safety and reaction efficiency have been coupled with the development of a variety of automated peptide synthesizers, leading to the widespread adoption of SPPS techniques and making available the synthetic peptides needed to drive current biological research. Despite these advances, sequence dependent and "difficult" syntheses are still encountered, leading to exploration of new methods for improving synthetic results.

Since its early investigation for organic synthesis, microwave radiation has been successfully applied to an ever-increasing number of organic reactions with a resulting reduction in synthesis time and/or improvement in yield (7).

Yu and coworkers first reported microwave-assisted SPPS in 1992 using a domestic microwave oven, making the conditions difficult to reproduce (8). Since then, commercial microwave reactors that modulate power input to maintain a constant reaction temperature have been developed (9). The polar reaction solvents (i.e., *N,N*-dimethylformamide (DMF)) and reagents employed in SPPS are amenable to microwave heating, accelerating reaction kinetics. Microwave irradiation may also disrupt the on-resin aggregation via intermolecular hydrogen bonding of growing oligopeptide chains, leading to the efficient synthesis of "difficult" sequences. We and others have found that application of microwave irradiation to SPPS reduces reaction time and increases the product purity of several classes of peptide products, including α-peptides, glycopeptides, β-peptides, phosphopeptides, peptaibols, and peptides ≥30 residues in length (10–16). Microwave-assisted SPPS has been extended to the parallel synthesis of peptide libraries for rapid structure–activity relationship elucidation (17–20). Though speculation of a "microwave effect" for SPPS has persisted in the literature, a recent investigation has shown that similar synthetic results are obtained using conventional thermal heating (21). Furthermore, careful reaction optimization has been necessary to avoid a resurgence of the chronic side reactions of racemization and aspartimide formation during microwave irradiation (22, 23). Consequently, microwave-assisted SPPS employs relatively low reaction temperatures (45–80°C) at atmospheric pressure in contrast to other microwave-assisted organic synthesis (MAOS) reactions. In this protocol, we report a general procedure for the preparation of synthetic peptides by microwave-assisted SPPS using either a manual or automated synthesis format. We demonstrate the manual SPPS of a difficult peptide sequence from the acyl carrier protein, ACP(65-74), with microwave irradiation in a multimode reactor (24). We also prepare the reduced linear precursor to human hepcidin, a 25-residue peptide containing 8 cysteines (25), in high initial purity using an automated microwave-assisted peptide synthesizer.

2. Materials

2.1. Manual Solid-Phase Peptide Synthesis of ACP (65-74), Using Microwave Irradiation

1. Solid Support: 0.2 mmol Fmoc-Gly-4-methylbenzhydryl-polystyrene resin (444 mg, 0.45 mmol/g loading, 100–200 mesh) (see Notes 1 and 2).
2. Reaction Vessel: 25 mL polypropylene solid-phase extraction (SPE) tube with polyethylene frit with top and bottom caps (Grace, Deerfield, IL) (see Note 3).
3. Wash Solvents: DMF (see Note 4) and dichloromethane (DCM) in separate 500 mL squirt bottles.
4. N^{α}-Fmoc Amino Acids: Calculate and weigh out 1 mmol of solid into separate 20 mL scintillation vials for each of the Fmoc-amino acids in the ACP(65-74) sequence, VQAAIDYING, excluding the preloaded C-terminal glycine (Fmoc-Val-OH, Fmoc-Gln(Trt)-OH, 2× Fmoc-Ala-OH, 2× Fmoc-Ile-OH, Fmoc-Asp(tBu)-OH, Fmoc-Tyr(tBu)-OH, and Fmoc-Asn(Trt)-OH) (see Notes 5 and 6).
5. Coupling Solution: 25 mL of 0.5 M *N*-[(1H-benzotriazol-1-yl)(dimethylamino)methylene]*N*-methylmethanaminium HBTU (4.73 g,) in DMF. Make solution fresh before synthesis, but it may be stored for up to 1 week at −20°C. Caution: HBTU is a sensitizer.
6. Base Solution: 25 mL of 1.0 M *N*,*N*-diisopropylethylamine ($i\mathrm{Pr}_2\mathrm{EtN}$, 3.23 g or 4.35 mL) in DMF. Make solution fresh before synthesis, but it may be stored for up to 1 week at room temperature.
7. Fmoc Removal Solution: 250 mL of 20% piperidine in DMF. Make solution beforehand; it may be stored indefinitely at room temperature.
8. Equipment: Multimode microwave reactor with turntable, fiber optic temperature probe, and magnetic stirrer (MARS™, CEM Corp.).
9. Equipment: 12-Port Vacuum manifold with waste collection (Honeywell Burdick & Jackson) and vacuum pump.

2.2. Solid-Phase Peptide Synthesis of Linear Human Hepcidin Using an Automated Microwave Peptide Synthesizer

1. Solid Support: 0.25 mmol Fmoc-Thr(tBu)-Wang-polystyrene resin (333 mg, 0.60 mmol/g loading, 75–150 μm.
2. Wash Solvents: DMF and DCM in separate 4 L bottles.
3. N^{α}-Fmoc Amino Acids: 10–50 mL of 0.2 M Fmoc-amino acid solutions in DMF for each residue in the human hepcidinsequence, DTHFPICIFCCGCCHRSKCGMCCKT, excluding the preloaded C-terminal threonine (Fmoc-Cys(Trt)-OH, Fmoc-Asp(tBu)-OH, Fmoc-Phe-OH, Fmoc-Gly-OH, Fmoc-His(Trt)-OH, Fmoc-Ile-OH, Fmoc-Lys(Boc)-OH,

Fmoc-Met-OH, Fmoc-Pro-OH, Fmoc-Arg(Pbf)-OH, Fmoc-Ser(tBu)-OH, and Fmoc-Thr(tBu)-OH.

4. Coupling Solution: 100 mL of 0.5 M benzotriazole-1-yl-oxy-tris-pyrrolidino-phosphonium hexafluorophosphate (PyBOP, 26 g) in DMF. Make solution fresh before synthesis, but it may be stored for up to 1 week at −20°C.
5. Base Solution: 50 mL of 2.0 M diisopropylethylamine (*i*Pr_2EtN, 12.92 g or 17.4 mL) in 1-methyl-2-pyrrolidinone (NMP). Make solution fresh before synthesis, but it may be stored for up to 1 week at room temperature.
6. Fmoc Removal Solution: 1 L of 20% piperidine in DMF (v/v). Make solution beforehand; it may be stored indefinitely at room temperature.
7. Equipment: Automated peptide synthesizer with monomode microwave reactor (Liberty™, CEM Corp.).

2.3. Peptide Cleavage with Side Chain Deprotection

1. Cleavage Reagent: 2 mL of triisopropylsilane.
2. Cleavage Reagent: 2 mL 3,6-dioxa-1,8-octanedithiol (DODT).
3. Cleavage Reagent: 50 mL of TFA. Caution: TFA is extremely corrosive.
4. Solvent: 1 L of cold, anhydrous diethyl ether (−20°C).
5. Equipment: VICI Mininert® Syringe Valve Luer tip syringes (Grace).
6. Equipment: rotary evaporator.

2.4. Reversed-Phase High Performance Liquid Chromatography (RP-HPLC) Analysis

1. Buffer A: 4 L of 0.1% TFA in high performance liquid chromatography (HPLC) grade water.
2. Buffer B: 4 L of 0.1% TFA in HPLC grade acetonitrile.
3. Analytical HPLC Column: Phenomenex Luna 5u C18(2) 100A, 50 × 2 mm.
4. Semipreparative HPLC Column: Phenomenex Luna 5u C18(2) 100A, 250 × 10 mm.
5. Equipment: analytical and/or semipreparative LC-MS with a fraction collector.
6. Equipment: lyophilizer.

3. Methods

The manual and automated preparation of ACP(65-74) and reduced, linear human hepcidin demonstrates the advantages of microwave-assisted over conventional SPPS of reduced synthesis time and higher initial purity of "difficult" peptides without increased side reactions. The application of microwave irradiation to SPPS shortens the time required for Fmoc removal from 15 to 30 min under conventional conditions to 4 min. Likewise, microwave-assisted amino acid coupling reactions are performed in 6 min rather than the 30–120 min incubation time required at room temperature. The cyclical nature of SPPS repeatedly takes advantage of these shorter reaction times to reduce the overall synthesis time from days to hours. Furthermore, microwave-assisted peptide synthesis has proven effective for disruption of the intermolecular hydrogen-bonded aggregation characteristic of "difficult" peptide sequences. This is demonstrated by the successful synthesis of ACP(65-74), wherein the coupling of Val65 is hindered by secondary structure formation after Fmoc removal from the penultimate glutamine. The ACP(66-74) deletion peptide is reduced from approximately 10% under single coupling conventional SPPS to less than 1% with microwave irradiation. Lastly, to address the concern that microwave irradiation and elevated reaction temperatures increase common SPPS side reactions, such as racemization, the linear precursor to human hepcidin, a 25-residue peptide containing 8 cysteines and 2 histidines has been prepared. We and others have previously found that utilization of PyBOP/DIEA or pentafluorophenyl ester activation chemistry or lowering the reaction temperature to 45–50°C efficiently incorporates cysteine and/or histidine residues with minimal epimerization (22, 23). Two synthesis protocols are described; the first may be adapted for use with any of the multimode microwave reactors common in today's organic synthesis laboratories (for a monomode reactor, please see the protocol of Bacsa and Kappe (26), while the second is specific for an automated microwave-assisted peptide synthesizer. Overall, combining the more recent technological advancement of MAOS with the historical chemical innovations has improved the convenience and efficiency of the SPPS technique.

3.1. Manual Solid-Phase Peptide Synthesis of ACP(65-74), Using Microwave Irradiation

3.1.1. Resin Preswell

1. Transfer 0.2 mmol of resin into the 25 mL polypropylene SPE tube.
2. Add a small magnetic stir bar to the SPE tube. Add 15 mL of DMF to the resin in the tube, and allow the resin to swell for 15 min.

3.1.2. Resin Wash

1. Remove the bottom cap from the filter tube, and quickly transfer the tube to the vacuum filtration manifold.
2. Drain the solvent from the tube by applying vacuum.
3. Close the valve to vacuum. Using a squirt bottle, rapidly add 5–10 mL of DMF to the tube, rinsing down the sides of the vessel and agitating the resin.

4. Repeat steps 2 and 3 four more times, then drain the solution a final time.
5. Remove tube from the vacuum manifold and replace the bottom cap.

3.1.3. Fmoc Removal

1. Add 10 mL of the Fmoc removal solution (20% piperidine in DMF) to the resin in the tube.
2. Place the tube in the turntable inside the multimode microwave cavity of the CEM MARS™ (Fig. 2).
3. Position the fiber optic temperature probe in the tube, ensuring that the tip of the probe is submerged in the reaction solution but above the magnetic stir bar (see Note 7). This can be accomplished by poking a hole in a spare top cap for the filter tube with a needle, inserting the temperature probe through the hole, and lightly placing the cap on the filter tube.
4. Irradiate the sample (600 W maximum power, 80°C, ramp 2 min, hold 2 min) with stirring (see Note 8).
5. Remove the tube from the microwave reactor, wipe the temperature probe clean, and wash the resin (5× DMF) as described in Subheading 3.1.2.

3.1.4. Amino Acid Coupling

1. To the vial containing preweighed solid Fmoc-Asn(Trt)-OH, add 2 mL of 0.5 M HBTU in DMF and 2 mL of DMF. Cap the vial and vortex the mixture for 5–20 s to initiate dissolution. Add 2 mL of 1.0 M $i\mathrm{Pr_2EtN}$ in DMF to the vial. Cap the

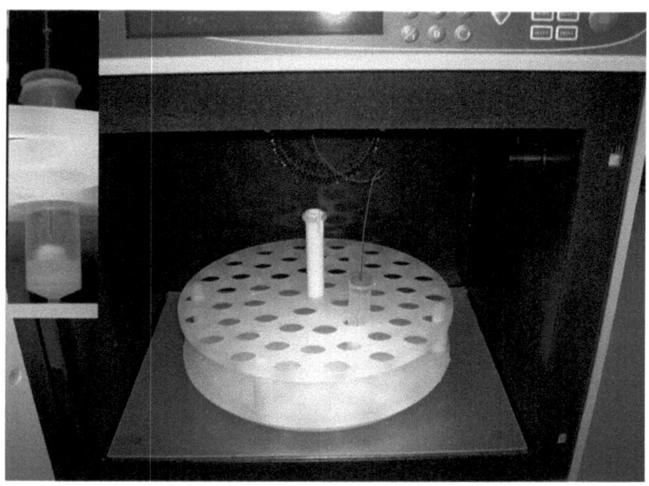

Fig. 2. Experimental set-up in the multimode microwave reactor with *inset* showing close-up of reaction vessel containing resin, solvent, stir bar, and properly positioned temperature probe.

vial and vortex the mixture for 60–90 s, ensuring that the Fmoc-amino acid has completely dissolved (see Note 9).

2. Transfer the preactivated amino acid solution to the resin in the tube.
3. Place the tube in the turntable inside the multimode microwave, and position the fiber optic temperature probe in the tube, ensuring that the tip of the probe is submerged in the reaction solution but above the magnetic stir bar (see Note 7).
4. Irradiate the sample (600 W maximum power, 70°C, ramp 2 min, hold 4 min) (see Note 10).
5. Remove the tube from the microwave reactor, wipe the temperature probe clean, and wash the resin (5× DMF) as described in Subheading 3.1.2.

3.1.5. Peptide Chain Elongation

1. Repeat the process of Subheadings 3.1.3 and 3.1.4 with Fmoc-Ile-OH.
2. Repeat the iterative Fmoc removal/coupling cycle (step 1), incorporating in order Fmoc-Tyr(tBu)-OH, Fmoc-Asp(tBu)-OH, Fmoc-Ile-OH, Fmoc-Ala-OH, Fmoc-Ala-OH, Fmoc-Gln(Trt)-OH, and Fmoc-Val-OH (see Note 11).
3. Perform the final Subheading 3.1.3 of Val65.
4. Wash the resin five times as in Subheading 3.1.2, except use DCM instead of DMF. After the final wash, dry the resin by leaving it open to vacuum for approximately 1 min, and proceed to Subheading 3.3.

3.2. Solid-Phase Peptide Synthesis of Linear Human Hepcidin Using an Automated Microwave Peptide Synthesizer

1. Open the Pepdriver™ (v 2.4.0) software. Within the Sequence Editor, import or input the amino acid sequence of the desired peptide (DTHFPICIFCCGCCHRSKCGMCCKT).
2. Within the Microwave Editor, program a "Coupling 6 min" standard method with power = 25 W, temperature = 75°C, time = 360 s (see Note 12). Program a "Coupling 45°C Temp" multistep method with step 1: power = 0 W, time = 120 s, temperature = 45°C and step 2: power = 15 W, time = 240 s, and temperature = 45°C. For all methods, set bubbling on = 3 s and off = 7 s and pressure = low.
3. Also within the Microwave Editor, program an "Initial Deprotect" standard method with power = 55 W, temperature = 75°C, and time = 30 s. Program a "Deprotection" standard method with power = 55 W, temperature = 75°C, and time = 180 s.
4. Within the Amino Acid folder in the Cycle Editor, program a "0.25 Single" coupling cycle as in Table 1.
5. Also within the Cycle Editor, program a "0.25 Single 45°C Temp" coupling cycle by changing the step 16 Microwave Method from "Coupling 6 min" to "Coupling 45°C Temp."

Table 1
"0.25 Single" coupling cycle

	Operation	Parameter	Volume	Drain	Cycles	Pause
1	Clean resin dip tube	*N*,*N*-dimethylformamide (DMF)		Yes	1	No
2	Wash – top	DMF	10	Yes	1	No
3	Add deprotection	20% Piperidine	10	No	1	No
4	Microwave method	Initial deprotection		Yes	1	No
5	Wash – top	DMF	5	Yes	1	No
6	Add deprotection	20% Piperidine	10	No	1	No
7	Microwave method	Deprotection		Yes	1	No
8	Wash – top	DMF	10	Yes	1	No
9	Wash – bottom	DMF	10	Yes	1	No
10	Wash – top	DMF	10	Yes	1	No
11	Clean resin dip tube	DMF		Yes	1	No
12	Wash – top	DMF	10	Yes	1	No
13	Add amino acid		5	No	1	No
14	Add activator	Benzotriazole-1-yl-oxy-tris-pyrrolidino-phosphonium hexafluorophosphate (PyBOP)	2	No	1	No
15	Add activator base	DIEA	1	No	1	No
16	Microwave method	Coupling 6 min		Yes	1	No
17	Wash – top	DMF	10	Yes	1	No
18	Wash – bottom	DMF	10	Yes	1	No
19	Wash – top	DMF	10	Yes	1	No

6. Within the Final Deprotection folder of the Cycle Editor, program a "0.25" Fmoc removal cycle as in Table 2.
7. Within the Cleaving folder of the Cycle Editor, program a "Non-cleavage" cycle as in Table 3.
8. Within the Method Editor, create a new method by selecting the sequence saved in step 4. Select the "0.25 Single" coupling cycle for all amino acid residues, except for cysteine and histidine, which should be incorporated using the "0.25 Single 45°C Temp" coupling cycle. Input the following parameters: Skip resin load = No, Scale = 0.25,

Table 2
"0.25" fluorenylmethoxycarbonyl (Fmoc) removal cycle

	Operation	Parameter	Volume	Drain	Cycles	Pause
1	Clean resin dip tube	DMF		Yes	1	No
2	Wash – top	DMF	10	Yes	1	No
3	Add deprotection	20% Piperidine	10	No	1	No
4	Microwave method	Initial deprotection		Yes	1	No
5	Wash – top	DMF	5	Yes	1	No
6	Add deprotection	20% Piperidine	10	No	1	No
7	Microwave method	Deprotection		Yes	1	No
8	Wash – top	DMF	10	Yes	1	No
9	Wash – bottom	DMF	10	Yes	1	No
10	Wash – top	DMF	10	Yes	1	No

Table 3
"Non-cleavage" cycle

	Operation	Parameter	Volume	Drain	Cycles	Pause
1	Wash – top	Dichloromethane (DCM)	10	Yes	1	No
2	Transfer product solid			No	2	No
3	Clean reaction vessel-unfiltered			No	2	No
4	Wash – top	DCM	10	Yes	1	No

C-Terminus = Acid, and Final Deprotection = Yes. Set the Default Cycles as follows: Resin = standard resin, Cleaving = Non-cleavage, and Final Depro = 0.25 (see Note 13). Save the method.

9. From the main page of Pepdriver™, load the saved method to position 1. Under Calculator\Usage, print the synthesizer set-up page. Prepare necessary volumes of amino acids and reagents.
10. Change out the dip tube filters for the amino acid and reagent solutions. Replace in-line Filters F1 and F2 and in-line filter in drain line.
11. Transfer 0.25 mmol of dry resin into a 50 mL polypropylene centrifuge tube.

12. Load resin to position 1 and amino acid solutions, reagent solutions, and solvents in appropriate positions on the instrument. Prime lines for the reagent solutions (Activator and Activator Base).
13. Press "Start" to initiate the synthesis. The instrument will preswell the resin and transfer it to the reaction vessel, then iteratively perform the sequence of programmed Fmoc removal and amino acid coupling reactions. Pause the synthesis as needed to refill the solvents.
14. At the end of the synthesis, the resin will be transferred from the reaction vessel to the original 50 mL centrifuge tube. Remove the tube from the instrument, and transfer the resin to a 25 SPE filter tube using DMF or DCM. Add a small magnetic stir bar to the tube.
15. Wash the resin five times as in steps 3–7, except use DCM instead of DMF. After the final wash, dry the resin by leaving it open to vacuum for approximately 1 min.
16. If the instrument is not going to be used immediately, then back flush all the reagents. Remove amino acid solutions from the instrument (see Note 14).

3.3. Peptide Cleavage with Side Chain Deprotection

1. Remove the bottom cap from the filter tube and attach the PTFE stopcock, ensuring that it is closed.
2. In a fume hood, add to the resin-bound peptide 1 mL of triisopropylsilane and 1 mL of water. If the peptide contains cysteine, i.e., human hepcidin, then also add 1 mL of DODT.
3. In a fume hood, add to the mixture 15–20 mL of TFA, leaving some headspace in the tube. Place the top cap on the tube lightly, and stir the cleavage solution for 2–3 h (see Note 15).
4. Position the filter tube over an empty 150 or 250 mL round bottom flask using a clamp. Open the bottom stopcock and remove the top cap to gravity filter the cleavage solution into the round bottom flask. Rinse the remaining resin with an additional 5 mL of TFA.
5. Concentrate the combined filtrate by rotary evaporation (40→8 mbar, 25°C) to a final volume of approximately 5 mL.
6. To a 50 mL centrifuge tube add 40 mL of cold diethyl ether. To the ether add in a dropwise manner the concentrated cleavage solution. A white precipitate should form. Vortex the mixture to ensure complete precipitation.
7. Centrifuge the mixture (2,000 × *g*, 4 min), and decant the supernatant. To the precipitated peptide add 40 mL of cold diethyl ether and mix thoroughly using a spatula. Centrifuge and decant. Dry the precipitated peptide under vacuum for 2 h.

3.4. Reversed-Phase High Performance Liquid Chromatography Analysis

1. Dissolve the dry peptide product mixture in a minimal volume of water/acetonitrile with stirring and/or sonication.
2. Assess the initial purity of the peptide product mixtures on an analytical LC-MS (Phenomenex Jupiter 20×2 mm, 100 Å, 5 μm column eluted with a 10–60% B over 10 min gradient at a 0.750 mL/min flow rate monitoring absorbance at 220 nm). Use the mass spectra to identify components of the peptide product mixture (see Note 16). Please see Figs. 3 and 4 for examples of LC-MS chromatograms and mass spectra of ACP(65-74) and reduced human hepcidin.
3. Purify the crude peptides using a semipreparative LC-MS (Phenomenex Jupiter 250×10 mm, 100 Å, 10 μm column eluted with a 10–60% B over 50 min gradient at an 8 mL/min flow rate), collecting the desired product using a UV absorbance (220 nm) or mass detection threshold.
4. Combine the HPLC fractions containing the purified product peptide, freeze the solution using a dry ice/isopropanol bath, and lyophilize to obtain the product.

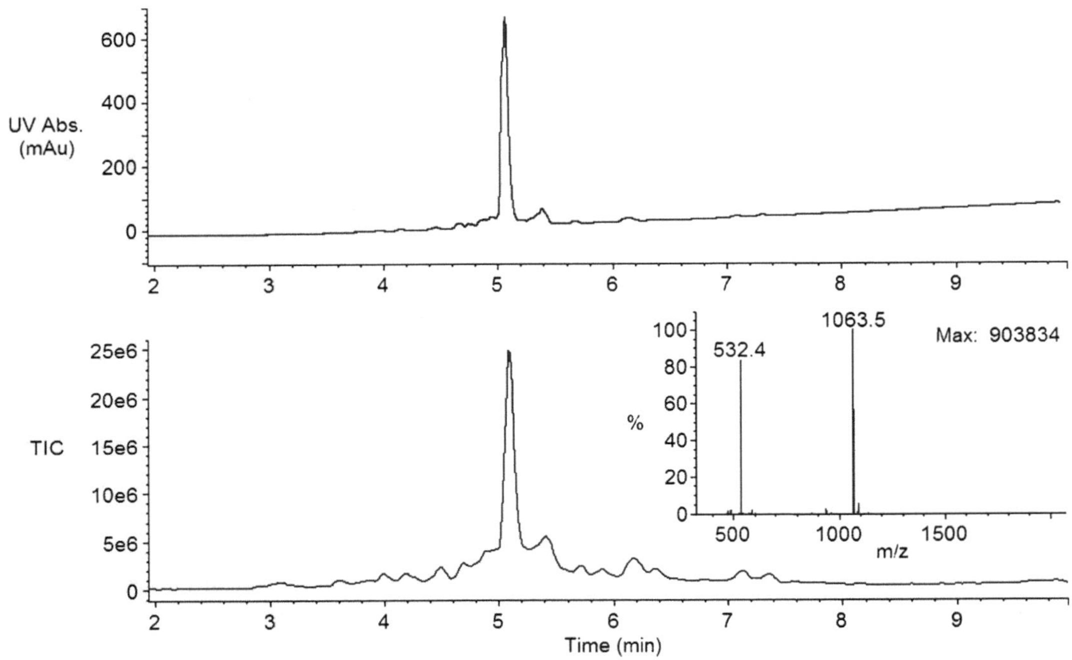

Fig. 3. High performance liquid chromatography (HPLC) chromatogram (*top*: UV absorbance at 214 nm and *bottom*: MS TIC) of crude ACP(65-74) prepared using manual microwave-assisted SPPS. The major peak eluting with $r_t = 5.1$ min has (m/z) = 1,063.5 (*inset*), corresponding to the $[M+H]^+$ of ACP(65-74) (monoisotopic MW = 1,062.64).

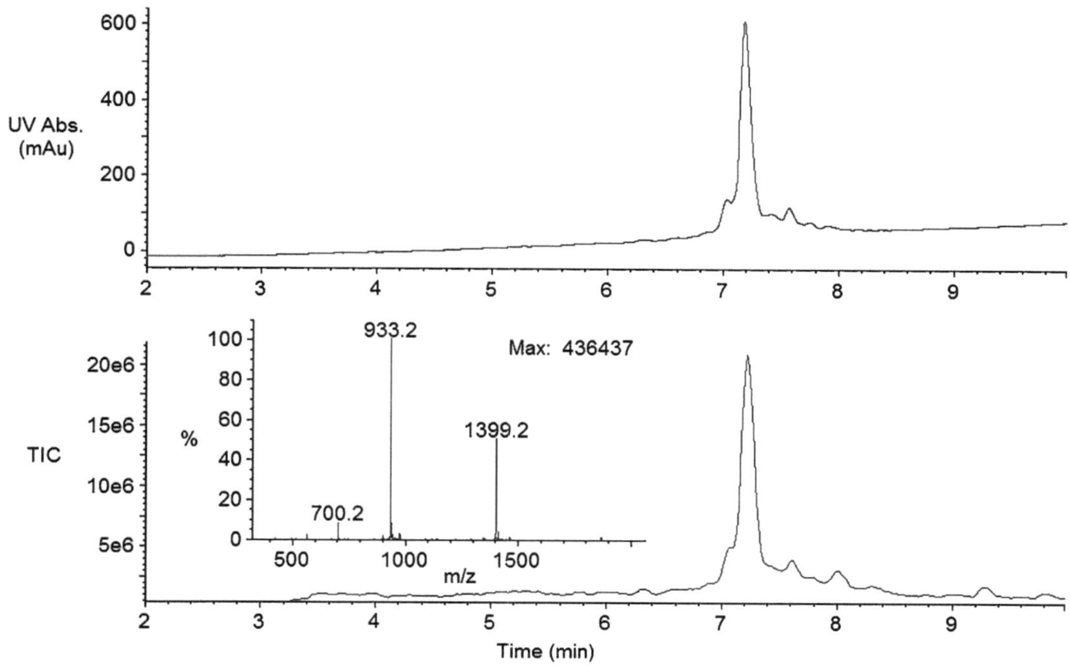

Fig. 4. HPLC chromatogram (*top*: UV absorbance at 214 nm and *bottom*: MS TIC) of crude linear human hepcidin prepared using automated microwave-assisted SPPS. The major peak eluting with r_t = 7.2 min has (*m/z*) = 1,399.6, 933.1, and 700.0 (*inset*), corresponding to the $[M+2H]^{2+}$, $[M+3H]^{3+}$, and $[M+4H]^{4+}$ of reduced human hepcidin (monoisotopic MW = 2,796.14).

4. Notes

1. Preloaded methylbenzhydryl (MBH) and Wang linkers should be employed for the preparation of C-terminal peptide acids, whereas a Rink amide linker provides the C-terminally amidated peptide. Microwave peptide synthesis may be performed on polystyrene (PS), polyethylene glycol (PEG)-PS, PEG (ChemMatrix, Matrix Innovation), and cross-linked ethoxylate acrylate (CLEAR, Peptides International) resin matrices.
2. The synthesis scale may be varied from 0.010 to 0.25 mmol depending on the amount of product desired [scale (mmol)/loading (mmol/g) = mass of resin (g), e.g., 0.2 mmol/0.45 mmol/g = 0.444 g].
3. A reaction vessel of the appropriate size should be selected based on the scale (25 mL SPE filter tubes, frits, and caps are available from Grace: 210425, 211416, 221006, and 220710).

4. Purchasing high quality DMF and storing over ion exchange resin eliminates the traces of dimethylamine that result from the decomposition of DMF; high concentrations of dimethylamine can lead to premature Fmoc-removal under microwave irradiation. Alternatively, reagent solutions can be prepared in NMP.
5. Select Fmoc-amino acids with the orthogonal side-chain protecting groups: Fmoc-Ala-OH, Fmoc-Cys(Trt)-OH, Fmoc-Asp(tBu)-OH, Fmoc-Glu(tBu)-OH, Fmoc-Phe-OH, Fmoc-Gly-OH, Fmoc-His(Trt)-OH, Fmoc-Ile-OH, Fmoc-Lys(Boc)-OH, Fmoc-Leu-OH, Fmoc-Met-OH, Fmoc-Asn(Trt)-OH, Fmoc-Pro-OH, Fmoc-Gln(Trt)-OH, Fmoc-Arg(Pbf)-OH,Fmoc-Ser(tBu)-OH,Fmoc-Thr(tBu)-OH, Fmoc-Val-OH, Fmoc-Trp(Boc)-OH, and Fmoc-Tyr(tBu)-OH. Fmoc-amino acids are available from a number of suppliers, including Novabiochem, CBL, and Midwest Biotech.
6. 5 Equivalents × scale (mmol) × MW (mg/mmol) = mass of amino acid (mg) [e.g., 5 × 0.20 mmol × 596.7 mg/mmol = 596.7 mg Fmoc-Asn(Trt)-OH].
7. Caution: if the fiber optic probe is not positioned inside the tube and in the solution, the microwave reactor will not accurately detect the increasing temperature of the solution. Since the air temperature being sensed by the probe does not increase, the reactor will continue to irradiate at full power for the entire length of the experiment, overheating the sample. If this occurs, the polyethylene frit of the filter tube is normally compromised. Transfer the reaction solution and resin to a new filter tube before draining and washing.
8. The medium stirring setting is sufficient. Excessive stir rates or stirring for long periods of time grinds the resin into a finer particle size that is much slower to filter during washes. If a filter tube becomes clogged, transfer to a new tube.
9. Preactivation of the Fmoc-amino acid (step 13) may be performed concurrently with the microwave-assisted Fmoc removal reaction (step 11) to reduce the overall cycle time.
10. Multiple microwave-assisted peptide coupling reactions may be carried out in parallel within the multimode microwave reactor, provided the scale is the same for each reaction and the same Fmoc-amino acid is being coupled. Different amino acids should be coupled sequentially to ensure controlled heating for each reaction. Fmoc removal reactions of the same scale may also be carried out in parallel (17–20).
11. After a coupling reaction is complete, the washed resin can be stored at room temperature for several hours or overnight.

12. The wattage setting will vary slightly from one microwave instrument to the next but will be calibrated in the factory for the standard methods.
13. For safety considerations and improved instrument longevity, do not perform cleavage reactions on the machine.
14. Leaving amino acid solutions on the instrument for more than a week can lead to precipitation in the lines. On a monthly basis run a sensor calibration and calibrate reagent deliveries for DMF, DCM, and piperidine solution.
15. Caution: TFA is extremely corrosive. Proper personal protective equipment (eye protection, a lab coat, and gloves) should be worn throughout this procedure, but extra precaution should be used during the cleavage process.
16. If analysis of the crude library members by LC-MS reveals that the product mixture contains a substantial amount of a deletion peptide side product resulting from an incomplete coupling reaction, then in a second synthesis consider repeating steps 8–12 to ensure that the Fmoc protecting group is completely removed from the preceding amino acid and/or repeating steps 13–17 two times (i.e., double coupling) for the difficult amino acid coupling step. Alternatively, modify step 16 of the difficult coupling step by subjecting the reaction mixture to multiple cycles (e.g., 3) of microwave irradiation, waiting about 10 min between cycles for the sample to cool to room temperature. A small amount of the resin can be removed, cleaved, and analyzed by LC-MS to ensure that coupling has gone to completion before proceeding with Fmoc removal. Alternatively, a small amount of the resin can be tested qualitatively by incubation in 1 mL of DMF, $i\text{Pr}_2\text{EtN}$ (30 μL of 1.0 M solution in DMF) and 2,4,6-trinitrobenzne sulfonic acid (TNBS, 30 μL of a 1% solution in DMF) for 5 min. Wash the resin with DMF (3 × 1 mL) and observe. Beads will be stained red, indicating the presence of free amino groups, if the coupling reaction is incomplete and should be repeated.

References

1. Merrifield, R. B. (1963) Solid phase peptide synthesis. I. The synthesis of a tetrapeptide *J Am Chem Soc.* **85**: 2149–2154.
2. Albericio, F. (2004) Developments in peptide and amide synthesis *Curr Opin Chem Biol.* **8**: 211–221.
3. Fields, G. B., Noble, R. L. (1990) Solid-phase peptide synthesis utilizing 9-fluorenylmethoxycarbonyl amino acids *Int J Pept Protein Res.* **35**: 161–214.
4. Konig, W., Geiger, R. (1970) A new method for synthesis of peptides: activation of the carboxyl group with dicyclohexylcarbodiimide using 1-hydroxybenzotriazoles as additives *Chem Ber.* **103**: 788–798.
5. Abdelmoty, I., Albericio, F., Carpino, L. A., Foxman, B. M., Kates, S. A. (1994) Structural studies of reagents for peptide bond formation: crystal and molecular structures of HBTU and HATU *Lett Pept Sci.* **1**: 52–67.

6. Garcia-Martin, F., Quintanar-Audelo, M., Garcia-Ramos, Y., Cruz, L. J., Gravel, C., Furic, R., Cote, S., Tulla-Puche, J., Albericio, F. (2006) ChemMatrix, a poly(ethylene glycol)-based support for the solid-phase synthesis of complex peptides *J Comb Chem.* **8**: 213–220.
7. Kappe, C. O. (2004) Synthetic methods. Controlled microwave heating in modern organic synthesis *Angew Chem Int Ed.* **43**: 6250–6284.
8. Yu, H.-M., Chen, S.-T., Wang, K.-T. (1992) Enhanced coupling efficiency in solid-phase peptide synthesis by microwave irradiation *J Org Chem.* **57**: 4781–4784.
9. Ferguson, J. D. (2003) Focused microwave instrumentation from CEM corporation *Mol Divers.* 7: 281–286.
10. Erdélyi, M., Gogoll, A. (2002) Rapid microwave-assisted solid phase peptide synthesis *Synthesis.* **11**: 1592–1596.
11. Matsushita, T., Hinou, H., Kurogochi, M., Shimizu, H., Nishimura, S.-I. (2005) Rapid microwave-assisted solid-phase glycopeptide synthesis *Org Lett.* 7: 877–880.
12. Murray, J. K., Gellman, S. H. (2005) Application of microwave irradiation to the synthesis of 14-helical β-peptides *Org Lett.* 7: 1517–1520.
13. Rizzolo, F., Sabatino, G., Chelli, M., Rovero, P., Papini, A. M. (2007) A convenient microwave-enhanced solid-phase synthesis of difficult peptide sequences: case study of gramicidin A and CSF114(Glc) *Int J Pept Res Ther.* **13**: 203–208.
14. Harris, P. W. R., Williams, G. M., Shepherd, P., Brimble, M. A. (2008) The synthesis of phosphopeptides using microwave-assisted solid phase peptide synthesis *Int J Pept Res Ther.* **14**: 387–392.
15. Hjoerringgaard, C. U., Pedersen, J. M., Vosegaard, T., Nielsen, N. C., Skrydstrup, T. (2009) An automatic solid-phase synthesis of peptaibols *J Org Chem.* **74**: 1329–1332.
16. Chi, Y., Zhang, H., Huang, W., Zhou, J., Zhou, Y., Qian, H., Ni, S. (2008) Microwave-assisted solid phase synthesis, PEGylation, and biological activity studies of glucagon-like peptide-1(7-36)amide *Bioorg Med Chem.* **16**: 7607–7614.
17. Murray, J. K., Sadowsky, J. D., Scalf, M., Smith, L. M., Tomita, Y., Gellman, S. H. (2008) Exploration of structure-activity relationships among foldamer ligands for a specific protein binding site via parallel and split-and-mix library synthesis *J Comb Chem.* **10**: 204–215.
18. Murray, J. K., Gellman, S. H. (2007) Parallel synthesis of peptide libraries using microwave irradiation *Nat Protoc.* **2**: 624–631.
19. Sadowsky, J. D., Murray, J. K., Tomita, Y., Gellman, S. H. (2007) Exploration of backbone space in foldamers containing α- and β-amino acid residues: developing protease-resistant oligomers that bind tightly to the BH3-recognition cleft of Bcl-xL *Chembiochem.* **8**: 903–916.
20. Murray, J. K., Gellman, S. H. (2006) Microwave-assisted parallel synthesis of a 14-helical β-peptide library *J Comb Chem.* **8**: 58–65.
21. Bacsa, B., Horvati, K., Bosze, S., Andreae, F., Kappe, C. O. (2008) Solid-phase synthesis of difficult peptide sequences at elevated temperatures: a critical comparison of microwave and conventional heating technologies *J Org Chem.* **73**: 7532–7542.
22. Aral, J., Long, J., Shah, A., Diamond, S., Holder, J. R., Miranda, L. (2005) Effects of coupling reagent, base, and solvent choice on microwave-assisted solid-phase peptide synthesis *Biopolymers.* **80**: 530.
23. Palasek, S. A., Cox, Z. J., Collins, J. M. (2007) Limiting racemization and aspartimide formation in microwave-enhanced Fmoc solid phase peptide synthesis *J Pept Sci.* **13**: 143–148.
24. Johnson, T., Quibell, M., Owen, D., Sheppard, R. C. (1993) A reversible protecting group for the amide bond in peptides. Use in the synthesis of difficult sequences *J Chem Soc Chem Commun.* **4**: 369–372.
25. Jordan, J. B., Poppe, L., Haniu, M., Arvedson, T., Syed, R., Li, V., Kohno, H., Kim, H., Schnier, P. D., Harvey, T. S., Miranda, L. P., Cheetham, J., Sasu, B. J. (2009) Hepcidin revisited, disulfide connectivity, dynamics, and structure *J Biol Chem.* **284**: 24155–24167.
26. Bacsa, B., Kappe, C. O. (2007) Rapid solid-phase synthesis of a calmodulin-binding peptide using controlled microwave irradiation *Nat Protoc.* **2**: 2222–2227.

Chapter 6

Fluorescent and Lanthanide Labeling for Ligand Screens, Assays, and Imaging

Jatinder S. Josan, Channa R. De Silva, Byunghee Yoo, Ronald M. Lynch, Mark D. Pagel, Josef Vagner, and Victor J. Hruby

Abstract

The use of fluorescent (or luminescent) and metal contrast agents in high-throughput screens, in vitro assays, and molecular imaging procedures has rapidly expanded in recent years. Here we describe the development and utility of high-affinity ligands for cancer theranostics and other in vitro screening studies. In this context, we also illustrate the syntheses and use of heteromultivalent ligands as targeted imaging agents.

Key words: Cy5, DELFIA, DTPA, DOTA, Dual-modal agents, Heteromultivalent ligands, Lanthaligands, PARACEST MRI, Solid-phase synthesis, Targeted imaging agents

Abbreviations

δ-OR	Delta-opioid receptor
Ado	8-Amino-3,6-dioxaoctanoyl
Arsenazo (III)	2,7-Bis(2-arsenophenylazo)-1,8-dihydroxyaphthalene-3, 6-disulfonic acid
BB	Bromophenol blue
Boc	*tert*-Butyloxycarbonyl
CCK(6)	Nle-Gly-Trp-Nle-Asp-Phe-NH_2
CCK(8)	Asp-Tyr-Nle-Gly-Trp-Nle-Asp-Phe-NH_2
CCK2R	Cholecystokinin receptor subtype 2
CDI	N,N′-carbonyldiimidazole
CEST	Chemical exchange saturation transfer
CH_3CN	Acetonitrile
CT	Computed tomography
Cy5	Cyanine 5 dye
DCM	Dichloromethane

Seetharama D. Satyanarayanajois (ed.), *Drug Design and Discovery: Methods and Protocols*, Methods in Molecular Biology, vol. 716, DOI 10.1007/978-1-61779-012-6_6,

DELFIA	Dissociation-enhanced lanthanide fluoroimmunoassay
DIC	N,N′-diisopropylcarbodiimide
DIEA	Diisopropylethylamine
DMBA	1,3-Dimethylbarbituric acid
DMEM	Dulbecco's modified eagle medium
DMF	N,N′-dimethylformamide
DMSO	Dimethylsulfoxide
Dmt	2′,6′-Dimethyl-l-tyrosine
DOTA	1,4,7,10-Tetraazacyclododecane-1,4,7,10-tetraacetic acid
DPLCE	c[DPen^2,Cys^5]enkephalin
DTPA	Diethylenetriamine-N,N,N′,N′,N″-pentaacetic acid
EDC	1-Ethyl-3-(3-dimethylaminopropyl) carbodiimide hydrochloride
EDT	1,2-Ethanedithiol
ESI-MS	Electrospray ionization-mass spectrometry
Fmoc	(9H-fluoren-9-ylmethoxy)carbonyl
FT-ICR	Fourier transform-ion cyclotron resonance
HBTU	2-(1H-benzotriazol-1-yl)-1,1,3,3-tetramethyluronium hexafluoro-phosphate
hMC4R	Human melanocortin-4 receptor
HOBt	N-hydroxybenzotriazole
HOCt	6-Chloro-1H-hydroxybenzotriazole
htBVLs	Heterobivalent ligands
htMVL	Heteromultivalent ligand
MALDI-TOF	Matrix-assisted laser desorption ionization-time of flight
MRI	Magnetic resonance imaging
MSH	Melanocyte-stimulating hormone
MSH-7	Ser-Nle-Glu-His-DPhe-Arg-Trp
Mtt	4-Methyltrityl
NDP-α-MSH	Ac-Ser-Tyr-Ser-Nle-Glu-His-DPhe-Arg-Trp-Gly-Lys-Pro-Val-NH_2
NHS	N-hydroxysuccinimide ester
NIR	Near-infrared
PARACEST	Paramagnetic chemical exchange saturation transfer
Pbf	2,2,4,6,7-Pentamethyl-dihydrobenzofuran-5-sulfonyl
PEG	Polyethyleneglycol
Pego	19-Amino-5-oxo-3,10,13,16-tetraoxa-6-azanonadecan-1-oic acid
RP-HPLC	Reverse-phase high-performance liquid chromatography
SPECT	Single photon emission computed tomography
SPPS	Solid-phase peptide synthesis
TA	Thioanisole
*t*Bu	*tert*-butyl
TFA	Trifluoroacetic acid
THF	Tetrahydrofuran
Tic	1,2,3,4-Tetrahydroisoquinoline-3-carboxylic acid
TIS	Triisopropylsilane
TRL	Time-resolved luminescence
Trt	Triphenylmethyl (trityl)

1. Introduction

The field of medical imaging is rapidly evolving towards the ability to visualize molecular events occurring at the cellular and whole animal level. High-throughput assays can utilize similar technology to rapidly screen cell populations for specific molecular phenotypes. We have applied the use of fluorescent and lanthanide-labeled monovalent and multivalent ligands (see Fig. 1 for examples) in the field of cancer "theranostics" (see Note 1). In this context, we have demonstrated the use of heteromultivalency to enhance by orders of magnitude the binding avidity and specificity to cells that express complementary receptors (1–3). Heteromultivalent ligands (htMVLs) are characterized by the presence of two or more different ligands linked together on a scaffold, which would bind with enhanced affinity only to cells that express complementary heterologous receptors on their surface. We hypothesize that a high degree of selectivity in tandem with high avidity could be achieved with these constructs (Fig. 2). Towards this end, we have tested two receptor pairs – human melanocortin type 4 receptor (hMC4R)/cholecystokinin-2 receptor (CCK-2R) and δ-opioid receptor (δOR)/hMC4R – as models of cell-surface receptor targeting by multivalent ligands. Using these two systems, we demonstrated an enhanced "apparent" binding affinity of heterobivalent ligands (htBVLs) to their complementary receptor pairs by 10–80-fold. The optimized bivalent ligands were then labeled with fluorescent (Cyanine 5 dye (Cy5) and lanthanide labels (e.g., Eu-DOTA) and were demonstrated to have high specific binding to cells expressing the cognate receptor pairs, but weak interaction with cells expressing the single receptor (Fig. 2).

1.1. In Vitro and In Vivo Fluorescence Imaging

The use of fluorescence detection is desirable because of its high sensitivity, excellent spatial and temporal resolution, and multiple detection capabilities by simultaneous use of several complimentary probes. Therefore, the use of fluorescently labeled agents has rapidly expanded in recent years for cell-based imaging (microscopy) and high-throughput assays (see Fig. 1 for representative structures). Fluorescence allows ready monitoring of superficial cancerous lesions in vivo (Fig. 3) and can detect targets at centimeter depths, though with decreased resolution (4). Extension into in vivo settings allows visualization of biology in its intact and native physiological state. However, there is a fundamental barrier to optical imaging in tissues due to autofluorescence and high absorption (e.g., hemoglobin ([Hb]) in the midvisible band. Tissue penetration is limited and depends upon wavelength. The use of red and near-infrared (NIR) light (wavelengths beyond

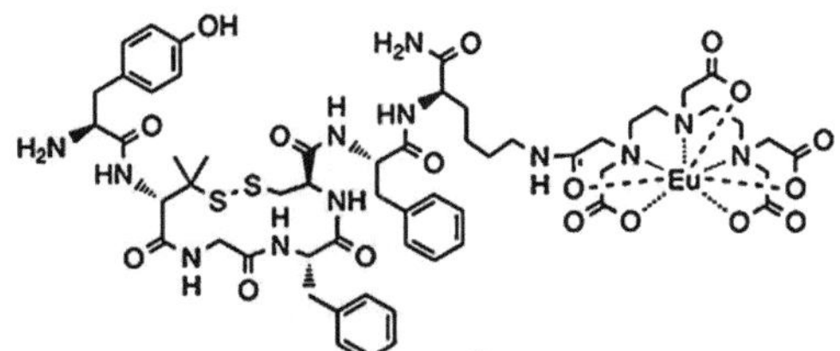

1
DPLCE-(Eu-DTPA)

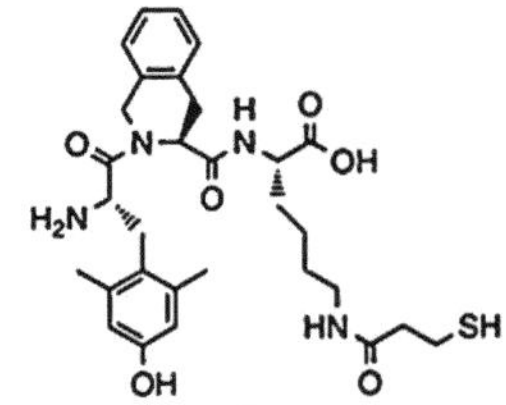

2
Dmt-Tic-Lys

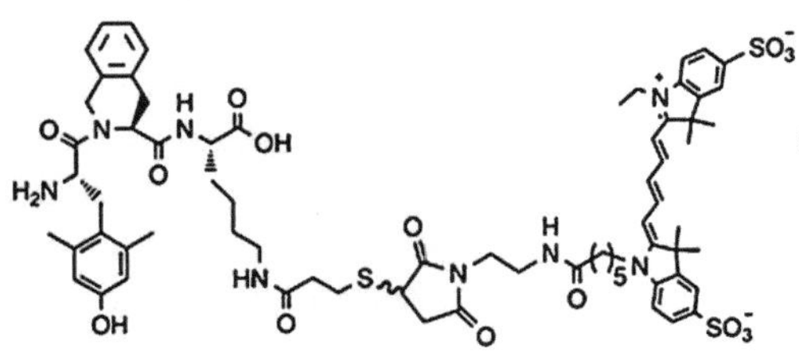

3
Dmt-Tic-Lys(Cy5)

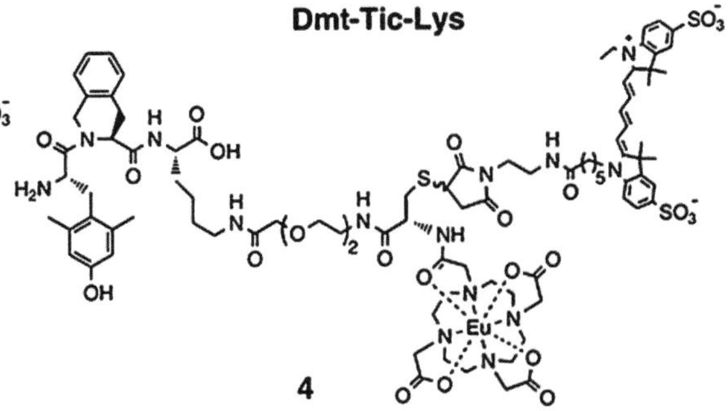

4
Dmt-Tic-Lys(Cy5/Eu-DOTA)

Ac-Ser-Tyr-Ser-Nle-Glu-His-DPhe-Arg-Trp-Gly-Lys-Pro-Val-NH_2

5
Ac-NDP-α-MSH

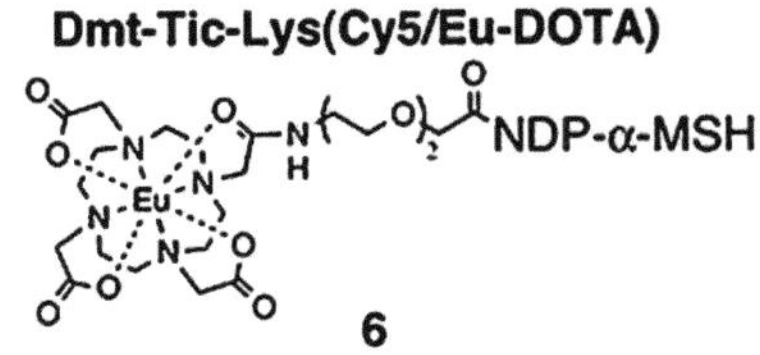

6
Eu-DOTA-NDP-α-MSH

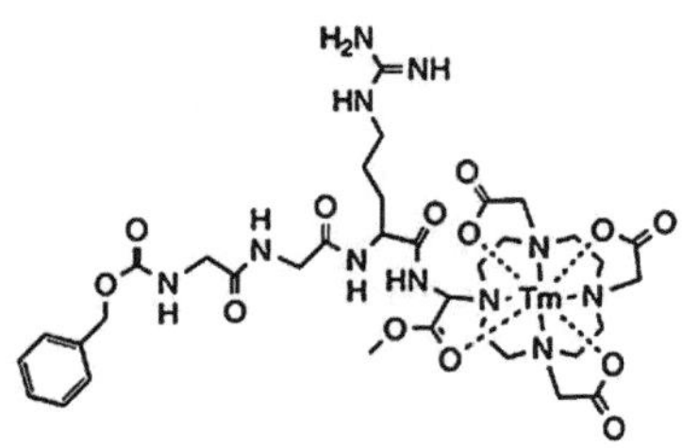

7
Z-GGR-(Tm-DOTA)

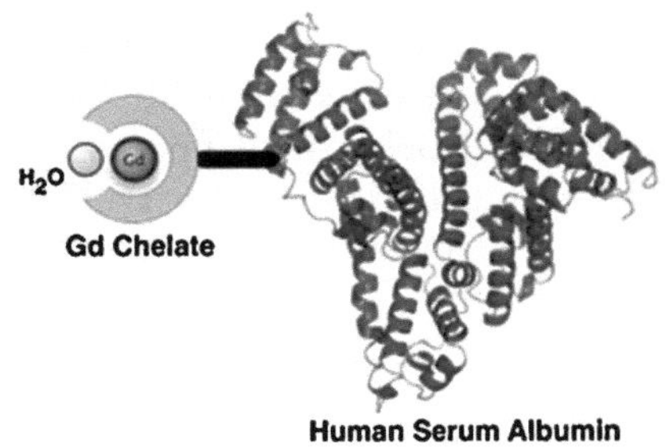

8
$(Ln\text{-}DOTA\text{-}Gly_4)_n$-HSA

BIVALENT LIGANDS

LEGEND
MSH(7): Ac-Ser-Nle-Glu-His-DPhe-Arg-Trp
CCK(6): Nle-Gly-Trp-Nle-Asp-Phe
$[PG]_3$: $(Pro\text{-}Gly)_3$, 18 atoms long linker
Pego:

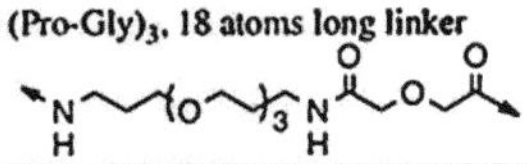

Ac-MSH(7)-Pego-$[PG]_3$-K(Cy5)-Pego-CCK(6)-NH_2
9 Cy5-htBVL

Ac-MSH(7)-Pego-$[PG]_3$-K-Pego-CCK(6)-NH_2

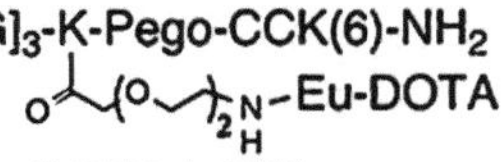

10 Eu-DOTA htBVL

Fig. 1. Examples of fluorescent and lanthanide-labeled ligands.

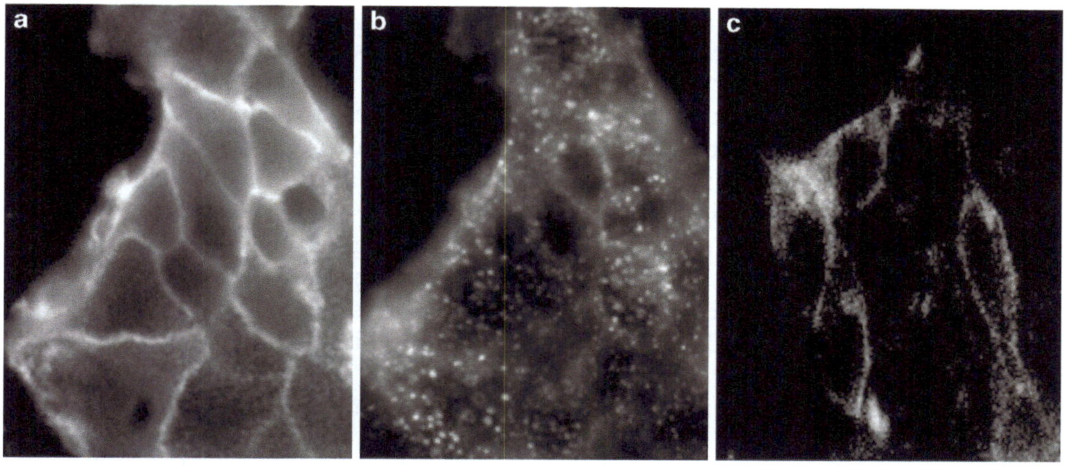

Fig. 2. In vitro imaging of Cy5-labeled htBVL 9 (conc.: 5 nM) of cells expressing both CCK-2R and hMC4R (**a**, **b**) or CCK-2R only (**c**). Images (**a**) and (**c**) were acquired 2 min following incubation with the ligand, while image (**b**) was acquired 10 min after ligand addition to the same cells shown in (**a**). The difference in fluorescence intensity levels between (**a**) and (**c**) is due to greater than 40-fold higher binding to the dual receptor expressing cells (**a**) than to the monoexpressing cells (**c**), at this ligand concentration. (**b**) Capping and endocytosis of ligand/receptor complex was nearly complete after 5 min at which time the addition of a saturating concentration of cold ligand to the media had no effect on the fluorophore intensity or distribution, i.e., the receptors were internalized.

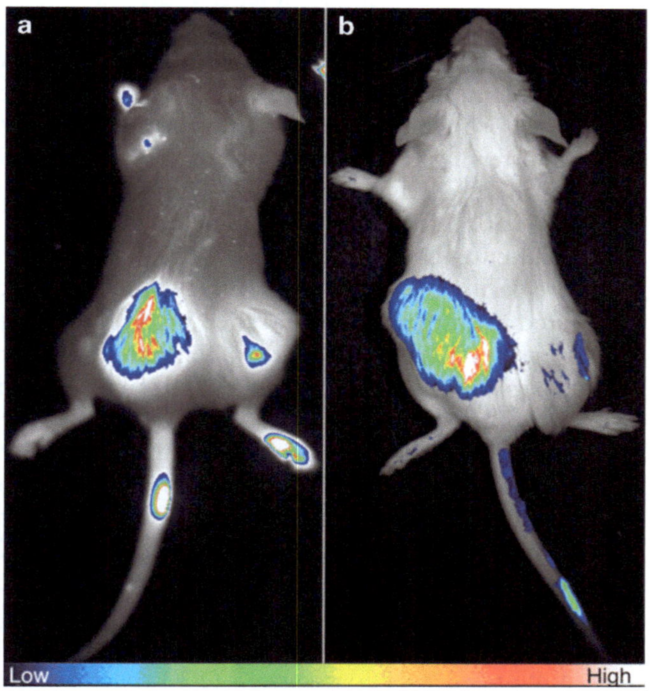

Fig. 3. Examples of in vivo imaging with optical agent. (**a**, **b**) Fluorescence imaging of Cy5-labeled targeted imaging agent 3. Mice were bilaterally implanted with HCT116 xenografts of cells overexpressing δOR (*left flank*) and control cells (*right flank*). (**a**) Mouse imaged 72 h postintravenous (i.v.) injection of 100 μg of ligand 3. (**b**) Mouse imaged 24 h post-iv injection of 10 μg of ligand 3 (reprinted with permission from Ref. 16: Josan et al., Organic Letters (2009), American Chemical Society).

650 nm) confers the advantage of less autofluorescence from tissues (mainly pyridine nucleotides, folates, and flavins) that are observed over lower bands. The most common organic NIR fluorophores are polymethines such as pentamethine and heptamethine cyanines. Their physical properties, biodistribution, pharmacokinetics, and applications for in vivo fluorescence imaging have been summarized in recent reviews (5–7). Briefly, the sulphonated cyanine dyes have good aqueous solubility, quantum yields greater than 0.1, and high extinction coefficients (e.g., ε_{650} for Cy5 >250,000). They are stable over a broad pH range (3–10) and exhibit low nonspecific binding to tissues and are more photostable than dyes like fluorescein (8). This allows repeated excitation cycles with limited loss of signal. Further, their small size (compared to fluorescent proteins) and spectral properties make them an excellent choice for whole cell assays including high-throughput screens.

1.2. Time-Resolved Fluorescence and DELFIA-Based Binding Assays

An additional approach for limiting the contributions of autofluorescence and improving the quantification of fluorescence signal is to utilize measurements of the fluorescence lifetime (9–11). Luminescent lanthanide chelates exhibit unusual spectral characteristics and are optimized for lifetime analyses making them useful as nonradiolabeled alternatives to organic fluorophores for screening and biodistribution analyses, particularly in applications where background autofluorescence is a significant problem. For luminescence, the lanthanide complex requires close proximity of a sensitizing chromophore, which is capable of transferring its excited state energy to the encapsulated lanthanide(III) ion (12, 13). This is essential since direct excitation of the Ln^{3+} ion is very inefficient, leading to low values of extinction coefficients ($\varepsilon \leq 1$ M/cm) as the relevant f-f transitions are parity forbidden. Alternatively, the lanthanide can be dissociated from the chelate and then incorporated into an in situ fluorescent chelate (see Note 2). Lanthanide emission bands are very sharp compared to organic fluorophores, typically with a full width at half maximum of ca. 10–20 nm. The detection limits of lanthanide chelates are conservatively in the range of 10^{-12} to 10^{-15} M (14). The two most important characteristics of lanthanide emission that make them very useful for bioassays are the extremely large Stokes' shift (often exceeding 200 nm) and the long-lived luminescence, which typically range from microseconds (Yb, Er, Nd) to milliseconds (Eu, Tb) (14). These long lifetimes immediately offer a signal/noise advantage as they allow time-resolved fluorescence (TRF) spectroscopy and microscopy to be used (see Note 3). The high sensitivity of these assays combined with the elimination of radiation and radioactivity disposal renders them amenable to easy automation and makes them

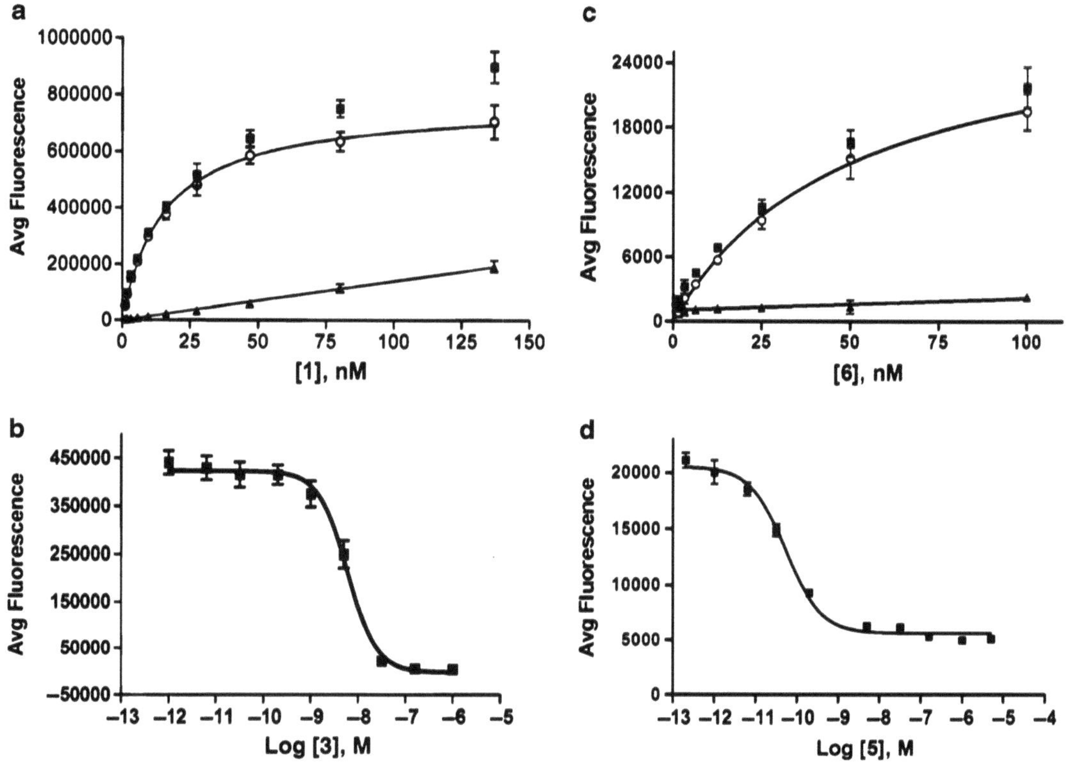

Fig. 4. Examples of DELFIA-based binding assays with Eu-DTPA/DOTA labels as an alternative to radiolabeled binding assays. (**a**) Saturation binding assay with DPLCE-(Eu-DTPA) ligand 1 binding to CHO cells overexpressing the δ-opioid receptor (δOR). (**b**) Competition binding assay of Dmt-Tic-Lys(Cy5) ligand 3 carried out with DPLCE-(Eu-DTPA) 1 on the same CHO cells. (**c**) Saturation binding study of Eu-DOTA-NDP-α-MSH (see text for modifications needed in DELFIA protocol for assaying Eu-DOTA labels) performed on HEK293 cells overexpressing hMC4R. (**d**) Competitive binding curve of NDP-α-MSH binding to HEK293/hMC4R using Eu-DOTA-NDP-α-MSH (Fig. 4a, b reprinted with permissions from Ref. 17: Heather et al. (2005), Analytical biochemistry, Elsevier Inc. Josan et al., Organic Letters (2009), American Chemical Society, respectively.)

highly attractive for high-throughput screening (HTS). Finally, some lanthanide ions display in vivo toxicity, but are considered nontoxic when complexed to a strong chelator (15).

An example of this luminescence-based technology is the dissociation-enhanced lanthanide fluoroimmunoassay (DELFIA®) (see Fig. 4 for examples of assays performed with DELFIA) (9, 10, 16, 17). This protocol requires the use of a lanthanide complex (e.g., DTPA) that is easily dissociable at acidic pH (~3.5). Our recent modifications to the DELFIA protocol have allowed its successful use with lanthanide chelates that are considerably more stable (e.g., DOTA, 1,4,7,10-tetraazacyclododecane-N,N′,N″,N‴-tetraacetic acid) (18). Lanthanide-DOTA chelates can be used to label peptides/ligands ("lanthaligands;" see Note 1) for in vivo applications with magnetic resonance imaging (MRI) and positron emission tomography/single photon emission computed tomography (PET/SPECT) techniques (19). For example, radioactive ^{153}Sm and ^{177}Lu lanthanides can be detected with SPECT and are used for radiotherapy (20). In addition, many radioactive metals such as ^{111}In, ^{99m}Tm, and ^{64}Cu can bind to the same chelators used for lanthanides, thereby expanding the scope of this tag's utility (20). Thus, modification of this DELFIA protocol for lanthanide-DOTA chelates provides a platform technology for vertical integration of this tag for in vitro and in vivo applications.

1.3. (PARACEST) Magnetic Resonance Imaging (MRI)

The lanthanides are also paramagnetic, which makes them useful as MRI contrast agents (such as gadolinium and dysprosium) by inducing the relaxation of water protons and, thus, decreasing T1 and/or T2 relaxation (21). More recently, lanthanide chelates have been used to create PARACEST MRI contrast agents for molecular imaging (22). PARACEST (PARAmagnetic Chemical Exchange Saturation Transfer) employs the ability of paramagnetic lanthanide ions to shift the MR frequencies of the protons of the chelator by as much as ±50 ppm (23). These extremely shifted frequencies (relative to the typical 0–10 ppm MR frequency range for nonparamagnetic molecules) facilitate selective saturation of an MR frequency of one PARACEST agent in the presence of other agents. This MR saturation procedure is similar to the fluorescence recovery after photobleaching (FRAP) used with optical imaging, in that the coherent MR signal is reduced or obliterated. Chemical exchange of the MR-saturated proton from the contrast agent to a water molecule transfers the saturation to water, which causes the MR signal of water to be reduced to levels that can be detected with standard MRI methods.

PARACEST MRI contrast agents provide advantages relative to T1/T2* MRI contrast agents for molecular imaging. Two or more PARACEST agents can be detected during the same experiment (similar to detecting multiple optical imaging dyes), which can be used to perform in situ comparative analyses with improved quantification (24). For example, the pharmacokinetics of two PARACEST agents with different sizes may be measured to investigate tumor vascular permeability characteristics (Fig. 5) (25). In addition, the chemical exchange rates of PARACEST agents can be very responsive to interactions with disease biomarkers (26). For example, we have created PARACEST agents that alter their chemical exchange rate after their peptidyl ligand is cleaved by an enzyme (24, 27, 28). The detection of a change in the PARACEST effect is used to detect the enzyme biomarker (Fig. 6). These examples demonstrate that lanthanide chelates that label peptides and other molecules are a useful platform technology for in vivo molecular imaging studies.

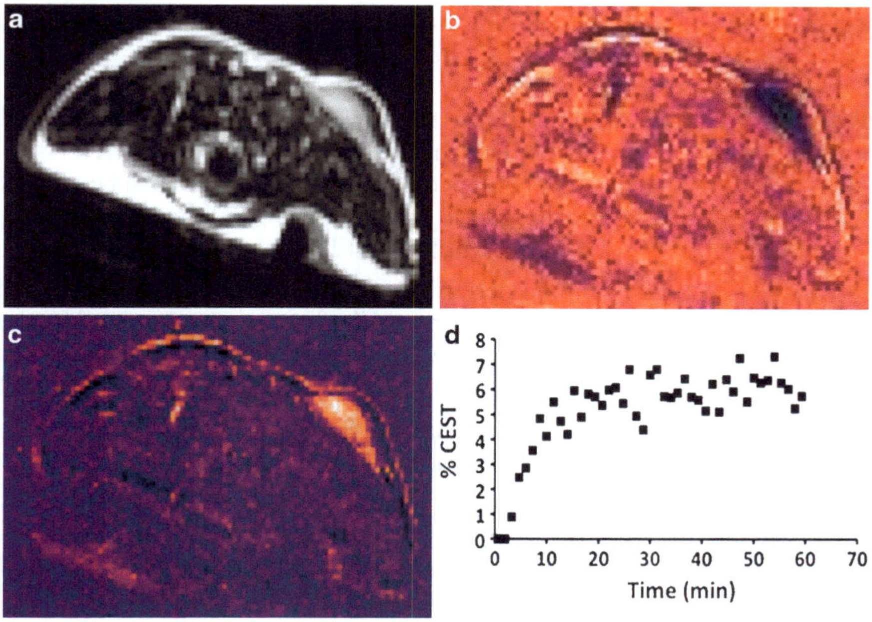

Fig. 5. Monitoring the pharmacokinetics of PARACEST-labeled albumin in a mouse model of mammary carcinoma. (**a**) An axial MR image showing the location of a subcutaneous flank MCF7 tumor on the back of an athymic nude mouse (*upper right side* of the image). The mammary fat pads on the front of the mouse were also clearly visible. (**b**) The change in MRI signal measured 60 min after injecting the PARACEST-labeled albumin into the tail vein of the mouse. The decrease in MRI signal in the tumor region indicated accumulation of the labeled albumin in this tissue. The periphery of the mouse showed increased and decreased MRI signals due to magnetic susceptibility artifacts. (**c**) The PARACEST map refined the analysis by reducing magnetic susceptibility artifacts and by normalizing the change in MRI signals after injection relative to the preinjection MRI signals. (**d**) The temporal evolution of the measured CEST effect showed an initial accumulation and subsequent retention of PARACEST-labeled albumin in the tumor. These results were used to assess tumor angiogenesis.

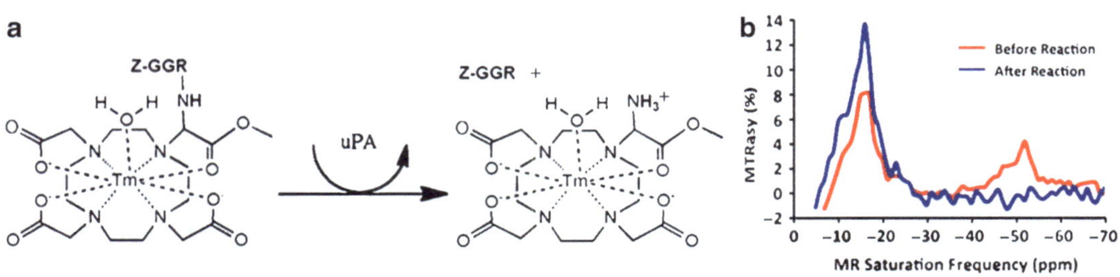

Fig. 6. Detection of urokinase plasminogen activator (uPA) with 7. (**a**) The proposed mechanism of uPA-mediated cleavage of the Z-GGR peptide ligand from the agent and showing conversion of an amide proton to an amine. (**b**) The MTRasy spectrum showed a CEST effect from the amide at −52 ppm before uPA was added (*red*). The disappearance of this CEST effect after uPA was added (*blue*) was used to detect uPA. An enzyme-unresponsive agent, Yb-DOTA-Gly, showed a CEST effect at −16 ppm before and after uPA was added, which served as an internal control.

2. Materials

2.1. Chemical Syntheses

1. An Fmoc/*t*Bu strategy is used here for the synthesis of peptides. For manual assembly of peptides, plastic syringe reactors equipped with a frit and piston can be employed. For manual multiple syntheses in a parallel fashion, use a Domino solid-phase synthesizer (Torviq, Niles, MI).
2. N^{α}-Fmoc derivatives of amino acids, N-hydroxybenzotriazole (HOBt), 6-chloro-1H-hydroxybenzotriazole (HOCt), N,N′-diisopropyl carbodiimide (DIC), and 2-(1H-benzotriazol-1-yl)-1,1,3,3-tetramethyluronium hexafluoro-phosphate (HBTU).
3. Rink amide Tentagel S resin (Rapp Polymere, Tubingen, Germany), Wang resin.
4. Polyethylene glycol-based flexible linkers – Fmoc-Ado-OH (Ado: 8-amino-3,6-dioxaoctanoyl; 9-atoms long linker) and Fmoc-Pego-OH (Pego: 19-amino-5-oxo-3,10,13,16-tetraoxa-6-azanonadecan-1-oyl; 20-atoms long linker) (Novabiochem, Gibbstown, NJ). Alternatively, Pego linker can be assembled with diglycolic anhydride (TCI America, Portland, OR), N,N -carbonyldiimidazole (CDI) (Sigma-Aldrich, Milwaukee, WI), and 4,7,10-trioxa-1,13-tridecane-diamine (PEG_3 diamine) (TCI America, Portland, OR) on the solid-phase.
5. 1,4,7,10-tetraazacyclododecane-1,4,7,10-tetraacetic acid mono N-hydroxysuccinimide ester (DOTA-NHS ester) (Macrocyclics, Dallas, TX). Diethylenetriaminepentaacetic dianhydride (DTPA dianhydride), Arsenazo(III) dye (Sigma-Aldrich).
6. A hydrogenator for hydrogenation reactions (Parr Instruments, Moline, IL).
7. Human serum albumin (HAS), benzylcarbamate, glyoxylic acid monohydrate, phosphorous tribromide, *tert*-butyl 2-bromoacetate, 10%-Pd/C, Fmoc-Cl, zinc dust, 1-ethyl-3-(3-dimethylaminopropyl) carbodiimide hydrochloride (EDC), N-hydroxysuccinimide (HOSu), 2-morpholinoethanesulfonic acid, bromophenol blue (BB), diisopropylethylamine (DIEA), N,N-dimethylbarbituric acid (DMBA), 1,2-ethandithiol (EDT), 2-mercaptoethanol, sodium diethyldithiocarbamate trihydride, tetrahydrofuran (THF), tetrakis(triphenylphosphine) palladium(0) [$Pd(0)TPP_4$], thioanisole (TA), trifluoroacetic acid (TFA), and triisopropylsilane (TIS).

2.2. Purification and Characterization

1. Analyze the purity of final products using high-performance liquid chromatography (HPLC) apparatus (Waters® HPLC used in this work) equipped with a C18 reverse-phase column

(e.g., Vydac column, diameter × length: 4.6 × 150 mm, pore size: 3 μm). A linear gradient of buffer B under various gradient conditions at a flow rate of 0.3–1 mL/min can be used. Monitor the separations at 220 and 280 nm. Achieve the purification of compounds using a preparative HPLC (Waters 600 HPLC apparatus) equipped with a C-18 reverse-phase column (e.g., Vydac column: 22 × 250 mm, 5 μm pore size) with similar buffers and 3–10 mL/min flow rate. Monitor the separations at 230 and 280 nm.

2. See Table 1 for HPLC conditions used.
3. Employ solid-phase extraction (SPE) where simple isolation of the final compounds is needed, with the C-18 Sep-Pak™ Vac RC cartridges (100 or 500 mg) (Waters, Milford, MA). Precondition the Sep-Pak cartridge with 5 column volumes (5 times the volume of packed column bed) each of acetonitrile, methanol, and water, in that order. After loading the compound, wash the column several times with water, and then gradually with 5, 10, 60, and 90% of aqueous acetonitrile to elute the peptide. Monitor the fractions for the required compound with analytical HPLC. The elution gradient here is designed such that most compounds will elute in the 60% fraction.
4. Size-exclusion chromatography (SEC) can be performed with a borosilicate glass column (2.6 × 250 mm) filled with medium-sized Sephadex G-25 or G-10 resin. Elute the compounds with an isocratic flow of 1.0 M aq. AcOH.
5. Cellulose membrane tubing with a molecular weight cut-off of 5,000 for dialysis purification (Pierce Biotechnology, Rockford, IL).
6. Mass spectra of positive or negative ions with a single stage reflectron matrix-assisted laser desorption ionization-time of flight (MALDI-TOF) mass spectrometer (Bruker Rexlex III, Bruker Daltonics, Billerica, MA; α-cyanocinnamic acid as a matrix) in reflectron mode or with a low resolution electrospray

Table 1
HPLC conditions used for various compounds

Phase A	Phase B
A1: 0.1% TFA in water	B1: 0.1% TFA in acetonitrile
A2: 0.1% TEA/AcOH (TEAA) in water (pH 6.0)	B2: 90% acetonitrile in Phase A2 (pH adjusted to 6.0 with AcOH)

Method A: 10–40% Phase B1 in Phase A1 in 30 min; Method B: 10–60% Phase B1 in Phase A1 in 50 min; Method C: 10–90% Phase B1 in Phase A1 in 30 min; Method D: 20–60% Phase B1 in Phase A1 in 50 min; Method E: 10–60% Phase B2 in Phase A2 in 50 min; Method F: 10–90% Phase B2 in Phase A2 in 40 min ionization (ESI) mass spectrometer (Finnigan, Thermoquest LCQ ion trap instrument, Lake Forrest, CA), and/or using a high-resolution Fourier transform mass spectrometer (FT-ICR MS, Bruker Apex Qh, Bremen, Germany) equipped with an ESI source. For internal calibration, use an appropriate mixture of standard peptides with an average resolution of ca. 10,000 and 60,000 on the Reflex III and the FT-ICR instrument, respectively.

2.3. Cell Cloning, Culture, and Binding Assays

1. HEK293 cells engineered to overexpress hMC4R (29). The coding region of hMC4R gene is cloned into a pcDNA3.1 vector (Invitrogen, V790-20). HEK293 cells overexpressing both hMC4 and CCK2 receptors for heterobivalent studies have also been reported previously (3, 30).
2. Cell culture media:

   For HEK293 cells: Add 50 mL of Super Calf Serum and 5 mL each of penicillin (Sigma; 1,000 units/mL) and streptomycin (Sigma; 1,000 μg/mL) to 500 mL of Dulbecco's modified eagle medium (DMEM) supplemented with 10% fetal bovine serum (FBS). Selection agents: 1% v/v of geneticin (Gibco) for hMC4R and 0.125% v/v of zeocin (Invitrogen) for Cholecystokinin receptor subtype 2 (CCK2R).

   For MCF-7 cells: Culture MCF-7 cells from ATCC (Manassas, VA) with RPMI-1640 medium with 5% FBS, and 1% Penicillin/Streptomycin.

   For tumor implantation, suspend MCF-7 cells in HEPES-buffered physiological salt solution (HBSS) medium and mix with Matrigel™ (BD Biosciences, Franklin Lakes, NJ).
3. To collect cells from a flask, incubate cells with 2–3 mL of RPMI-1630 medium containing 0.25% trypsin and 1 mM EDTA for 2–5 min.
4. Ligand binding assay medium: 2 g of bovine serum albumin, 5.97 g of HEPES pH 7.4, 2.2 g of $NaHCO_3$, 1 mL of 1,10-phenanthroline stock (1 g of 1,10-phenanthroline in 5.045 mL of ethanol), 1 mL of leupeptin stock (1 mg in 2 mL of water), and 1 mL of bacitracin stock (0.715 g in 3.75 mL of water) (Sigma) in 1,000 mL of DMEM, pH 7.4 adjusted with 1 N HCl or NaOH, if needed.
5. TRIS wash buffer (10×): 10 g of BSA, 9 g of NaCl, 250 mL of 1 M Tris–HCl in distilled water (total volume 500 mL), pH 7.6 adjusted with 1 M HCl or 1 M NaOH.
6. Enhancement solution (Perkin Elmer Lifesciences: #1244-105).
7. Black CoStar 96-well plates (Perkin Elmer Lifesciences: (#3503).

2.4. In Vitro Live Cell Imaging Microscopy

1. An inverted Olympus IX70 microscope equipped with a 40× 1.4 NA ultrafluor objective, and a 200 W Hg lamp as the excitation source.
2. Matching excitation and emission filters for the fluorophore of interest. For Cy5, select the excitation light at 650 nm to focus onto the cell, and filter the emitted light at 670 nm (10 nm BP) prior to imaging onto a CCD camera.
3. HBSS Buffer: 5 mM KCl, 0.3 mM KH_2PO_4, 138 mM NaCl, 0.2 mM $NaHCO_3$, 0.3 mM Na_2HPO_4, 20 mM HEPES, 1.3 mM $CaCl_2$, 0.4 mM $MgSO_4$, and 5.6 mM glucose, pH 7.3 at 37°C.
4. A coverslip containing cells into a chamber held at 37°C on the stage of the microscope in 1 mL of HBSS.

2.5. PARACEST MR Imaging

1. Construct a customized MRI cradle, similar to a standard tube rack, for study of PARACEST MRI contrast agents in biochemical solutions. This cradle can be crafted from a PVC pipe, sheets of polycarbonate, electrical tape, and a Dremel drilling and shaping tool (see Note 4).
2. For in vivo imaging, construct a customized MRI compatible "mouse sled" with a nosecone for gas anesthetic for study of PARACEST MRI contrast agents within in vivo models. This can be crafted from sheets of polycarbonate, a 30 mL syringe, electrical tape, and a Dremel drilling and shaping tool.
3. For in vivo MRI, anesthetize the mice with isofluorane (Aerrane™, Henry Schein Animal Health, Inc., Melville, NY) in 100% Oxygen gas (Praxair, Inc.).
4. To perform in vivo MR imaging, use physiological monitoring instrumentation (SA Instruments, Stony Brook, NY), syringes, needles, PE20 tubing, suture thread, tape and a Gaymar heat pad (Henry Schein Animal Health, Inc., Melville, NY), a 150 W heat lamp (PetSmart, Inc.), and a 9.4T Biospec MRI Scanner (Bruker Biospin Corp., Billerica, MA) for in vivo MR imaging.
5. Gd-DTPA (Magnevist™, Bayer Health Pharmaceuticals, Inc.) for in vivo MR imaging without further purification.

3. Methods

The following subheadings describe in detail the individual steps necessary to incorporate Cy5 dye, chelates, and lanthanide labels (Eu, Yb, and Tm) into ligands. The solid-phase strategy was favored for labeling, wherever possible. Also, many ligands need a free N-terminus to preserve the high binding affinity and potency to their cognate receptors, such as endorphins to the δ-opioid receptor. This requires orthogonal protection schemes during synthesis (e.g., Fmoc/*t*Bu/Aloc or Mtt). Thus, if a free N-terminal amine is needed, an orthogonal group is introduced at the C-terminus, either on the amino acid side chain or on the linker coupled to the C-terminus (final product as secondary amide). This group can then be selectively cleaved to label via solid-phase procedures (see Subheadings 3.2 and 3.3). For lanthaligands, DTPA solid-phase labeling procedures are simple, but very few published procedures are available that describe the efficient reduction of dimer products often seen with DTPA dianhydride reagent. Most of these protocols require selective protection of the carboxylates. Since we routinely prepare many lanthaligands by these methods, we will describe here an efficient and yet simple route for DTPA coupling (31). Whereas DTPA is desirable for in vitro applications, in vivo settings require a stronger chelator such as DOTA. Standard solid-phase synthesis methods can easily couple the DTPA/DOTA chelates to the amine terminus of a resin-bound peptide during solid-phase peptide synthesis. However, conjugation on carboxyl terminus requires some modifications and is usually done by introducing a C-terminus residue (e.g., lysine) or a linker coupled on the C-terminus (see Subheadings 3.2 and 3.3 for examples). We have developed an alternative method to create a resin-bound amine-derivatized DOTA, which has an amine that can couple to the carboxyl terminus of amino acids during standard Fmoc solid-phase synthesis (24). The synthesis of a resin-bound α-amino-DOTA for Fmoc chemistry is described in Subheading 3.5.

3.1. General Solid-Phase Synthesis

1. Solid-phase syntheses can be carried out in polypropylene syringes (5–20 mL) fitted with polyethylene porous disks (32). Solvents and soluble reagents can be removed with a syringe fitted with piston or by vacuum if using a manual solid-phase synthesizer. The compounds described here can be synthesized on a Tentagel Rink amide resin (the initial loading 0.2–0.26 mmol/g) using N^{α}-Fmoc protecting groups and a standard DIC/HOCt or HBTU/HOBt activation strategy, unless otherwise noted. An on-resin BB test can be used for qualitative and continuous monitoring of reaction progress. For quantitative analyses, a Kaiser test can be performed (see Note 5).
2. Swell the resin in THF for an hour, and wash with N,N′-dimethylformamide [DMF] (2×). Remove Fmoc group with 20% piperidine in DMF (2 + 20 min), followed by washing the resin with DMF (3×), dichloromethane [DCM] (3×), 0.2 M HOBt in DMF (2×), and finally with DMF (3×).

3. Couple the first amino acid using preactivated 0.3 M HOCt ester in DMF or DMF-DCM 1:1 mixture (3 eq of N^{α}-Fmoc amino acid, 3 eq of HOCt, and 3 eq of DIC). To avoid deletion sequences, perform a double coupling at all steps with 3 eq of amino acid, 3 eq of HBTU, and 6 eq of DIEA or 2,4,6-collidine in DMF. If the Kaiser test is positive at this stage, perform a third coupling using the symmetric anhydride method (stir 4 eq of amino acid and 2 eq of DIC in DCM or DMF-DCM mixture for 5 min, and add it to resin). Cap any unreacted NH_2 groups on the resin using 50% acetic anhydride in pyridine for 5 min. Following completion of coupling reaction, wash the resin with DMF and repeat the same procedure for the next amino acid until all the amino acids have been coupled.
4. Frequently during the synthetic steps, cleave a small amount of the peptide from the resin (see Subheading 3.1, step 6) and analyze by HPLC and MS to monitor the synthesis and purity of the peptide intermediates.
5. After the final amino acid has been incorporated, cleave N^{α}-Fmoc groups and acetylate or label the free N^{α}-termini as required. If free N-termini are desired, use a Boc-protected amino acid for the last residue coupling.
6. For cleavage of the peptide from the resin, wash the resin with DCM (3×), DMF (5×), THF (2×), DCM (2×), and dry it over vacuum. A cleavage cocktail (10 mL per 1 g of resin) of 82.5% TFA, 5% water, 5% TIS, 5% TA, and 2.5% EDT can be used, unless otherwise noted. Inject the TFA cocktail into the resin-containing vessel and stir for 3–6 h at room temperature. Isolate the crude peptides from the resin by filtration, reduce the filtrate to low volume by evaporation using a stream of nitrogen, and precipitate the peptides in ice-cold diethyl ether, centrifuge, wash several times with ether, dry the crude mass, dissolve in 1.0 M (6%) aq. acetic acid, and then lyophilize to give solid powders that can be stored as solid or 2 mM solution in dimethylsulfoxide [DMSO] at −20°C. Purify the peptides by preparative HPLC and/or gel-filtration.

3.2. Synthesis of DPLCE-Lys (Eu-DTPA) Lanthaligand 1

This example (Fig. 7) illustrates the synthesis of a cyclic ligand with free N-terminus (required for opioid binding in this case) and a DTPA chelate assembled on the C-terminus using a lysine side chain as a functional handle. The Aloc group has been used as an orthogonal protection that is cleaved after the completion of peptide sequence and prior to DTPA coupling. Lanthanide complexation is then accomplished in solution following purification of linear peptide and disulfide formation.

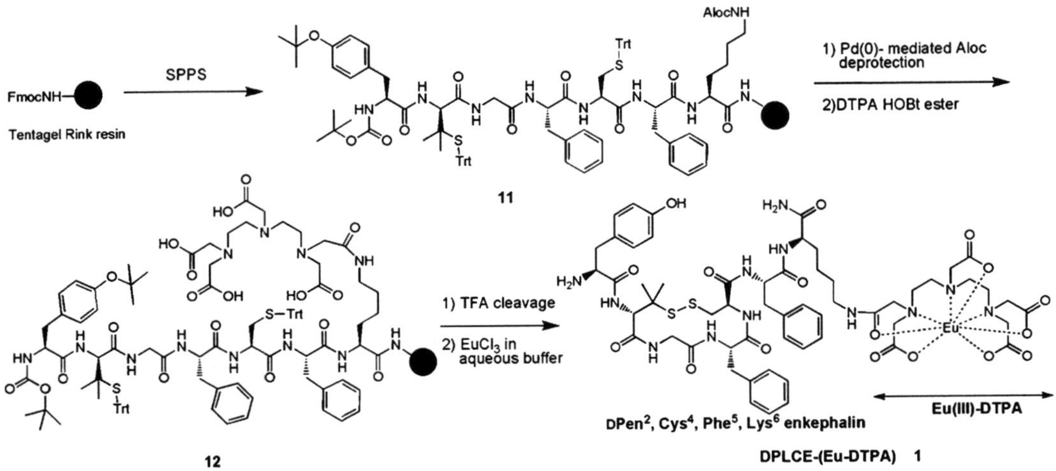

Fig. 7. Synthesis of Eu-DTPA-labeled DPLCE lanthaligand 1.

1. The chelate-derivatized c[DPen²,Cys⁵]enkephalin (DPLCE) peptide can be synthesized on a Tentagel Rink amide resin (initial loading: 0.2–0.26 mmol/g) using N^{α}-Fmoc protecting groups and a standard DIC/HOCt or HBTU/HOBt activation strategy as described in Subheading 3.1 (Fig. 7). Introduce the last residue as Boc-Tyr(*t*Bu)-OH to obviate a subsequent deprotection step. These protecting groups (Boc/*t*Bu) will be removed upon cleavage of entire product off the resin.
2. Carefully wash the resin-bound peptide 11 with dry, oxygen-free DCM (argon-flushed), and introduce an argon atmosphere using a Domino block (see Note 6).
3. The Aloc deprotection can be carried out with Pd[0] reagents under argon and oxygen-free solvents as follows (33, 34): dissolve 0.5% w/v of tetrakis(triphenylphosphine) palladium(0) [Pd(0)TPP_4] and 3% w/v of dimethylbarbituric acid (DMBA) in DCM (10 mL per 1 g of resin). Treat the resin with the deprotection reagent mixture (2×30 min). Wash the resin with DCM (3×), DMF (3×), 5% DIEA in DMF (3×), DMF (2×), 1% sodium diethyldithiocarbamate trihydride in DMF (2×, 5 min; this step removes the resin-bound palladium), DMF (2×), 5% piperidine in DMF (2×), DMF (3×), 0.2 M HOBt in DMF (2×), DMF (2×), and DCM (3×).
4. DTPA coupling: In a glass scintillation vial, dissolve 20 eq of DTPA dianhydride (in final concentration of 0.6 M) and 40 eq of HOBt in dry DMSO by heating it to 50°C, followed by stirring for another 20 min at room temperature. If precipitation occurs, briefly heat the reagent mixture again to 80°C and stir until cooled to room temperature. Add the

HOBt diester mixture to the resin and vortex for 30 min (see Notes 7 and 8).

5. Wash the resin in the following sequence: DMSO (3×), THF (3×), 20% aq. THF (3×, 5 min), 10% DIEA and 10% water in THF (2×, 5 min), 20% aq. THF (2×, 1 min), THF (3×), and DCM (3×). It is necessary to comply with this washing protocol and at no stage must the resin be exposed to DMF (see Note 7).
6. Cleave the peptide off the resin 12 using TFA-scavenger cocktail (91% TFA, 3% water, 3% EDT, and 3% TA). Wash the resin with neat TFA, pool the collected filtrates, and evaporate TFA under a stream of nitrogen. Precipitate the peptide with cold Et_2O (add 2% of 2-mercaptoethanol to prevent premature oxidation). Follow the Subheading 3.1, step 6, to achieve a lyophilized product.
7. For disulfide formation, dissolve the purified peptide (0.1 mg/mL) in 0.1 M ammonium acetate buffer (pH 8) and stir in an open jar with a few drops of DMSO (see Note 9).
8. For europium chelation to DTPA, add 3 eq of $EuCl_3 \cdot 6H_2O$ to the reaction above and stir the solution overnight (see Note 10). Purify the final product using SPE with a C-18 Sep-Pak™ cartridge.

3.3. Synthesis of Labeled Dmt-Tic-Lys Derivatives

This procedure illustrates a solid-phase synthetic methodology devised for coupling labels on-resin or in-solution as desired. The applicability of this synthetic approach is demonstrated by derivatizing a Dmt-Tic-Lys(R)-OH with the lanthanide chelator on a solid-phase support, and the Cy5 label in solution.

1. In a 50 mL bottle containing 1 g of Wang resin (0.93 mmol/g) and equipped with a magnetic stir bar, add dry DCM to swell the resin for 1 h. Carefully decant the solvent, close the bottle with a septum, and flush with nitrogen. Add DIEA (9 eq, 1.4 mL) in 15 mL of DCM. Cool the resin slurry to 0°C and add dropwise mesyl chloride (MsCl, 8 eq, 0.57 mL) in 2 mL of DCM. Stir the reaction for 20 min, remove the ice bath, and continue the stirring for another 20 min at room temperature. Transfer the resin to a 20 mL syringe reactor and wash with dry DCM (5×) and dry DMF (3×). Add Fmoc-Lys(Mtt)-OH (2 eq, 1.2 g), CsI (2 eq, 0.5 g), and DIEA (2 eq, 0.32 mL) in 10 mL of dry DMF and stir the reaction overnight at room temperature.
2. Wash the resin with DMF (3×), DCM (2×), and remove N^{α}-Fmoc with 20% piperidine in DMF (2 + 20 min). Subsequently, wash the resin with DMF (3×), DCM (3×), 0.2 M HOBt in DMF (2×), and DMF (3×). Add Fmoc-Tic-OH (3 eq), HOCt (3 eq), and DIC (3 eq) in DMF and stir the resin for 2 h.

3. Wash the resin above and cleave N^{α}-Fmoc protection with 20% piperidine in DMF (2 + 5 min). A shorter deprotection time should be used here to prevent dioxopiperazine-mediated cyclative cleavage of the unprotected dipeptide from the resin. Wash the resin with DMF (3×), DCM (3×), 0.2 M HOBt in DMF (2×), and DMF (3×). Add Boc-Dmt-OH (3 eq), HBTU (3 eq), and DIEA (6 eq) in DMF to the resin. Heat the reaction in a household microwave for 3 s, followed by stirring until it cools to room temperature; repeat the heating/cooling agitation (5×) and stir the resin for another 2 h at room temperature. A small amount of 2′,6′-dimethyl-l-tyrosine (Dmt) oligomers (acylated via unprotected phenol) is formed. To remove these oligomers, treat the resin with 50% piperidine in DCM:MeOH (1:1) to conveniently convert back this side product to desired compound (see Note 11).
4. After coupling completion, wash the resin with DMF (3×) and DCM (7×) and dry over vacuum. Cleave the peptide from the resin with 82.5% TFA, 5% TIS, 5% water, 5% TA, and 2.5% EDT.
5. For Cy5 labeling, we prefer the more cost-effective conjugation of the dye in solution via a thiol–maleimide reaction. Cleave the Mtt protection on lysine by repetitive treatment with 3% TFA and 5% TIS in DCM (2 min each). Between steps, wash the resin with 5% TIS in DCM (2×). Following final cleavage treatment, wash the resin with 5% TIS in DCM (3×), DCM (2×), 5% DIEA in DCM (3×), DMF (3×), and finally with DCM (3×). Couple TrtS-CH_2CH_2COOH (Trt-Mpr-OH) to 15 using the HOCt/DIC protocol and then cleave the peptide with acidic cocktail (82.5% TFA, 5% H_2O, 5% TIS, 5% TA, and 2.5% EDT) to give 2 (Fig. 8). Purify the compound by preparative HPLC. To carry out Cy5 dye conjugation to obtain compound 3, dissolve the lyophilized product in DMSO and add 1.3 eq of Cy5-maleimide in DMSO. Stir the reaction and monitor every hour with analytical HPLC (see Note 12).
6. For the synthesis of the dual-modal agent 4, we have employed a bifunctional handle for labeling. This is comprised of a short 8-amino-3,6-dioxaoctanyl (Ado) linker with an orthogonally protected Cys residue (Fmoc-Cys(Mmt)-OH) incorporated at the end of the Ado linker. Couple Fmoc-Ado-OH and Fmoc-Cys(Mmt)-OH using a standard HOCt/DIC coupling protocol to give intermediate 16. For coupling DOTA on-resin, we have chosen the amine group of Cys for coupling. This can be accomplished by reacting the free amines with DOTA-NHS ester (2 eq) and DIEA (8 eq) in DMF for overnight to give 17 (alternatively, the thiol group can be used for

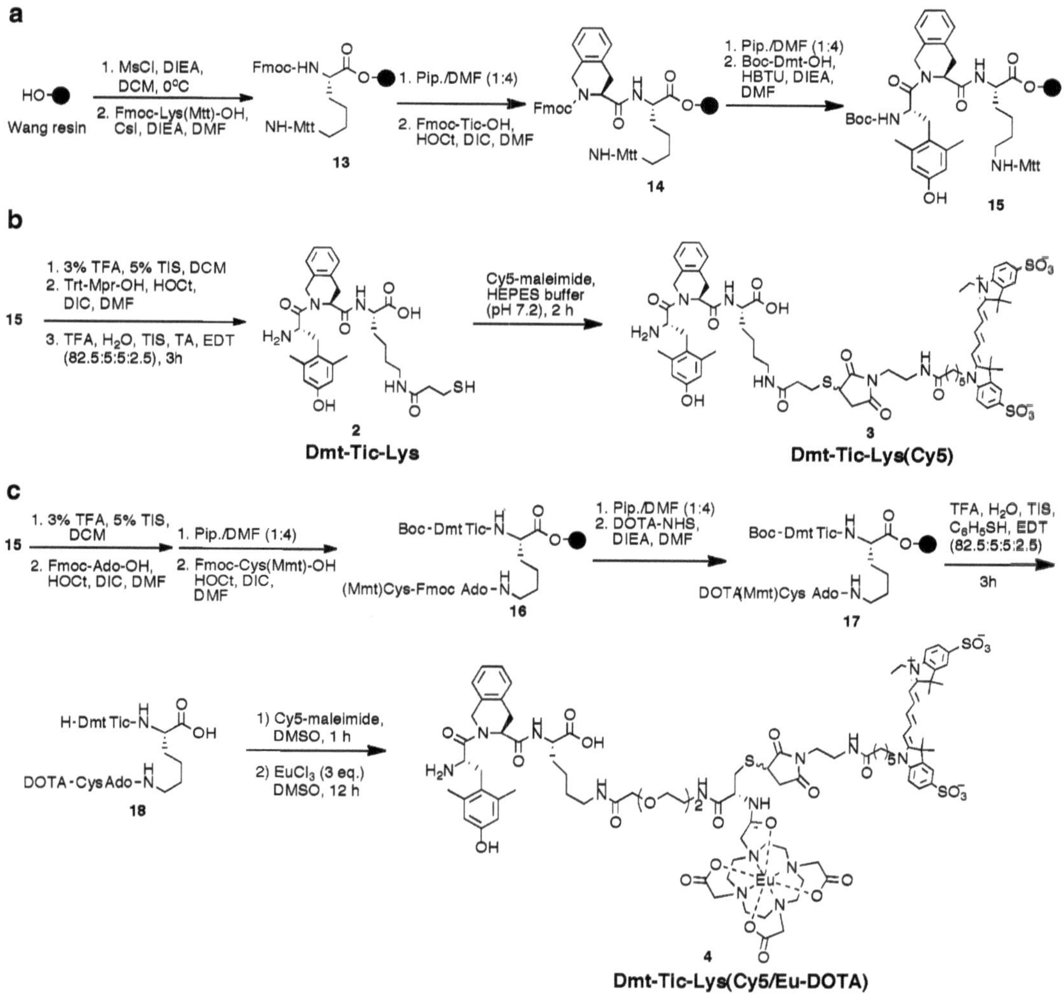

Fig. 8. Synthesis of Cy5-labeled and/or Eu-DOTA-labeled derivatives of Dmt-Tic 3 and 4.

conjugation with DOTA–maleimide compound, if the amine group is desired for other conjugations). Cleave the peptide from the resin using 82.5% TFA, 5% water, 5% TIS, 5% TA, and 2.5% EDT. Following purification of the peptide, both Cy5 conjugation and europium chelation can be carried out in a one-pot reaction. Add 1.1 eq of Cy5-maleimide to the purified peptide in DMSO and monitor the reaction with HPLC every hour. Add additional aliquots of dye, if necessary, until HPLC indicates complete conversion to Cy5 product. For Europium chelation to DOTA, add 3 eq of $EuCl_3.6H_2O$ in DMSO to the reaction above and stir the solution overnight (see Note 10). Purify the final product using SPE with C-18 Sep-Pak™ cartridge.

3.4. Synthesis of Labeled Heterobivalent Ligands (htBVLs)

In lieu of the utility of htMVLs vis-à-vis monovalent ligands described earlier in the text, examples of an htBVL labeled with either a lanthanide chelator or a dye label are demonstrated. These ligands, composed of both peptide and nonpeptide building blocks, illustrate feasibility and successful assembly of complex ligands with the labels attached in the middle of a long sequence. We have previously reported the syntheses of these htBVLs using a modular strategy based on parallel solid-phase synthesis (1). Representative examples of two labeled htBVLs are shown in Fig. 1 and their syntheses shown in Fig. 9.

1. Assemble the htBVL peptides using the N^{α}-Fmoc/*t*Bu strategy on Tentagel Rink amide resin (initial loading: 0.2 mmol/g). To avoid deletion sequences and slower coupling rates, perform double coupling (HOCt/DIC and HBTU/HOBt/DIEA) and N-capping at each step as described in Subheading 3.1. The Pego linkers and other modifications to incorporate labels are discussed below.

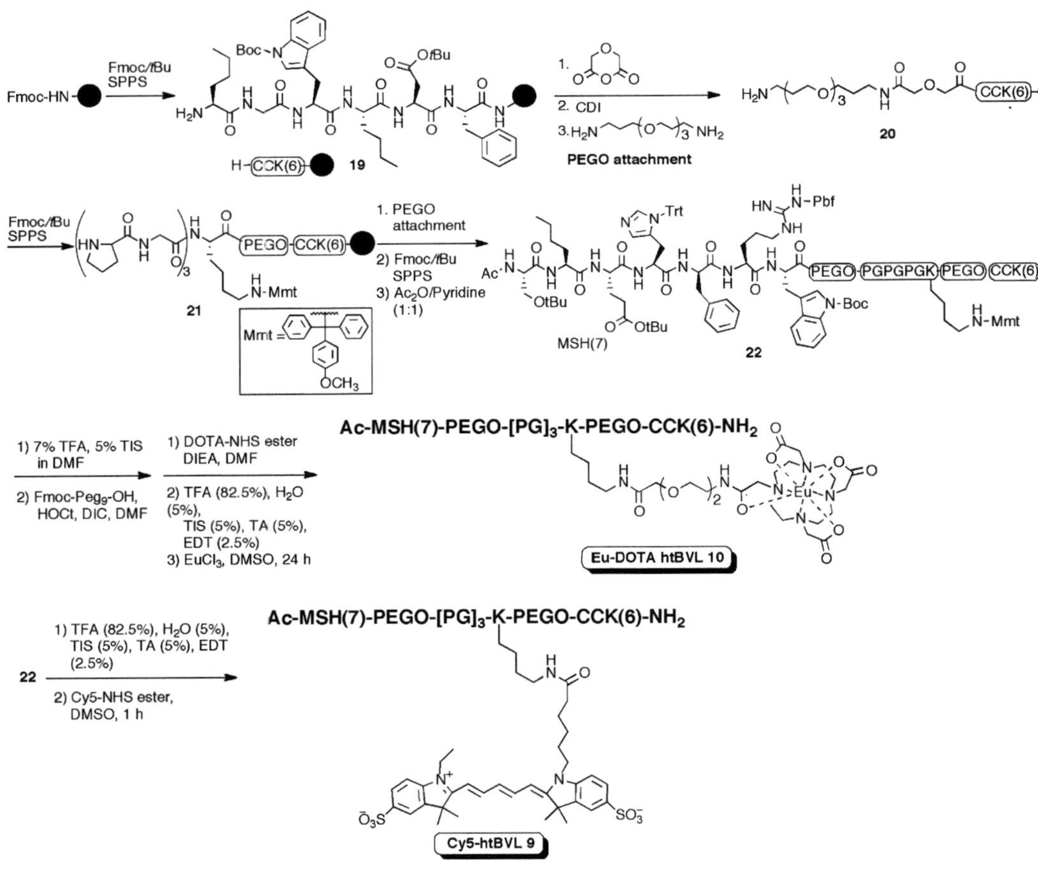

Fig. 9. Synthesis of Cy5 and Eu-DOTA-labeled heterobivalent ligands 9 and 10.

For parallel library generation (see refs. (1, 2) for examples), complete the assembly of first ligand (CCK6 ligand in this case), then split the resin into appropriate units, continue the assembly of different linkers and linker length on each, incorporate an orthogonally protected functional handle, wherever appropriate, for later derivatization, and finally assembly the second ligand.

2. *Pego coupling*: The Pego spacers can be introduced in the following manner. Couple the N-terminus of 19 with the glycolic acid spacer using 50 eq of diglycolic anhydride in DMF (10 mL per 1 g of resin; 1 M concentration of reagent) for 5 min (see Note 13). Wash the resin with DMF (3×), with the last washing with dry DMF (1×). Activate the free carboxylic acid groups using 10 eq of carbonyldiimidazole (CDI) in dry DMF for 30 min. Wash the resin with dry DMF (3×), couple the PEG_3 diamine using excess of 50% 4,7,10-trioxa-1,13-tridecanediamine in dry DMF, and stir the resin for 30 min (vigorous vortexing for first 5 min).
3. For later modifications of these ligands with various labels/payloads, we have incorporated an orthogonally protected Lys residue as a functional handle (the N-terminal of melanocyte-stimulating hormone [MSH] ligand is acetylated and no other free amine-bearing group is present in the multivalent ligand). This handle can be incorporated in between Pego and poly(Pro-Gly) linker region, in order to keep an adequate spacing between the tag and the ligands, thus minimizing any influence on ligand binding. After the first Pego linker assembly on the resin, couple Fmoc-Lys(Mmt) to the peptide, followed by coupling as many Pro and Gly residues as are needed to build the required poly(Pro-Gly) linker.
4. Following poly(Pro-Gly) linker construction on the resin, couple another Pego unit as described above. Continue the addition of amino acid residues to complete the synthesis of second ligand, MSH (7). Finally, deprotect the N-terminus and acetylate with an excess of acetic anhydride/pyridine (1:1).
5. For Cy5-labeled htBVL 9, cleave the peptide from the resin using TFA-scavenger cocktail (see Subheading 3.1), and purify with preparative HPLC. Add 1.1 eq of Cy5-NHS ester to a solution of purified compound 9 in DMSO and monitor the reaction as described in Subheading 3.3, step 6.
6. For Eu-DOTA-labeled htBVL 10, cleave the side chain Mmt protection from Lys by repetitive treatment with 10% TFA, 5% TIS in DCM (see Note 14). Wash the resin with 5% TIS in DCM (2×). Following final cleavage treatment, wash the resin with 5% TIS in DCM (3×), DCM (2×), 5% DIEA in DCM (3×), DMF (3×), and finally with DCM (3×). Couple

the Ado linker with 3 eq of Fmoc-Ado-OH, 3 eq of HBTU, 3 eq of HOBt, and 6 eq of DIEA in DMF, and stir the resin overnight. Remove the Fmoc protection from Ado linker with 20% piperidine in DMF, and couple the DOTA chelator with 2 eq of DOTA-NHS ester, 8 eq of DIEA in DMF, and stir the resin overnight.

7. Following acidic cleavage of peptides from the resin and HPLC purification, the Europium complexation to the DOTA chelate can be carried out in solution. Add 3 eq of $EuCl_3 \cdot 6H_2O$ to a solution of DOTA-labeled peptide in DMSO (see Note 10), and stir the solution for 24 h. Check the completion of chelation reaction with analytical HPLC (Methods E and F in Table 1). Purify the final product from excess of Eu ions using SPE with a C-18 Sep-Pak™ cartridge (see Note 15).

3.5. Synthesis of Peptidyl-PARACEST MRI Agents

The following procedure provides flexibility in assembly of DOTA chelate to either terminus of the peptide or within the peptide backbone, in contrast to many other procedures that label DOTA to the N-terminus of the peptide. Further, various DOTA derivatives have been described in the literature for various imaging needs/properties. The synthesis below provides a representative template for making such DOTA contrast agents, in this case with a derivatized glycine for the PARACEST effect.

1. Prepare Z-Gly(Br)-OMe (methyl 2-(benzyloxycarbonylamino)-2-bromoacetate) as follows (35): combine an equimolar ratio of benzyl carbamate and glyoxylic acid monohydrate in diethylether for 7 days. Filter the precipitate and use the crude product for further reaction. Add 0.5 mL of concentrated sulfuric acid to an ice-cooled solution of 3 g of N-(benzyloxycarbonyl)-α-hydroxyglycine in anhydrous methanol (50 mL). Allow the reaction to warm to room temperature and stir for 2 days. Quench the reaction with ice-saturated $NaHCO_3$ and extract with EtOAc (3×), dry the pooled organic phase over Na_2SO_4, filter, and concentrate in vacuo to obtain N-(benzyloxycarbonyl)-α-methoxyglycinate. To a suspension of the latter in chloroform, under a N_2 atmosphere, add 3 eq of phosporus tribromide. Stir the reaction for 7 days. Concentrate the reaction mixture in vacuo and triturate with dry pentane for 24 h. Filter the reaction mixture to obtain the final racemic product, Z-Gly(Br)-OMe (see Fig. 10).
2. Add 3 eq of *tert*-butyl 2-bromoacetate and 6 eq of triethylamine to selectively trialkylate cyclen in chloroform to give compound 23 (36).
3. Prepare a suspension of Z-Gly(Br)-OMe (2.66 g, 8.8 mmol), compound 23 (4.52 g, 8.8 mmol), and K_2CO_3 (12.02 g, 88 mmol) in 100 mL of dry acetonitrile and heat to 60°C

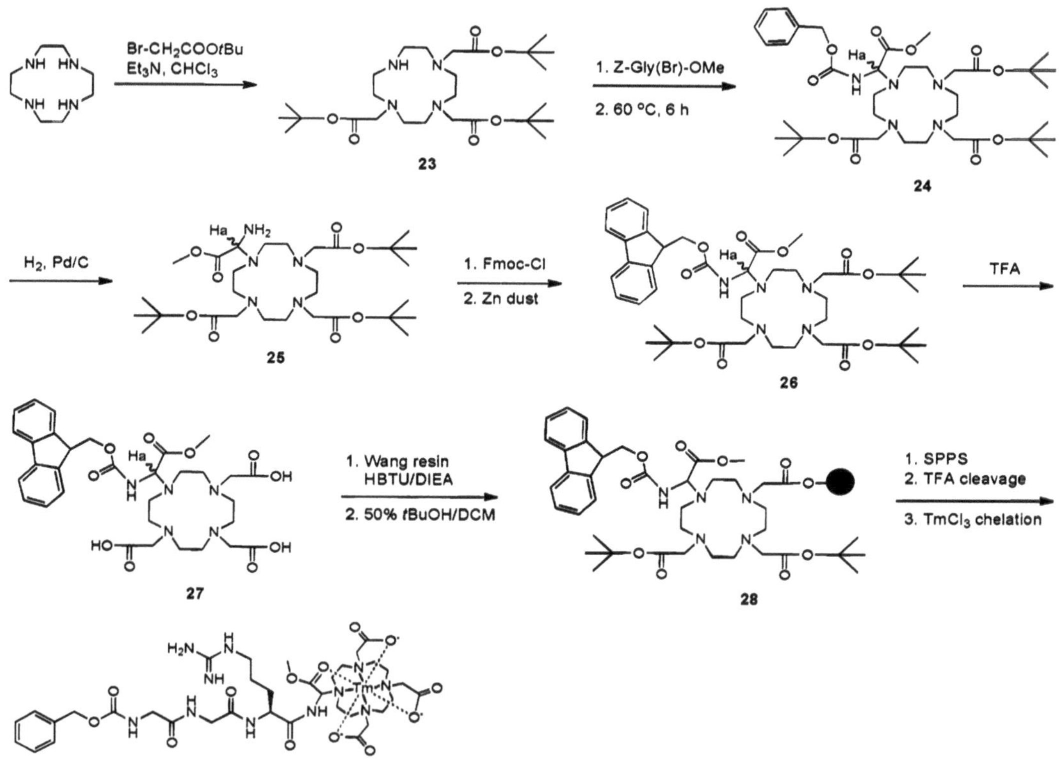

Fig. 10. Synthesis of a peptidyl-PARACEST MRI contrast agent.

for 6 h. Remove solids by filtration, and evaporate the solvent to obtain compound 24 in 83% yield.

4. Dissolve compound 24 (5.15 g, 7.0 mmol) in 50 mL of absolute ethanol, and add a dispersion of 10% Pd/C (1.4 g, 1.3 mmol). Hydrogenate the reaction mixture for 4 h at 40 psi. Remove the catalyst and solvent to obtain compound 25 in quantitative yield.
5. Compound 26 can be prepared from 25 by use of Fmoc-Cl with zinc dust. Add activated zinc dust (100 mg) to a solution of 25 (6.6 mmol) in 20 mL of anhydrous acetonitrile. The reaction mixture attains a neutral pH. Add a solution of Fmoc-Cl (1.78 g, 6.6 mmol) in 5 mL of acetonitrile in one portion and stir the reaction mixture for 20 min. Wash the dibenzofulvene with diethyl ether and dry the product to yield a white solid 26 (87%).
6. Deprotect *tert*-butyl ester from compound 26 using 95% TFA in DCM for 4 h, producing a quantitative yield of a pale yellowish compound 27.

7. Couple compound 27 (3.63 g, 5.54 mmol, 1.5 eq) to the Wang resin (4 g, 3.72 mmol; initial resin loading: 0.93 mmol/g) using the HBTU procedure overnight (see Subheading 3.1, step 3). Wash the resin with NMP (3×), DCM (3×), then treat with 50% *tert*-butanol in DCM for 2 h. Wash the resin again with DCM (3×), then acetylate (3 mL of acetic anhydride in 50 mL DCM for 20 min) to cap unreacted hydroxyl groups. Determine the resin loading using a Fmoc release method (0.41 mmol/g; 71% in this case), or using a picric acid titration, correcting for the effect of tertiary amines on DOTA (0.44 mmol/g; 76% with this method) (see Note 16).
8. Assemble the Z-GGR peptide onto the α-amino group of the resin-bound DOTA resin 28 using the solid-phase synthesis procedure listed in Subheading 3.1. Perform the last coupling reaction with Z-Gly-OH to gain the Z-peptidyl-resin. Finally, cleave the peptide from the resin with 95% TFA in DCM, yielding white solid (1.2 g, 1.4 mmol, 88% vs. amine contents on the resin).
9. To chelate the final product 7, add 1 eq of Tm(III) triflate to peptidyl-DOTA in acetonitrile and stir the solution at 50°C for 12 h. Maintain a neutral pH during the chelation by periodically adding DIEA. Raise the pH to 9–10 with concentrated NaOH to precipitate free lanthanide ions, which then can be removed by filtration. Lyophilize the final product to yield 7 as a fluffy powder.

3.6. Synthesis of PARACEST-Labeled Albumin

This procedure is described to produce a contrast agent with a high molar ratio of contrast moiety on the biocompatible nanocarrier. For the specific PARACEST application, the use of Gly on DOTA further increases the high molar ratio of amide groups, while also acting as a spacer between albumin and the contrast moiety.

3.6.1. Synthesis of DOTA-Gly$_4$ (see Fig. 11)

1. Dissolve ethyl glycinate hydrochloride (H-Gly-OEt·HCl, 14 g, 0.1 mol) and pyridine (20 mL, 0.25 mol) in DCM, and cool the solution to 0°C. Add 2-bromoacetyl bromide (10.5 mL, 0.12 mol) in dropwise manner for 1 h and stir for 3 h at 0°C followed by 1 h stirring at room temperature. Wash the solution with 1 N HCl (150 mL×3), water (150 mL×2), and brine (150 mL×2) sequentially, and dry in vacuo to give N-(2-bromoacetyl) ethyl glycinate.
2. Couple N-(2-bromoacetyl) ethyl glycinate (9.19 g, 41 mmol) to cyclen (1,3,5,7-tetraazacyclododecane, 1.72 g, 10 mmol) in the presence of K_2CO_3 (11.06 g, 80 mmol) in acetonitrile. Heat the reaction to 70°C for 6 h under N_2 purging. Cool the solution to room temperature and remove any undissolved materials by filtration. Evaporate the solvent to obtain DOTA-Gly$_4$-OEt (7.40 g, quantitative yield).

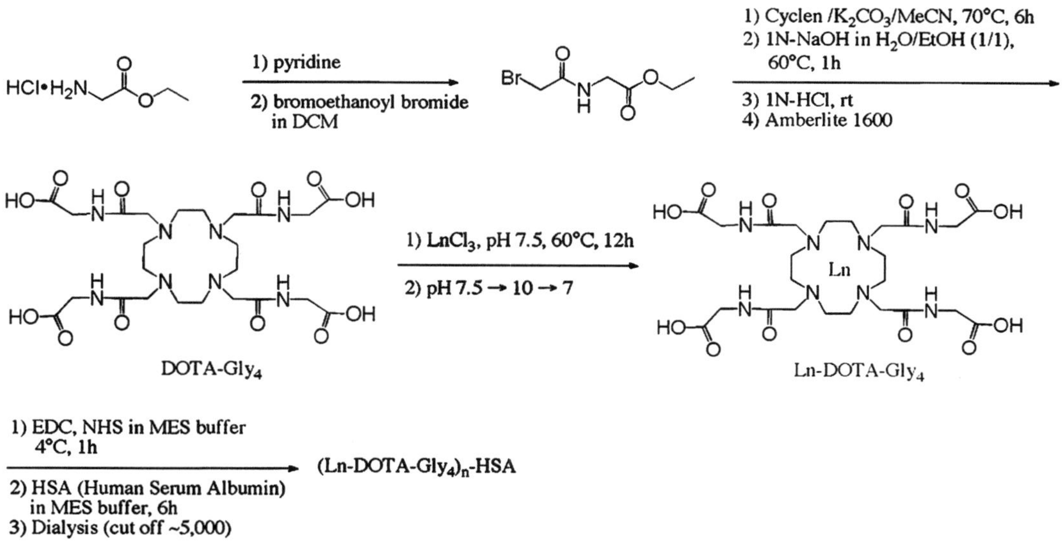

Fig. 11. Synthesis of a PARACEST-labeled albumin 8.

3. In order to hydrolyze the ester from DOTA-Gly_4-OEt, adjust the pH to ~11 with 1 N NaOH solution in ethanol/water (1:1), and heat at 60°C for 1 h. Trace the reaction with TLC to verify the reaction completion after 1 h. Acidify the cooled reaction mixture to pH 3 with 1 N HCl. Lyophilize the product and purify with ion-exchange chromatography using Amberlite® XAD-1600 (eluent: water, 5.04 g, yield: 80%).

3.6.2. Lanthanide Complexation (Yb-DOTA-Gly_4)

1. Dissolve DOTA-Gly_4 (633 mg, 1 mmol) in 5 mL of water (pH 6.5) at 60°C. Add $YbCl_3$ (273 mg, 1 mmol) in 3 mL of water dropwise for 1 h and adjust the pH to 7.5 with 0.1 N NaOH. Stir this solution for 12 h at 60°C and adjust to pH 7.5 whenever the pH drops below 5.
2. Cool the reaction mixture to room temperature and adjust the pH to 10 to precipitate the residual lanthanides in a lanthanide–hydroxide complex. Remove this precipitate by filtration.
3. Evaluate the final product for the presence of free lanthanide ions with an Arsenazo III color test (see Note 17). If free lanthanide ions are present, repeat the previous steps. If free lanthanide ions are absent, lyophilize the final product (755 mg, yield: 94.5%).

3.6.3. Yb-DOTA-Gly_4 Conjugation to Human Serum Albumin (HSA)

1. Dissolve 400 mg of Yb-DOTA-Gly_4 (0.5 mmol), 0.15 g EDC, and 30 mg of NHS in 5 mL of MES (2-morpholinoethanesulfonic acid) buffer (pH 5) and stir at 4°C for 1 h.
2. Dissolve HSA (0.34 g) in MES buffer in an ice bath with stirring.

3. Add the activated Yb-DOTA-Gly_4-EDC adduct in a dropwise manner to the HSA solution for 30 min. Stir the solution for 6 h. Dialyze the product by adding the solution of labeled HSA to cellulose membrane tubing with a molecular weight cut-off of 5,000, immersing the tubing in a larger container of water (with at least a 1:20 ratio of tubing volume to container volume) and gently stirring the water and tubing in the container.
4. Lyophilize the dialyzed solution to obtain $(\text{Yb-DOTA-Gly}_4)_n$-HSA as white fluffy solid (0.63 g, yield: 79%).
5. The coupling efficiency (the ratio of Yb-DOTA-Gly_4:HAS) can be measured with MALDI-mass spectrometry and compared with MALDI-MS results with unlabeled HSA as a control. Typical coupling efficiencies range from 8 to 15 Yb-DOTA-Gly_4 labels per HSA.

3.7. Lanthanide-Based Cell Binding Assays

The protocols below provide a comprehensive methodology to screen ligands on whole cells using DELFIA technology. DELFIA methods have been widely employed to study receptor binding of ligands labeled with DTPA derivatives. These lanthaligands can be employed for both saturation binding (direct read-outs) and competitive binding schemes (indirect read-outs). Further, examples from our recently modified DELFIA protocol for DOTA-labeled ligands (a stronger chelator than DTPA) are also described.

3.7.1. Plating Cells

1. Grow cells in T75 sterilized flasks containing 250 mL SCS media and incubate at 37°C with 5% CO_2. At 90% cell confluency (determined by microscopy), split the cells for passage or harvest for plating into 96-well plates. Aspirate the growth media and cover the cells with 2 mL of trypsinization solution for 2–5 min at 37°C to detach the cells from the plastic surface (see Note 18). Add 5 mL of cell culture medium to stop the trypsin digestion, and transfer the cell containing media to 15 or 50 mL falcon tubes. Collect the cells by centrifugation for 3 min at $750 \times g$, followed by aspirating the media and replacing it with 5 mL of fresh cell culture media (see Note 19). Detach cells from each other by gentle pipetting. Count the cell density on a hemocytometer. For passage, dilute the media to about 1×10^5 cells/mL of media and then transfer to a sterile T75 flask. Change the media every third day or as per cell requirement (see Note 20). For plating in 96-wells, dilute the cell containing media to 200,000 cells/mL.

3.7.2. Saturation Binding Assay Using Eu-DTPA Ligand 1 on CHO/δOR Cells (see Note 21)

1. Plate cells in black Costar 96-well plates (white translucent walls and bottom) at a density of 20,000 cells/well by adding 100 μL of cell containing culture media. Incubate the cells at 37°C and under 5% CO_2 atmosphere for 3 days, and monitor for growth and morphology by light microscopy (see Note 22).

2. Prepare requisite dilutions of the Eu-DTPA ligand 1 in binding buffer in a deep well dilution plate. For initial assay, a concentration range of 10^{-5} to 10^{-12} M can be used. Make dilutions across a row (e.g., from A12 to A1, right to left) and repeat in eight rows from A to H using an 8-channel micropipette. For instance, for a 1:3 dilution scheme, add 200 μL of binding buffer to each well from A1 to H11 (first 11 columns). To the 12th column (A12–H12), add 250 μL of 10 μM ligand solution. Transfer 100 μL of the solution from 12th column wells to 11th column wells, mix properly by aspiration, and continue the dilutions until 1st column is reached (see Note 23).
3. On the day of the experiment, aspirate the cell culture medium from all wells containing cells prior to the addition of the ligand to be tested (see Note 20). Add 50 μL of 20 μM cold competitive ligand (naloxone in this experiment) to rows E–H (to test nonspecific binding), and 50 μL of binding buffer to rows A–D (to test total binding), and preincubate for 15 min at 37°C (see Note 24).
4. Add increasing concentrations of the Eu-labeled peptide (50 μL/well) to all wells, and incubate the cells again for 1 h at 37°C.
5. Gently aspirate the ligand-containing binding buffer using a vacuum manifold, without disturbing the cell monolayer (see Note 20).
6. Wash each well three times with 100 μL of wash buffer by adding buffer to each well and immediately removing by vacuum aspiration.
7. Add the enhancement solution to the wells (100 μL/well) and incubate the plates for at least 30 min at 37°C.
8. Read the plates on a Wallac VICTOR^3 instrument using the standard Eu time-resolved luminescence (TRL) measurement (340 nm excitation, 400 μs delay, and emission collection for 400 μs at 615 nm).
9. Analyze the data with GraphPad Prism or other appropriate software using nonlinear regression analyses (Fig. 4).

3.7.3. Saturation Binding Assay Using Eu-DOTA Ligand 6 on HEK293/hMC4R Cells

1. Follow steps 1–6 in Subheading 3.7.2, with a modification of the cold ligand (100 μL of NDP-α-MSH, ligand 5, in this case). Then follow the procedure for the detection of DOTA-bound Eu(III) as follows.
2. Following ligand incubation and washings (Subheading 3.7.2, step 6), add 50 μL of 2.0 M HCl to each well and incubate the plate at 37°C for 2 h.
3. Neutralize the acidic solution with addition of 55 μL of 2.0 M NaOH to each well. Subsequently, add 115 μL of the

DELFIA enhancement solution to each well (see Note 25), followed by incubation for 30 min at 37°C.

4. Perform the Eu TRF measurements and analysis as described above.

3.7.4. Competition Binding Assay of Ligand 5 Using Eu-DOTA Ligand 6 on HEK293/hMC4R Cells

1. Competitive binding assays can be performed using variable concentrations of nonlabeled ligand and a fixed concentration of Eu-DOTA (or Eu-DTPA)-labeled ligand, using otherwise identical assay conditions provided above. In a 96-well plate format, two assays (of the same or different ligands) can be performed with rows A–D and E–H (quadruplicate measurements for each).
2. Prepare the dilutions of the nonlabeled ligand in binding buffer and concentrations ranging from 1×10^{-5} to 1×10^{-12} M, in an identical fashion as described in Subheading 3.7.2, step 6 above (also see Note 23), taking note of the fact that each concentration will be halved upon addition of Eu-labeled ligand during the assay.
3. The choice of concentration for the Eu-labeled ligand is based on its K_d value and the sensitivity of the DELFIA (see Note 26). For Eu-DOTA-labeled NDP-α-MSH, 10 nM concentration can be used for adequate signal/noise ratio. Thus, prepare 20 nM of ligand 6 in binding buffer considering the 1:1 dilution during the assay.
4. Aspirate the cell culture medium and add 50 μL of nonlabeled ligand ("cold") dilution, followed by addition of 50 μL of 20 nM Eu-DOTA-labeled ligand 9 ("hot") to each well (see Note 24).
5. Incubate the plates at 37°C for 1 h under 5% CO_2.
6. Follow the above detailed wash steps and Eu(III) count measurement protocols (see Subheadings 3.7.2 and 3.7.3). (If DTPA-labeled ligand is used instead, the extra acidification and neutralization step is not necessary; follow Subheading 3.7.2.)

3.8. In Vitro Single Cell Imaging

1. Split the cells from 75 mm culture flasks in 3 mL, and place 100 μL of the suspension onto the center of a 25 mm round #1 coverslip housed in a well of a 6-well plate.
2. After approximately 30 min, add 5 mL of fresh incubation media to each well, and maintain the cells under CO_2-controlled incubator until the cover-slips are 40–60% confluent.
3. Dilute an aliquot of the labeled (Cy5) ligand into 0.5 mL of HBSS to make a solution that is 2× the final required concentration (see Note 27).

4. Remove a single coverslip and place it into a chamber held at 37°C on the stage of the microscope (3, 30), and add 0.5 mL of a HBSS (see Subheading 2.3 for materials).
5. Acquire several images at equally spaced intervals (~ every 3 min) to provide a background for subsequent subtraction following addition of the labeled ligand.
6. Add 0.5 mL of the solution containing the 2× ligand media to the incubation chamber.
7. Acquire images at regular intervals (see Notes 28 and 29).
8. Remove the ligand-containing media after 2–3 min, and replace it with 1 mL of media without the ligand to decrease out-of-cell background.
9. Continue to acquire images at regular intervals.

3.9. In Vitro PARACEST MR Imaging

This procedure is intended to correlate the detected PARACEST effect with concentration of the agent, in order to establish a calibration that can be used for in vivo studies. The calibration establishes the minimum concentration for detection of the agent during in vivo studies. To perform PARACEST MRI studies with biochemical solutions:

1. Place the solutions in multiple 200 μL PCR tubes, and position the tubes in a customized cradle in a vertical orientation.
2. Insert the cradle into a horizontal-bore MRI magnet.
3. Acquire the MR image slices in a coronal orientation to show the contents of each tube as a filled circle that has a minimal surface-to-volume ratio, in order to minimize magnetic field susceptibilities within the image of each solution (37).

3.10. Preparation for In Vivo PARACEST MR Imaging

Research with animal models must be conducted with the highest standards of care. This procedure has been devised to ensure these standards, and improve the reproducibility of results among greatly variable in vivo conditions (37).

1. To ensure the safety of the mouse, secure the mouse to a customized sled with masking tape. This type of tape ensures that the mouse is immobilized without compromising the long-term health of the mouse.
2. Attach the respiration, ECG, and temperature probes to the mouse to monitor physiology. Changes in respiration rate are often the first sign of physiological changes during the MRI study. Monitoring and maintaining core body temperature and ECG are essential for ensuring hemodynamic consistency.

3. Position the mouse and sled in a customized cradle, and place the latter into an MRI magnet.
4. Warm an anesthetized mouse with either an electrical pad, a water pad, or a heat lamp, and/or with warm air until the core body temperature is at least 37°C.
5. Warm the tail with hot water (45–50°C) or hot air, or temporarily coat it with Oil of Wintergreen to dilate the tail veins. Installation of a catheter in the tail vein is facilitated by first dilating the veins with heat or a vasodilator.
6. Insert a catheter (consisting of a 0.5-in., 27 g needle attached to PE20 tubing) into a tail vein prior to inserting the mouse into the magnet (37) (also see Note 30).
7. Apply a temporary tourniquet to the base of the tail to retain high blood volume in the tail veins. This tourniquet can be constructed by inserting both ends of the PE20 tubing in a syringe without a plunger and then reinserting the plunger into the syringe to hold the tubing in place, with a loop of tubing protruding from the needle-end of the syringe and the two tubing ends protruding from the plunger end of the syringe.
8. Verify that the catheter is patent, and then secure the catheter to the tail with suture ties and/or tape. The tubing is designed to hold a solution of contrast agent near the catheter needle and should be long enough to stretch from the center of the MRI magnet to a place outside the magnet where a blunt-needle syringe can be connected to the tubing. Small ~2 μL air bubbles can be used to separate the contrast agent solution in the PE20 tubing from the rest of the tubing, but otherwise the tubing should be devoid of air to prevent cardiac arrest upon injection of the tubing contents into the mouse.
9. Acquire preinjection images, and then inject the contrast agent into the mouse through the tail vein catheter. No more than 300 μL of fluid should be injected into the mouse (smaller injections volumes are preferred), and no faster than 10 μL/s.

3.11. Acquisition of PARACEST MR Images

Prepend a period of selective saturation to a standard MRI acquisition scheme as described previously (38). A saturation power of 20 μT provides sufficient power to generate a strong chemical exchange saturation transfer (CEST) effect while minimizing sample heating. When the T_1 MR relaxation time of the sample with the contrast agent is greater than 1 s, then a saturation time period ≥2 s and a multiple-echo acquisition scheme provide a good CEST detection in a reasonable experiment time. If the T_1 MR relaxation time is less than 1 s, then a saturation time period ≤300 ms and a single-echo acquisition scheme provide a good

CEST detection within a practical time frame. Three methods may be employed to measure CEST as follows:

1. Selectively saturate the MR frequency of the exchangeable proton of the PARACEST agent (+ω relative to the MR frequency of water that is conventionally defined to be 0). Then selectively saturate the opposite MR frequency (−ω) as a control. Calculate the percent decrease in MR water signal with saturation at +ω relative to saturation at −ω. This method works well for static biochemical solutions that have negligible magnetic field susceptibilities (39).
2. Selectively saturate the +ω MR frequency before and after injecting the contrast agent. Calculate the percent decrease in MR water signal after injection relative to before injection. This method works well for in vivo studies with negligible magnetic field susceptibilities and negligible changes in T2* relaxation times following the injection (37).
3. Selectively saturate a series of MR frequencies to acquire a Z-spectrum (a.k.a. a CEST spectrum). This series of MR frequencies ranges beyond +ω and −ω to ensure that the full spectrum has been acquired. Then analyze the CEST spectrum using line-fitting methods to measure the percent decrease in MR water signal. This method works well for samples with magnetic field susceptibilities (in which the MR frequency of water is not necessarily at 0 ppm) or those have dynamic changes in T2* relaxation times during the experiment (25).

4. Notes

1. Terminology: *Theranostics* (var. *theragnostics*) – The term denotes the fusion of therapeutics and diagnostics, an emerging trend in healthcare management. Recent progress in targeted therapies will provide individualized medicines in the future according to the genotype-–phenotype of the patient and the underlying pathology (pharmacogenomics). The key is to identify patients who respond or do not respond (or adversely respond) to a treatment, monitor the response to a treatment, and determine the most effective, nontoxic drug dosage for a given patient. In this context, in vivo diagnostic imaging is being combined with therapy to provide rational therapeutic choices for individual patients. *Lanthaligands* (40) – The term has been used here to denote lanthanide-chelate labeled ligands such as Eu-DTPA, Gd-DOTA, etc., which is suitable for diagnosis, therapy, or for research-oriented biomolecular studies.

2. This is usually accomplished with a buffered solution containing a polyanion (typically a polyacid such as nitrilotriacetic acid to dissociate the lanthanide from the chelate), an enhancer reagent, i.e., a fluorophoric antenna for excitation (such as 2-naphthoyltrifluoroacetone), and a synergistic detergent to enhance fluorescence by forming micelles and shielding the complex from water (typically a Lewis base such as trioctylphosphine oxide, TOPO) (10, 41, 42).
3. The introduction of a time delay (say 400 μs) prior to detection of the emitted light eliminates the interference from light scattering and autofluorescence. This greatly enhances the signal/noise ratio with further signal amplification by multiple read-outs, thus increasing the reliability of detection and monitoring during automated HTS.
4. A cradle can hold multiple 200 μL PCR tubes in a vertical orientation in a horizontal-bore MRI magnet. An MR image slice in a coronal orientation can show the contents of each tube as a filled circle that has a minimal surface-to-volume ratio, which minimizes magnetic field inhomogeneities within the image of each solution.
5. The BB on-resin color test was used to monitor the progress of amino acid coupling reaction (32). Add a few drops of 0.01% w/v solution of BB in N,N-dimethylacetamide to 0.2 M solution of HOBT/DMF (yellow color is produced). Inject the solution into the syringe reactor containing resin, stir for few seconds when a dark blue color develops, and wash with DMF to remove excess BB. Free amino groups yield blue color to beads and remove yellow color from solution. The blue resin beads turn yellow as the coupling proceeds (no basic amino groups available). Note that if the resin contains a trace of base (e.g., DIEA), the resin cannot be properly colorized and the solution turns blue. Therefore, this method cannot be used for HBTU/base coupling protocols. For quantitative determination of coupling efficiency, perform a Kaiser test by heating a few resin beads to 100°C for 2 min with a mixture of one drop each of Reagent A (40 g phenol in 10 mL of dry ethanol), Reagent B (0.2 mM KCN in pyridine; dilute 2 mL of 10 mM aq. KCN stock solution in 100 mL of pyridine), and Reagent C (6% w/v of ninhydrin in ethanol). An intense blue color is generated with free primary amines, and a slight yellow coloration appears when the coupling is complete (level of sensitivity: 1 μmol/g resin ≈ 99.5% coupling).
6. If a Domino block is not available, fill the syringe with DCM up to the full capacity of the reactor, then puncture with a stainless steel needle close to the orifice but in front of the piston. Remove the solvent with a stream of argon, preferably

in a vertical position. When the needle is removed, the syringe can still function as a reactor because the puncture is outside of the piston's working range.

7. The reaction of DTPA dianhydride with free N-terminus of peptides has to be carried out in DMSO. DTPA dianhydride is sparingly soluble in organic solvents, except in DMSO and DMF. However, DMF leads to severe side reactions, especially when trace impurities of dimethylamine are presented. Therefore, the resin must be washed with DMSO prior to reaction, and all postreaction washings should be without DMF. Use THF, 20% aq. THF, 10% DIEA and 10% water in THF, and 20% aq. THF for hydrolysis. Finally wash with THF and DCM and dry the resin in vacuo. If DTPA dianhydride is insoluble at 0.6 M concentration in DMSO after rigorous stirring even at 80°C, the dianhydride is likely decomposed resulting in inefficient coupling. Therefore, store DTPA dianhydride stock under argon to minimize decomposition.
8. It is absolutely imperative to vigorously agitate the resin when the DTPA reagent mix is added. Initial attempts led to high content of peptide head-to-head dimer cross-linked by DTPA. Therefore, the DTPA reaction was optimized, and the side reaction was suppressed by vigorous agitation, selection of leaving group (HOBt = HONSu = HOCt < anhydride), nature of resin (Tentagel < PS/DVB), lower resin substitution (0.6 < 0.2 ≈ 0.1 mmol/g), higher DTPA concentration, and higher DTPA stoichiometry (up to 20-fold excess). The lower ratio of HOBt/DTPA (such as 1 eq each) and higher temperature did not suppress this side reaction. Optimized condition did not eliminate this side reaction completely, but suppressed it to a reasonable level ~5%. Antiparallel DTPA-dimer can be efficiently separated with SEC (Sephadex G25, 1.0 M aq. acetic acid).
9. The detailed procedures for solution-phase disulfide formation in peptides have been reviewed before (43). Alternatively, the on-resin oxidation can be carried out prior to the Aloc deprotection and DTPA coupling step (44, 45). However, this alternative approach is limited to peptides that do not need thiol scavengers during acidic cleavage (e.g., peptides not containing Trp, Arg, etc.).
10. Europium chelation: Europium chelation to DTPA is relatively fast (~4 h). However, Eu-DOTA chelation is quite slow and needs 12–48 h. In either case, the completion of chelation reaction must be verified with analytical HPLC using a relatively basic solvent system (such as Method E in Table 1; cf. TFA system). A TFA-based gradient should be avoided as it results in removal of the metal from the chelate. Also, note that the amount of $EuCl_3$ salt required in the described procedures

is usually very small and can be conveniently handled by first dissolving an easily weighable quantity in 1–5 mL of solvent and adding an appropriate aliquot of it to the reaction.

11. The coupling of Boc-Dmt-OH with an unprotected side chain (free phenol) leads to limited oligomerization. Up to four Dmt oligomers can be noticed in MS with decreasing intensities. However, the formed phenolic esters can be readily cleaved with 50% piperidine in MeOH:DCM (1:4). In this particular sequence, Boc-Dmt-Tic-Lys, the extent of oligomerization is relatively high because of stronger coupling condition (HBTU/DIEA) needed for the sterically hindered secondary amine of Tic.
12. For ease in handling of costly Cy5 dyes, dissolve the stock amount (usually 5 mg) in 5 mL of water or 20% acetonitrile/water mixture, aliquot them into 1 mL (or as appropriate) vials, and lyophilize and store them under argon for later use. For Cy5 coupling in the cited example, weigh 1.3 eq of Cy5-NHS ester or use the aliquot as directed above. Add 1.1 eq of dye to the reaction and stir it for 1 h. Run an analytical HPLC on a small amount. If unreacted starting material is noticed, add additional 0.2 eq of dye. Repeat until full conversion is obtained. Typically, the conjugation is fairly rapid and reacts to completion within an hour of addition of the dye to the free amine of ligand.
13. Avoid the use of a base during diglycolic anhydride reaction because a diglycolic imine can be formed that terminates the peptide elongation on the resin.
14. It was noticed that the usually recommended 1–3% TFA concentration for cleavage of Mmt group was insufficient to deprotect lysine side chain in the htBVLs, resulting in partially unprotected peptides (~25% still Mmt-protected). This can be checked by acetylating the free amine groups of lysine followed by cleavage of the peptide from resin and comparing the HPLC chromatogram of acetylated and unacetylated peptide products.
15. Before loading the peptide on the C-18 Sep-Pak cartridge, dilute the 1 mL solution with 50 mL of water. This is done to reduce the DMSO concentration to less than 5% and thus prevent elution of peptide from the column.
16. To measure the loading of an amine-derivatized DOTA on the resin, remove the Fmoc group from the amino group and measure the Fmoc concentration spectrophotometrically (46). Alternatively, perform a picric acid titration by treating the amine-containing resin with picric acid to form an adduct between the picrate and the amines. After washing to remove excess picric acid, treat the resin with a base to release the picrate from the amine groups and measure the concentration of the picrate spectrophotometrically (47).

17. Perform an Aresenazo (III) dye test to detect the presence of free lanthanide ions (48). Add a few drops of the chelation product to a ~0.2 mL volume of 25 μM Arsenazo (III) in 2 mM-Tris/1 mM-acetate buffer. Measure absorbance at 655 nm to quantify the concentration of free lanthanide ions at concentrations of ≥20 μM. A qualitative visual change from red/pink to blue/aqua indicates the qualitative presence of free lanthanide ions. The absence of absorbance at 655 nm or the absence of a color change indicates that free lanthanide ions are present at <20 μM. Alternatively, a similar spectrophotometric test with xylenol orange can be conducted, although xylenol orange is more sensitive to variations in physiological pH and the presence of cations (49).
18. Addition of too much trypsin can inhibit the cell attachment to the wells or cover-slips. The time required for the detachment of cells from the flask depends on the cell type.
19. The volume of the culture media used to suspend the cells can be adjusted depending on cell confluency.
20. HEK293 cells are weakly adherent and all medium changes should be performed with extreme care and minimal agitation. If vacuum aspiration (adjust suction to as low as possible) removes the adherent cells, manual pipetting can be used instead. This precaution should be taken until the ligand incubation and washings (Subheading 3.7.2, step 6) during the assay have been completed when no additional buffer removals are needed. The cells are likely compromised after this stage when the enhancement solution (acidic pH) is added.
21. All binding assays were carried out in quadruplicate, unless otherwise noted.
22. For observing cell growth and morphology and evaluating confluency, use a 96-well plate with clear bottom (with translucent white walls) for binding assays, or a separate 96-well clear plate for better visualization (plate a sample row).
23. For initial assays, a general range of 10^{-5} to 10^{-12} M ligand concentration is appropriate. Alternative 1:2 or 1:4 dilution scheme, instead of the 1:3 dilution scheme described, can be used to increase or decrease this range. Once hysteresis is established, narrow the concentration range (e.g., 0.1–100 nM) in follow-up assays for more conclusive results. While preparing dilutions, take note of the fact that each ligand concentration will be diluted in half during addition to the plate (with either 50 μL of binding buffer or cold ligand for saturation binding assay; and 50 μL of labeled ligand for competition binding assay).
24. Disposable polystyrene reagent reservoirs (Cole Parmer) can be used for multipipetting stock solutions and binding buffers during the assay. For example, for saturation binding assay,

prepare 6 mL of 20 μM cold ligand, and using a 12-channel pipette, add 50 μL of ligand to each well (one row at a time).

25. Neutralization must be tested using 2.0 M HCl and 2.0 M NaOH before using them in binding assay protocols (with Eu(III)-DOTA-labeled peptides) as the detection of Eu ions cannot be accomplished at pH less than 2. Extreme care must be taken during the neutralization and enhancement steps to prevent the contamination among wells. It is recommended to use fresh micropipette tips during each reagent transfer.
26. For competition binding assays, it is best to keep the concentration of labeled ligand as low as possible (well below Kd), while binding no more than 20% of the ligand (ideally, below 10% to minimize ligand depletion effects). Since the nonspecific background usually increases linearly with concentration, this is necessary to keep an adequate signal/noise (S/N) ratio (~4–10) to generate data of good precision.
27. A larger volume of ligand stock solution can be made at the appropriate concentration if multiple experiments are to be performed.
28. As shown in Fig. 2, binding occurred rapidly with substantial internalization within 3 min. The ligand was fully internalized within 10 min. A standard time course for image acquisition should be selected to allow for combination of data from multiple experiments over the full time course.
29. An acquisition time should be selected that provides a signal/background of at least 2.5:1, based on initial image sets acquired at the selected ligand concentration.
30. The MRI study must be conducted by acquiring the images before and after administration of the contrast agent. The mouse must not be moved before and after to facilitate the comparison of images. A catheter is installed in the tail vein for administering the contrast agent while the mouse is inside the MRI scanner.

Acknowledgments

The authors would like to thank Prof. Robert J. Gillies and his team for development of various cell lines and animal model for δOR tumor animal model described in this work. This work was supported by the National Cancer Institute through NIH Grant R21CA133455-01, R01 CA09736, and R01 CA 123547, and by the U.S. Army Medical Research and Materiel Command under W81XWH-04-1-0731. This work was also supported by the Northeastern Ohio Animal Imaging Resource Center, an NIH-funded program, R24CA110943.

References

1. Josan, J. S., Vagner, J., Handl, H. L., Sankaranarayanan, R., Gillies, R. J., and Hruby, V. J. (2008) Solid-phase synthesis of heterobivalent ligands targeted to melanocortin and cholecystokinin receptors. *Int J Pep Res Ther.* **14**: 293–300.
2. Vagner, J., Xu, L., Handl, H., Josan, J. S., Morse, D. L., Mash, E. A., Gillies, R. J., and Hruby, V. J. (2008) Heterobivalent ligands crosslink multiple cell-surface receptors: the human melanocortin-4 and delta-opioid receptors. *Angew Chem Int Ed.* **47**: 1685–1688.
3. Xu, L., Vagner, J., Josan, J., Lynch, R. M., Morse, D. L., Baggett, B., Han, H., Mash, E. A., Hruby, V. J., and Gillies, R. J. (2009) Enhanced targeting with heterobivalent ligands. *Mol Cancer Ther.* **8**: 2356–2365.
4. Sokolov, K., Follen, M., and Richards-Kortum, R. (2002) Optical spectroscopy for detection of neoplasia. *Curr Opin Chem Biol.* **6**: 651–658.
5. Ballou, B., Ernst, L. A., and Waggoner, A. S. (2005) Fluorescence imaging of tumors in vivo. *Curr Med Chem.* **12**: 795–805.
6. Frangioni, J. V. (2003) In vivo near-infrared fluorescence imaging. *Curr Opin Chem Biol.* **7**: 626–634.
7. Sevick-Muraca, E. M., Houston, J. P., and Gurfinkel, M. (2002) Fluorescence-enhanced, near infrared diagnostic imaging with contrast agents. *Curr Opin Chem Biol.* **6**: 642–650.
8. Mujumdar, R. B., Ernst, L. A., Mujumdar, S. R., Lewis, C. J., and Waggoner, A. S. (1993) Cyanine dye labeling reagents: sulfoindocyanine succinimidyl esters. *Bioconjug Chem.* **4**: 105–111.
9. Handl, H. L., Vagner, J., Yamamura, H., Hruby, V. J., and Gillies, R. J. (2004) Lanthanide-based time-resolved fluorescence of in cyto ligand–receptor interactions. *Anal Biochem.* **330**: 242–250.
10. Handl, H. L., and Gillies, R. J. (2005) Lanthanide-based luminescent assays for ligand-receptor interactions. *Life Sci.* **77**: 361–371.
11. Pandya, S., Yu, J., and Parker, D. (2006) Engineering emissive europium and terbium complexes for molecular imaging and sensing. *Dalton Trans.* **23**: 2757–2766.
12. Selvin, P. (2002) Principles and biophysical applications of lanthanide-based probes. *Annu Rev Biophys Biomol Struct.* **31**: 275–302.
13. Steinkamp, T., and Karst, U. (2004) Detection strategies for bioassays based on luminescent lanthanide complexes and signal amplification. *Anal Bioanal Chem.* **380**: 24–30.
14. Parker, D. (2004) Excitement in f block: structure, dynamics and function of nine-coordinate chiral lanthanide complexes in aqueous media. *Chem Soc Rev.* **33**: 156–165.
15. Thunus, L., and Lejeune, R. (1999) Overview of transition metal and lanthanide complexes as diagnostic tools. *Coord Chem Rev.* **184**: 125–155.
16. Josan, J. S., Morse, D. L., Xu, L., Trissal, M., Baggett, B., Davis, P., Vagner, J., Gillies, R. J., and Hruby, V. J. (2009) Solid-phase synthetic strategy and bioevaluation of a Labeled δ-opioid receptor ligand Dmt-Tic-Lys for in vivo imaging. *Org Lett.* **11**: 2479–2482.
17. Handl, H. L., Vagner, J., Yamamura, H. I., Hruby, V. J., and Gillies, R. J. (2005) Development of a lanthanide-based assay for detection of receptor–ligand interactions at the δ-opioid receptor. *Anal Biochem.* **343**: 299–307.
18. De-Silva, C. R., Vagner, J., Lynch, R., Gillies, R. J., and Hruby, V. J. (2010) Optimization of time-resolved fluorescence assay for detection of Eu-DOTA labeled ligand-receptor interactions. *Anal Biochem.* **398**: 15–23.
19. Leon-Rodriguez, L. M. D., and Kovacs, Z. (2008) The synthesis and chelation chemistry of DOTA-peptide conjugates. *Bioconjug Chem.* **19**: 391–402.
20. Uusijärvi, H., Bernhardt, P., Rösch, F., Maecke, H. R., and Forssell-Aronsson, E. (2006) Electron- and positron-emitting radiolanthanides for therapy: aspects of dosimetry and production. *J Nucl Med.* **47**: 807–814.
21. Merbach, A. F., and Toth, E. (2001) The chemistry of contrast agents in medical magnetic resonance imaging. Wiley, New York.
22. Zhang, S., Merritt, M., Woessner, D. E., Lenkinski, R. E., and Sherry, A. D. (2003) PARACEST agents: modulating MRI contrast via water proton exchange. *Acc Chem Res.* **36**: 783–790.
23. Aime, S., Barge, A., Delli Castelli, D., Fedeli, F., Mortillaro, A., Nielsen, F. U., and Terreno, E. (2002) Paramagnetic lanthanide (III) complexes as pH sensitive chemical exchange saturation transfer (CEST) contrast agents for MRI applications. *Magn Reson Med.* **47**: 639–648.
24. Yoo, B., Sheth, V., and Pagel, M. D. (2009) An amine-derivatized, DOTA-loaded polymeric support for Fmoc solid phase peptide synthesis. *Tet Lett.* **50**: 4459–4462.
25. Ali, M. M., Liu, G., Shah, T., Flask, C. A., and Pagel, M. D. (2009) Using two chemical

exchange saturation transfer magnetic resonance imaging contrast agents for molecular imaging studies. *Acc Chem Res.* **42**: 915–924.

26. Yoo, B., and Pagel, M. D. (2008) An overview of responsive MRI contrast agents for molecular imaging. *Front Biosci.* **13**: 1733–1752.
27. Yoo, B., and Pagel, M. D. (2006) A PARACEST MRI contrast agent to detect enzyme activity. *J Am Chem Soc.* **128**: 14032–14033.
28. Yoo, B., Raam, M., Rosenblum, R., and Pagel, M. D. (2007) Enzyme-responsive PARACEST MRI contrast agents: a new biomedical imaging approach for studies of the proteasome. *Contrast Media Mol Imaging.* **2**: 189–198.
29. Grieco, P., Lavecchia, A., Cai, M., Trivedi, D., Weinberg, D., MacNeil, T., Van der Ploeg, L. H., and Hruby, V. J. (2002) Structure-activity studies of the melanocortin peptides: discovery of potent and selective affinity antagonists for the hMC3 and hMC4 receptors. *J Med Chem.* **45**: 5287–5294.
30. Martinez-Zaguilan, R., Tompkins, L. S., Gillies, R. J., and Lynch, R. M. (1999) Simultaneous analysis of intracellular pH and Ca^{2+} from cell populations. *Meth Mol Biol.* **114**: 287–306.
31. Edwards, W. B., Fields, C. G., Anderson, C. J., Pajeau, T. S., Welch, M. J., and Fields, G. B. (1994) Generally applicable, convenient solid-phase synthesis and receptor affinities of octreotide analogs. *J Med Chem.* **37**: 3749–3757.
32. Krchnák, V., Vágner, J., and Lebl, M. (1988) Noninvasive continuous monitoring of solid-phase peptide synthesis by acid-base indicator. *Int J Pept Prot Res.* **32**: 415–416.
33. Bräse, S., Kirchhoff, J. H., and Köbberling, J. (2003) Palladium-catalysed reactions in solid phase organic synthesis. *Tetrahedron.* **59**: 885–939.
34. Gomez-Martinez, P., Dessolin, M., Guibé, F., and Albericio, F. (1999) N^{α}-Alloc temporary protection in solid-phase peptide synthesis. The use of amine–borane complexes as allyl group scavengers. *J Chem Soc Perkin Trans.* **1**: 2871–2874.
35. Williams, R. M., Aldous, D. J., and Aldous, S. C. (1990) General synthesis of β, γ-alkynylglycine derivatives. *J Org Chem.* **55**: 4657–4663.
36. Moore, D. A. (2008) Selective trialkylation of cyclen with tert-butyl bromoacetate. *Org Synth.* **85**: 10–14.
37. Ali, M., Yoo, B., and Pagel, M. D. (2009) Tracking the relative in vivo pharmacokinetics of nanoparticles with PARACEST MRI. *Mol Pharm.* **6**: 1409–1416.
38. Liu, G., Ali, M. M., Yoo, B., Griswold, M. A., Tkach, J. A., and Pagel, M. D. (2009) PARACEST MRI with improved temporal resolution. *Magn Reson Med.* **61**: 399–408.
39. Liu, G., Li, Y., and Pagel, M. D. (2007) Design and characterization of a new irreversible responsive PARACEST MRI contrast agent that detects nitric oxide. *Magn Reson Med.* **58**: 1249–1256.
40. Josan, J. S. (2008) Heteromultivalent ligands directed targeting of cell-surface receptors – implications in cancer diagnostics & therapeutics. Ph.D. dissertation. The University of Arizona, Tucson.
41. Dakubu, S. (1992) Method of determining a biological substance involving labelling with a metal chelate. *US Patent 5,124,268.*
42. Wilkinson, D. (1999) A one-step fluorescent detection method for lipid fingerprints; $Eu(TTA)_3$.2TOPO. *Forensic Sci Int.* **99**: 5–23.
43. Albericio, F., Annis, I., Royo, M., and Barany, G. (2000) Preparation and handling of peptides containing methionine and cysteine. In: Chan, W. C., White P. D. (eds) Fmoc solid phase peptide synthesis, 1st ed., Oxford University Press, Oxford, pp 77–114.
44. Annis, I., Hargittai, B., and Barany, G. (1997) Disulfide bond formation in peptides. *Meth Enzymol.* **289**: 198–221.
45. Chen, L., Annis, I., and Barany, G. (2001) Disulfide bond formation in peptides. *Curr Protocols Prot Sci.* 18.16.11–18.16.19.
46. Fields, G. B., Lauer-Fields, J. L., Liu, R., and Barany, G. (1992) Principles and practice of solid phase peptide synthesis. In: Grant, G. A. (ed) Synthetic Peptides: A User's Guide, 2nd ed., Oxford University Press, Oxford, pp 93–219.
47. Gisin, B. F. (1972) The monitoring of reactions in solid-phase peptide synthesis with picric acid. *Anal Chim Acta.* **58**: 248–249.
48. Rowatt, E., and Williams, R. J. (1989) The interaction of cations with the dye Arsenazo III. *Biochem J.* **259**: 295–298.
49. Barge, A., Cravotto, G., Gianolio, E., and Fedeli, F. (2006) How to determine free Gd and free ligand in solution of Gd chelates. A technical note. *Contrast Media Mol Imaging.* **1**: 184–188.

Chapter 7

DNA-Directed Assembly Microarray for Protein and Small Molecule Inhibitor Screening

Ng Jin Kiat, Fritz Simeon, Too Heng Phon, and Parayil Kumaran Ajikumar

Abstract

A robust high-throughput and high-fidelity screening platform for identifying and validating potential target molecules is the key for drug development. During the past decade, microarray platforms have demonstrated enormous potential for developing robust tools for small molecules as well as protein-based drug discovery and analysis. Recently, we developed a DNA-directed assembly microarray platform with improved screening and immobilization strategies. In contrast to conventional microarray platforms, our technique allows the solution phase interaction of the probes and analytes in a biological environment and further the detection through the directed assembly of specific DNA probes on a dendrimer-modified glass surface. Herein, we describe the detailed experimental protocols in performing the DNA-directed assembly platform for antibody microarray, a RNA polymerase-DNA binding microarray, and a drug-screening microarray.

Key words: CRE recombinase, Dendrimer, DNA-directed assembly platform, Drug-screening microarray, Protein microarray, RNA polymerase, ssDNA–dsDNA conjugate

1. Introduction

Development of microarray platforms enables unveiling of the functional roles of many biological molecules in a high-throughput and a cost-effective manner (1). Microarray platforms such as DNA array, protein array, carbohydrate array, and peptide array have been successfully applied for the global analysis of relative changes in various biomolecules concentration and formation of complexes, and for the dynamic overview of intermolecular networks and activities in diverse cellular events (2). Among the various platforms, protein microarray is an important tool for screening

Seetharama D. Satyanarayanajois (ed.), *Drug Design and Discovery: Methods and Protocols*, Methods in Molecular Biology, vol. 716, DOI 10.1007/978-1-61779-012-6_7,

the formation of protein complexes and interactions of proteins with other molecules (e.g., carbohydrates, nucleic acids, and drug molecules) (3–6). The key considerations in the development and application of protein microarrays include (a) the overall experimental design and strategy for capturing the target analytes from complex cellular samples and (b) detecting them quantitatively in an array format with spatial addressability (1). Such microarray techniques are key tools for high-throughput screening of small molecules and protein-based drug molecules (1).

Herein, we describe the experimental protocols of strategic design of a DNA-directed assembly microarray that uses single-stranded DNA (ssDNA) conjugated with fluorophore allowing a specific hybridization onto the slides with the complimentary strand (7). The key advantage of this design is that it allows various possible analyte interactions to take place in a homogenous solution phase. Another advantage in our DNA-directed microarray platform is the use of quasi-three-dimensional surfaces generated using dendrimers (8). Glass surface derivatives with carboxyl-terminated polyamidoamine (PAMAM) dendrimers allow the fabrication of high-density immobilization surface of complimentary ssDNA, while reducing nonspecific binding by using negatively charged surfaces. With the simple concept of DNA-directed assembly platform, we developed protein microarrays using protein–DNA conjugated probes (7) and protein–DNA binding microarray using de novo designed DNA probes (9). Our spatially addressable protein microarray was used for the detection of fluorophore-labeled rabbit immunoglobulin G from fluorophore-labeled cell lysate with a detection limit of as low as 1 pM (about 150 pg/mL) without amplification (Fig. 1) (7).

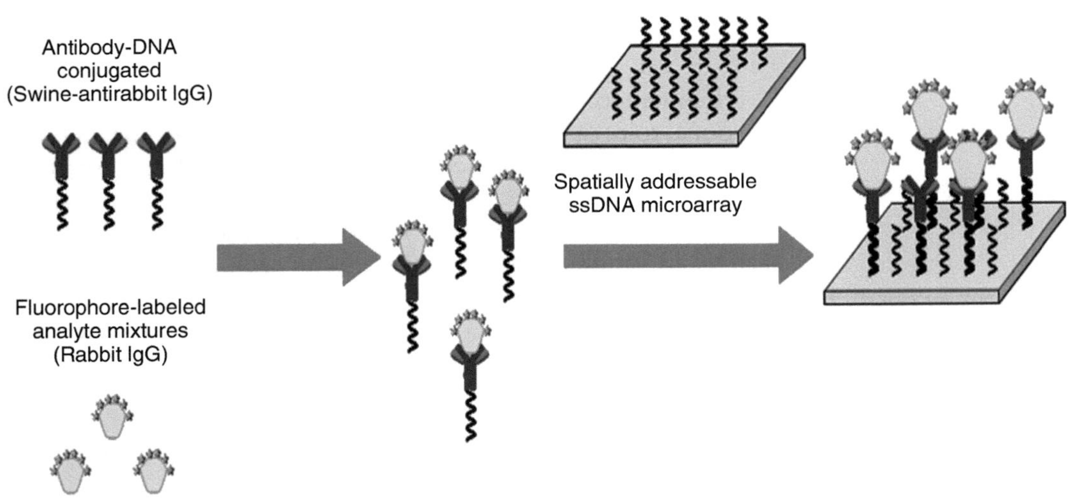

Fig. 1. Schematic illustration of DNA-directed assembly for antibody microarray.

DNA–protein interactions are central processes to many cellular functions, such as regulating gene transcription (10), DNA repair (11), enzymatic restriction (12), and genomic replication (13). Herein, we describe the versatility of the DNA-directed assembly platform for analyzing RNA polymerase (RNAP) binding to DNA. In this platform, a probe containing an ssDNA address linked to a dsDNA, which spanned the intergenic region and protein-coding sequence of the *Lac* operon and bound specifically to RNAP binding sequence, was generated using polymerase chain reaction (PCR). The probe was then allowed to bind the polymerase in a solution under optimal binding conditions. After binding, we separated the bound probes from unbound probes using gel electrophoresis and recovered the RNAP–probe complex. They are then hybridized DNA–probe complex and analyzed through the fluorophore tag on the DNA probe molecules (Fig. 2).

We further extend the protein–DNA binding microarray platform to screen for inhibitors against DNA-modifying enzymes that suppress viral replication (14). Recombinase is a highly specific enzyme that binds to a specific DNA sequence and catalyzes

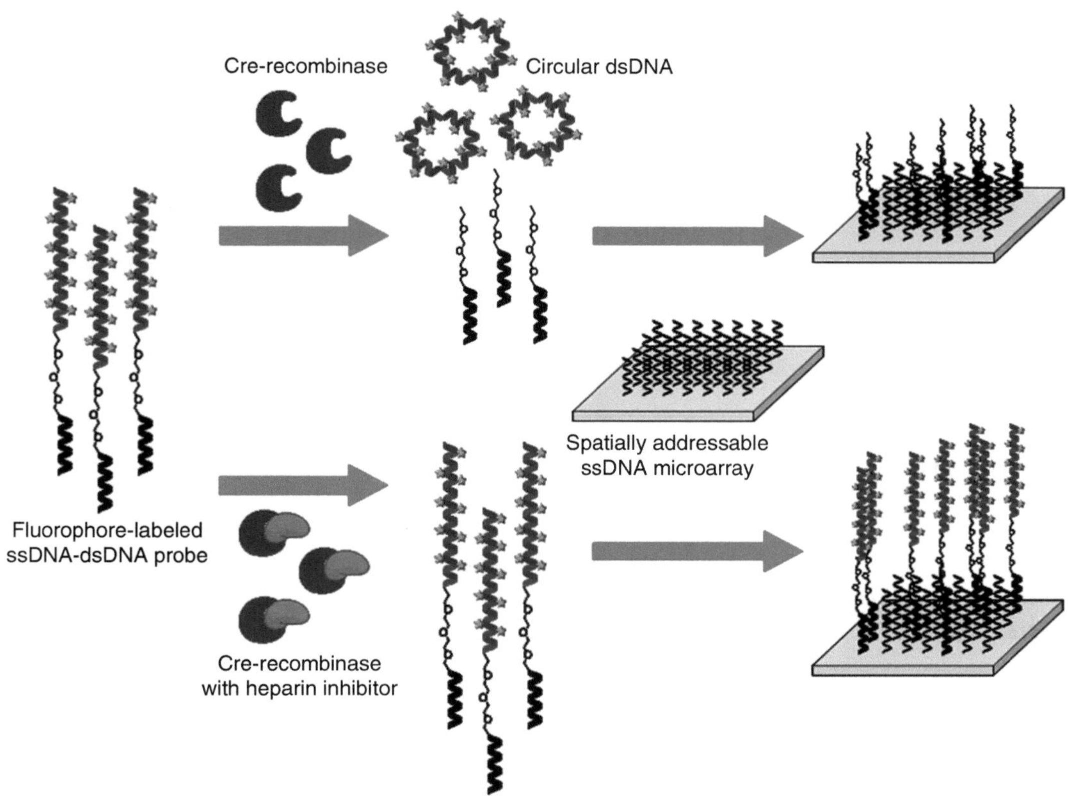

Fig. 2. Schematic illustration of DNA-directed assembly for RNA polymerase-DNA binding microarray.

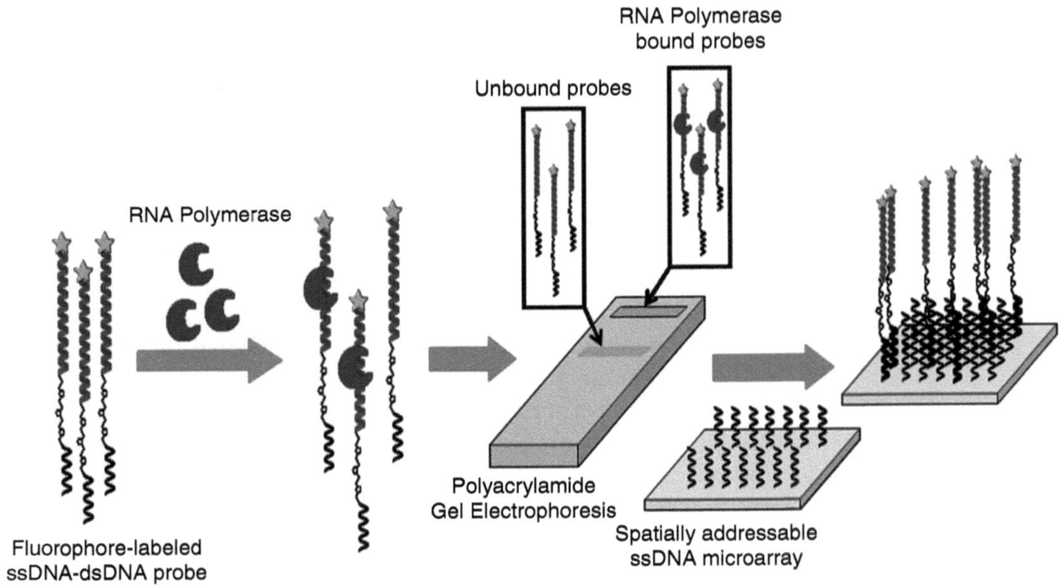

Fig. 3. Schematic illustration of DNA-directed assembly for drug-screening microarray.

both excision and integration without any supporting cofactors. The activity of recombinase is crucial in the life cycle of bacteriophages and viruses. The inhibition of its activity could potentially prevent the integration of viral DNA into the genome of the host cell and terminate viral replication (15, 16). Using the DNA-directed assembly microarray, we develop a biological assay to screen the activity of a recombinase in the presence of an inhibitor molecule, heparin as a model drug (14). A probe containing an ssDNA address linked to a double-stranded DNA (dsDNA) Cre-recombinase binding sequence was generated using PCR. Our approach allows the Cre recombinase to catalyze DNA recombination in a solution phase, followed by fluorescence detection on a DNA microarray surface (Fig. 3).

2. Materials

2.1. DNA-Directed Assembly for Antibody Microarray (7)

2.1.1. Preparation of Carboxyl-Terminated Dendrimer-Coated Slides (8)

1. Carboxyl-terminated poly(propyleneimine) (PAMAM) Generation 4.5 (10% solution in methanol).
2. 1-ethyl-3-(3-dimethylaminopropyl)carbodiimide hydrochloride (EDC).
3. *N*-hydrozysuccinimide (NHS).
4. Reaction buffer 1: 0.1 M 2-(*N*-morpholino)ethanesulfonic (MES) buffer pH 6.3.
5. Amine-silylated slides (Genetix Int., UK).
6. Absolute ethanol.

2.1.2. Immobilization of NH_2-ssDNA over the Activated Dendrimer-Coated Slides

1. 4-hydroxy-3-nitrobenzenesulfonic acid (HNSA).
2. 1-ethyl-3-(3-dimethylaminopropyl)carbodiimide hydrochloride.
3. *N*-hydroxysuccenimide.
4. 5′-amino-terminated ssDNA, 5′-NH_2-polyT_{20}-3′ (NH_2-ssDNA).
5. Reaction buffer 2: 500 mM sodium chloride (NaCl) in 0.1 M 2-(*N*-morpholino) ethanesulfonic (MES) buffer pH 6.3.
6. Reaction buffer 3: 0.1 M sodium bicarbonate ($NaHCO_3$) buffer pH 8.5 containing 10% glycerol.
7. *Quenching buffer 1*: 1 M 2-Amino-2-hydroxymethyl-propane-1,3-diol (Tris) buffer pH 9.0.
8. Absolute ethanol.

2.1.3. Labeling Swine Rabbit IgG

1. Swine rabbit IgG.
2. Pierce protein A/G column.
3. Protein desalting spin column.
4. Cy5 fluorescent monoreactive dyes (Amersham Biosciences, Piscataway, NJ).
5. Dimethylsulfoxide.
6. *Labeling buffer 1*: 50 mM NaCl in 0.1 M $NaHCO_3$ buffer pH 9.0.
7. *Deactivating buffer 1*: 0.1 M 2-Amino-2-hydroxymethyl-propane-1,3-diol (Tris) pH 8.0. The buffer pH was adjusted by adding hydrochloric acid (HCl).
8. *Equilibration buffer 1*: phosphate-buffered saline (PBS) pH 7.4, containing 137 mM NaCl, 2.7 mM potassium chloride (KCl), 10 mM disodium hydrogen phosphate (Na_2HPO_4), and 2 mM potassium dihydrogen phosphate (KH_2PO_4).
9. Micro BCA™ Protein Assay Kit (Pierce Chemicals, Rockford, IL).

2.1.4. Preparation of ssDNA-Antibody Conjugates

1. Swine antirabbit IgG.
2. Pierce protein A/G column.
3. Protein desalting spin column.
4. Sulfosuccinimidyl 4-[*N*-maleimidomethyl]cyclohexane-1-carboxylate (sulfo-SMCC) cross-linkers.
5. 3′-thiol-terminated ssDNA, 5′-polyA_{20}-SH-3′ (ssDNA-SH).
6. Dithiothreitol (DTT).
7. *Reaction buffer 4*: 0.1 M $NaHCO_3$ buffer, pH 8.5 containing 10% glycerol.
8. *Equilibration buffer 2*: PBS pH 7.4, containing 137 mM NaCl, 2.7 mM KCl, 10 mM Na_2HPO_4, and 2 mM KH_2PO_4.

9. *Storage buffer 1*: PBS pH 8.0, containing 137 mM NaCl, 2.7 mM KCl, 10 mM Na_2HPO_4, and 2 mM KH_2PO_4.
10. *Printing buffer 1*: 10% glycerol in 0.1 M $NaHCO_3$ buffer at pH 8.5.
11. *Washing buffer 1*: 0.1% TritonX-100 in PBS pH 8.0, containing 137 mM NaCl, 2.7 mM KCl, 10 mM Na_2HPO_4, and 2 mM KH_2PO_4.
12. Polyacrylamide gel (acrylamide:bisacrylamide = 19:1) (20% w/v).
13. PAGE Gel-electrophoresis system.
14. *Running buffer 1*: 1× Tris–Acetate EDTA (TAE) buffer.
15. BioOdyssey calligrapher MiniArrayer quipped with solid pin (Bio-Rad Laboratories, Hercules, CA).

2.1.5. Swine Rabbit IgG Capture and Detection in DNA-Directed Assembly for Antibody Microarray

1. *Hybridization buffer 1*: PBS pH 7.4, containing 137 mM NaCl, 2.7 mM KCl, 10 mM Na_2HPO_4, 2 mM KH_2PO_4, 0.1% milk, and 0.1% TritonX-100.
2. *Washing buffer 2*: 0.1% TritonX-100 in PBS pH 7.4, containing 137 mM NaCl, 2.7 mM KCl, 10 mM Na_2HPO_4, and 2 mM KH_2PO_4.
3. *Washing buffer 3*: PBS pH 7.4, containing 137 mM NaCl, 2.7 mM KCl, 10 mM Na_2HPO_4, and 2 mM KH_2PO_4.
4. High speed centrifuge.
5. GenePix 4000B, Axon laser scanner.

2.2. DNA-Directed Assembly for RNA Polymerase-DNA Binding Microarray (9)

2.2.1. Isolation of E. coli Genomic DNA

1. K12 *E. coli* DH5α.
2. Luria-Bertani Broth Medium (LB medium).
3. HRHZP-98/100 Incubator shaker.
4. High speed centrifuge.
5. Wizard® Genomic DNA purification kit (Promega Corp, Madison, WI).
6. UV/Vis Spectrophotometers.

2.2.2. Synthesis of ssDNA–dsDNA Probes

1. Primers.
2. DNAman version 4.15 Lynnon Biosoft (Vaudreuil-Dorion, Quebec, Canada).
3. Taq-polymerase PCR mix.
4. QIAquick PCR purification kit (Qiagen, Valencia,CA).
5. SYBR gold (Invitrogen Corp., CA).
6. UV light,UVP Imaging system.

2.2.3. RNAP-DNA Binding Assay

1. RNA polymerase.
2. Polyacrylamide gel (acrylamide:bisacrylamide = 19:1) (20% w/v).

3. PAGE Gel-electrophoresis system.
4. *Running buffer 2*: 1× Tris–Acetate EDTA (TAE) buffer.
5. *Hybridization buffer 2*: 0.1% TritonX-100 in PBS pH 7.4, containing 137 mM NaCl, 2.7 mM KCl, 10 mM Na_2HPO_4, and 2 mM KH_2PO_4.
6. GenePix 4000B, Axon laser scanner.

2.3. DNA-Directed Assembly for Drug-Screening Microarray (14)

2.3.1. Synthesis of ssDNA–dsDNA Probes

1. Primers
2. DNAman version 4.15, Lynnon Biosoft (Vaudreuil-Dorion, Quebec, Canada).
3. pLOX2+ plasmid.
4. Taq-polymerase Polymerase Chain Reaction (PCR) mix.
5. QIAquick PCR purification kit.
6. SYBR gold.
7. UV light from UVP Imaging system.

2.3.2. RNA Polymerase-DNA Inhibition Assay

1. Cre recombinase.
2. Hybridization buffer 3: 0.1% TritonX-100 in PBS pH 7.4, containing 137 mM NaCl, 2.7 mM KCl, 10 mM Na_2HPO_4, and 2 mM KH_2PO_4.
3. Microarray microplate (TeleChem International Inc., Sunnyvale, CA).
4. Washing buffer 4: 0.1% TritonX-100 in PBS pH 7.4, containing 137 mM NaCl, 2.7 mM KCl, 10 mM Na_2HPO_4, and 2 mM KH_2PO_4.
5. Genepix 4000B microarray scanner.
6. GenePix 3.0 software.

3. Methods

3.1. DNA-Directed Assembly for Antibody Microarray (7)

3.1.1. Preparation of Carboxyl-Terminated Dendrimer-Coated Slides

Carboxyl-terminated dendrimer-coated slides were prepared using amino-silylated glass slides. The terminal carboxylic acid of PAMAM dendrimer was activated with a solution of EDC/NHS (100 mM EDC and 100 mM NHS) in *reaction buffer 1*, layered onto the amine slides, and incubated for 2 h. The slides were then washed with double-distilled water followed by absolute ethanol and then air-dried. The dried dendrimer-coated slides were kept in vacuo until use.

3.1.2. Immobilization of NH_2-ssDNA over the Activated Dendrimer-Coated Slides

To immobilize the amino terminal ssDNA onto the carboxyl-terminated dendrimer-coated slides, the slides were activated by EDC/HNSA active ester method (1:1; 100 mM) in *reaction buffer 2*. The activated slides were quickly washed with double-distilled water and ethanol and dried by centrifugation on a slide holder (see Note 1).

For the covalent immobilization of the 5′ NH_2-polyT$_{20}$ 3′, 600 pL of a solution of the NH_2-ssDNA in *reaction buffer 3* was arrayed on to the HNSA-activated slides and incubated for 3 h in a humid chamber (see Note 2). The slides were then washed with distilled water and subsequently incubated in quenching buffer 1 for another 1 h at 42°C to quench remaining activated groups. The slides were then dried by spinning in a centrifuge with a slide holder (1,500×*g*, 5 min at 27°C) and further dried under a stream of nitrogen.

3.1.3. Labeling Swine Rabbit IgG

Swine rabbit IgG was purified using a Pierce protein A/G column using standard protocols and concentrated using YM-30 spin column (Millipore, USA). 1 mg/mL of Swine antirabbit IgG was prepared in *labeling buffer 1*. Cy5™ monofunctional NHS ester was prepared at a concentration of 10 mg/mL in dimethylsulfoxide. The volume required was calculated according to the desired ratio of Cy5 NHS ester to antibody (e.g., 20–1). The dye was added gradually to the antibody solution while stirring and then incubated with intermittent shaking at room temperature for 60 min in the dark. Unbound Cy5 dyes were deactivated by adding *deactivating buffer 1*; the mixture was incubated for 10 min at room temperature and then placed on protein desalting column to remove the deactivated unbound dyes. The column was preequilibrated in *equilibration buffer 1*. The column was placed in a fresh collection tube and 100 μL of the mixture was applied to the center of the compacted resin. The column was then centrifuged at 1,500×*g* for 2 min. The swine antirabbit IgG concentration was measured by Micro BCA™ Protein Assay Kit. For protein quantification, Bovine Serum Albumin (BSA) was used as protein standards, ranging from 200 to 0.5 μg/mL. 150 μL of each standards and the labeled antibody solution were pipetted into a microplate well. Working reagents were prepared by mixing 25 parts of MicroBCA Reagent MA and 24 parts of Reagent MB with 1 part of Reagent MC. 150 μL of the working reagent was added to each well, plate mixed thoroughly on a plate shaker for 30 s and incubated at 37°C for 45 min. The plate was then cooled to room temperature and the absorbance at 562 nm on a plate reader was measured. The standard curve was used to determine the protein concentration in the cell lysates.

3.1.4. Preparation of ssDNA-Antibody Conjugates

Swine antirabbit IgG antibody was purified using Pierce protein A/G column by standard protocols and concentrated using YM-30 spin column (Millipore, USA). The sulfuhydryl group of a thiol-modified ssDNA (5′-polyA$_{20}$-SH-3′) was linked to the amine group on the antibody using a bifunctional cross-linker, sulfo-SMCC. The protected thiol-modified ssDNA was decapped by reduction of the disulfide bond with 10 mM DTT to generate a free sulfuhydryl group and purified by precipitation with acetone and 0.3 M sodium acetate. The purified Swine antirabbit IgG was reacted with sulfo-SMCC cross-linker at a 50 molar excess in *reaction buffer 4* for 30 min at room temperature. Unreacted cross-linker was removed using protein desalting (see Note 3) column. The column was preequilibrated in *equilibration buffer 2*. The column was placed in a fresh collection tube and 100 μL of the mixture was applied to the center of the compacted resin. The column was then centrifuged at 1,500 ×*g* for 2 min. Purified products were reacted with thiol-modified ssDNA in a 1:10 molar equivalent for 1 h at 4°C. Excess ssDNA was separated from the conjugates by native polyacrylamide gel at 120 V for 10 min. The antibody-conjugated ssDNAs not migrating in the gel were recovered from the well by careful pipetting. These conjugates were diluted in *storage buffer 1* solutions and stored at 4°C.

Antibodies diluted in *printing buffer 1* were microspotted (~600 pL for each spot) on the activated slides using a BioOdyssey calligrapher MiniArrayer equipped with solid pin. The coupling reaction was allowed to proceed overnight at 25°C in a humid chamber. The arrayed slides were then washed with *washing buffer 1* for 20 min and then incubated in blocking buffer for 4 h.

3.1.5. Swine Rabbit IgG Capture and Detection in DNA-Directed Assembly for Antibody Microarray

ssDNA-labeled Swine antirabbit IgG antibody was prepared in *hybridization buffer 1* and incubated onto the ssDNA printed slides for 1 h at 37°C. The slides were then washed with *washing buffer 2* for 30 min, *washing buffer 3* for 1 min, and air-dried by spinning in a centrifuge with a slide holder ~100 ×*g* for 5 min at 27°C under a stream of nitrogen. The fluorescence intensity of the hybridized probe was measured using GenePix 4000B, Axon laser scanner.

3.2. DNA-Directed Assembly for RNA Polymerase-DNA Binding Microarray (9)

3.2.1. Preparation of DNA Microarray Slides

Carboxyl-terminated PAMAM dendrimer slides were prepared using amino-silylated glass slides. The carboxylic acid of the PAMAM dendrimer was activated with a solution of EDC/ NHS (1:1, 100 mM) in *reaction buffer 1*, layered onto the amine slides and incubated for 2 h. The slides were then washed with double-distilled water, ethanol, and air-dried. In order to immobilize the oligonucleotide address, the PAMAM slides were further activated by EDC/HNSA active ester (1:1; 100 mM) in *reaction buffer 2*. Activated slides were washed with double-distilled water, ethanol, and air-dried by centrifugation (1,500 ×*g*, 5 min at 27°C). The oligonucleotides with terminal amino group (250 μM) in *printing buffer 1* were spotted onto the activated slides using a

BioOdyssey Calligrapher MiniArrayer equipped with solid pin. The coupling reaction was allowed to proceed overnight at room temperature in a humid chamber. The arrayed slides were then blocked with *deactivating buffer 1* for 2 h followed by a quick wash in *washing buffer 1*.

3.2.2. Isolation of E. coli Genomic DNA

K12 *E. coli* was cultured overnight in LB broth at 37°C in a shaker incubator at 250 rpm. The cells were centrifuged for 5 min at 10,000 × *g*. The genomic DNA was then isolated using Wizard® Genomic DNA purification kit. The concentrations of the DNA solutions were determined using the UV/Vis Spectrophorometers.

3.2.3. Synthesis of ssDNA–dsDNA Probes

The DNA sequences were designed with computer program DNAman and listed in Table 1. The dsDNA fragment of the probe was 239 bp PCR-amplified DNA that contained 147 bp upstream and 92 bp downstream of the transcription start point (+1) of LacP1. The probe encompassed not only the main promoter site LacP1 but also the pseudopromoter sites LacP2-4.

PCR reaction mix (50 μL) contained 2 μg E. *coli* genomic DNA or DNA plasmid template, 1× reaction buffer, 0.2 mM dNTP, 1.2 μM of each primer, and a *Taq*-polymerase mix of approximately 2 U. The mixture was incubated at 94°C for 5 min. 40 cycles of denaturing (94°C, 30 s), annealing (58°C, 30 s), and

Table 1
Primer sequences for synthesizing the ssDNA–dsDNA probe for RNA Polymerase-DNA Binding Microarray

Set	Sequence
Cloning probe	
Oligo 1 SmaI LacP forw.	5′ CTTTATTCGCTTTTAACTTA<Int Spacer 9>TCCCCCGGGTT TCCCAGTCACGACGTTGTAA
Oligo 2 StuI LacP forw.	5′ TAAATACGTATAATAAGTTT<Int Spacer 9>AAAAGGCCT TTTCCCAGTCACGACGTTGTAA
Oligo 3 LacZ forw.	5′ CTTTATTCGCTTTTAACTTA <Int Spacer 9>CAATCAACTG TTTACCTTGTGGAGC
Oligo 4 LacZ forw.	5′ CTTTATTCGCTTTTAACTTACAATCAACTGTTTACCTTGT GGAGC
Cy5 LacP rev.	5′ Cy5-TTGGCCGATTCATTAATGCAG
Cy5 LacZ rev.	5′ Cy5-TTCTGTATGAACGGTCTGGTCTTTG
Microarray experiment	
Oligo 1 Amino	5′ TAAGTTAAAAGCGAATAAAG – Amine 3′
Oligo 2 Amino	5′ AAACTTATTATACGTATTTA – Amine 3′
Oligo 3 Amino	5′ AATCTATTTATCAGCCTAAG – Amine 3′

extension (72°C, 30 s) were conducted to amplify the probe. Final incubation at 72°C for 1 min ensured that all DNA were fully extended. The PCR product was then purified using QIAquick PCR purification kit. Purity of the probe was determined by performing agarose gel (2%) electrophoresis. Poststaining of DNA with SYBR gold allowed visualization under (see Note 4) UV light.

3.2.4. RNAP-DNA Binding Assay

The DNA probes were incubated with RNAP at 37°C for 30 min. Subsequently, the solution was loaded on a polyacrylamide gel and ran at 100 V for 4~6 min in *running buffer 2*. The mobility of DNA probe bound with the repressor was retarded allowing the separation of the bound from the unbound probes. The optimized electrophoresis parameters ensure that the free probe migrated into the gel, while the DNA–protein complex was retained in the loading wells of polyacrylamide gel. The probe–protein complex was then extracted by pipetting the solution from the wells of the gel into a sterile Eppendorf tube (see Note 5). The recovered DNA probes were mixed in *hybridization buffer 2* before incubated on the microarray. No RNAP was added with DNA probes for control. Fluorescence intensity of probe recovered was detected by microarray scanner.

3.3. DNA-Directed Assembly for Drug-Screening Microarray (14)

The microarray slides are prepared as described in Subheading 3.2.1.

3.3.1. Synthesis of ssDNA–dsDNA Probes

The DNA sequences were designed with computer program DNAman and listed in Table 2. A 24-bp flanking sequence was introduced in the forward primer in order to use the product DNA as templates in subsequent probe synthesis through PCR. The dsDNA fragment of the probe with two LOX1 sequences was 435 bp PCR-amplified that contained 23 bp upstream and 343 bp downstream of linearized pLOX2+ plasmid (3.65 kbp).

PCR reaction mix (50 μL) contained LOX DNA plasmid template, 1× reaction buffer, 0.2 mM dNTP, 5 μM of Cy3-dCTP, 1.2 μM of each primer, and a *Taq*-polymerase mix of approximately 2 U. The mixture was incubated at 94°C for 5 min. 40 cycles of denaturing (94°C, 30 s), annealing (58°C, 30 s), and extension (72°C, 30 s) were conducted to amplify the probe. Final incubation at 72°C for 1 min ensured that all DNA were fully extended. The PCR product was then purified using QIAquick PCR purification kit. Purity of the probe was determined by performing agarose gel (2%) electrophoresis. Poststaining of DNA with SYBR gold allowed visualization under UV light.

Table 2
Primer sequences for synthesizing the ssDNA–dsDNA probe for RNAP-DNA binding assay

Set	Sequence
Lox template	
Oligo 1	5′CTTTTGCTCACATGTTCTTTCCTGTCACTAGTCCATGGATAACTTCG
Oligo 2	5′CAATCAACTGTTTACCTTGTGGAGCTCACTAGTCCATGGATAACT TCG
Oligo 3[a]	5′ATATAACTTCGTATAGCATACATTATACGAAGTTATGCTATGTGGCG CGGTATT
Probe synthesis	
Oligo 4 Lox forw.	5′CTTAGGCTGATAAATAGATT<Int Spacer 9>CTTTTGCTC ACATGTTCTTTCCTG
Oligo 5 Lox forw.	5′TAAATACGTATAATAAGTTT<Int Spacer 9>CTTTTGCTCA CATGTTCTTTCCTG
RT-PCR primer	
RT Lox forw.	5′ TAGTGTATGCGGCGACCGA
RT Lox rev.	5′ CCACGATGCCTGCAGGAAT
Microarray experiment	
Oligo 1 Amino	5′ AATCTATTTATCAGCCTAAG – Amine 3′
Oligo 2 Amino	5′ AAACTTATTATACGTATTTA – Amine 3′

[a]Oligo 3 was used as the reverse primer for synthesis of ssDNA–dsDNA probe

3.3.2. Cre Recombinase-DNA Inhibition Assay

Cre recombinase activity assay was performed by mixing 100 ng of DNA probes and various concentrations of Cre recombinase in 50 μL solution for 90 min. To denature the enzyme, 5 μL of the reacted solution was diluted with 45 μL of water and incubated at 70°C for 20 min. The solution was then mixed with equal volume of *hybridization buffer 3*. Forty microliters of the sample were further incubated onto the microarray at 30°C for 2 h. The microarray slide was partitioned into 24 compartments using microarray microplate. The slide was then rinsed and washed (3 × 10 min) with *washing buffer 4* at room temperature. Subsequently, the slides were dried by centrifugation at 1,500 × *g* for 5 min at 27°C. Fluorescence intensity from the hybridized probe was measured using Genepix 4000B microarray scanner and analyzed using GenePix 3.0 software. Activity of the Cre recombinase was determined by comparing the reduction of fluorescence intensity from probes incubated with and without Cre recombinase. The standard curve of DNA concentration was obtained by incubating 0.035–1 nM of probes on the microarray.

4. Notes

1. The active ester groups are easily hydrolyzed under ambient conditions. Thus, we recommend to activate the slides just before the immobilization of NH_2-ssDNA; alternatively, for later usage, the dried slides should be kept in desiccators under nitrogen atmosphere.
2. The arraying chamber should be as humid as possible to ensure efficient coupling of oligos to activated slides. The small volume in the arrayed spots could evaporate in a short time.
3. Addition of sulfo-SMCC to antibody (mole ratio <1,000:1) should be kept as minimal as possible to prevent denaturation of the active sites. Western blot or immuno-cytochemistry could be used to determine whether the conjugated antibody has been denatured.
4. The primers/primer dimers should be avoided as much as possible from the ssDNA–dsDNA probe to prevent low assay sensitivity. DAN gel electrophoresis could be performed to verify the purification process.
5. The page gel should be removed from the gel tank when extracting the probe–protein complex from the well of the gel. The final volume should be fixed for all samples to prevent skewing of result.

References

1. Tang, Y.C., Wan, G.Q., Ng, J.K., Ajikumar, P.K., Too, H.P. (2008) DNA-directed assembly of protein microarrays. *Front Biosci.* **13**: 5755–5771.
2. Mueller, M., Martens, L., Apweiler, R. (2007) Annotating the human proteome: Beyond establishing a parts list. *Biochim Biophys Acta.* **1774**: 175–191.
3. Wingren, C., Borrebaeck, C.A.K. (2004) High-throughput proteomics using antibody microarrays. *Expert Rev Proteomics.* **1**: 355–364.
4. Wingren, C., Borrebaeck, C.A.K. (2006) Antibody microarrays: Current status and key technological advances. *Omics.* **10**: 411–427.
5. Uttamchandani, M., Wang, J., Yao, S.Q. (2006) Protein and small molecule microarrays: powerful tools for high-throughput proteomics. *Mol Biosyst.* **2**: 58–68.
6. LaBaer, J., Ramachandran, N. (2005) Protein microarrays as tools for functional proteomics. *Curr Opin Chem Biol.* **9**: 14–19.
7. Ng, J.K., Ajikumar, P.K., Tang, Y.C., Lee, J.Y., Stephanopoulos, G., Too, H.P. (2007) Spatially addressable protein array: ssDNA-directed assembly for antibody microarray. *Electrophoresis.* **28**: 4638–4644.
8. Ajikumar, P.K., Kiat, J., Tang, Y.C., Lee, J.Y., Stephanopoulos, G., Too, H.P. (2007) Carboxyl-terminated dendrimer-coated bioactive interface for protein microarray: High-sensitivity detection of antigen in complex biological samples. *Langmuir.* **23**: 5670–5677.
9. Ng, J.K., Ajikumar, P.K., Stephanopoulos, G., Too, H.P. (2007) Profiling RNA polymerase-promoter interaction by using ssDNA-dsDNA probe on a surface addressable Microarray. *ChemBioChem.* **8**: 1667–1670.
10. Kumar, A., Grimes, B., Fujita, N., et al. (1994) Role of the sigma(70)-subunit of *Escherichia coli* RNA-polymerase in transcription activation. *J Mol Biol.* **235**: 405–413.

11. Craig, N.L. (1988) The mechanism of conservative site-specific recombination. *Annu Rev Genet.* **22**: 77–105.
12. Fliess, A., Wolfes, H., Seela, F., Pingoud, A. (1988) Analysis of the recognition mechanism involved in the Ecorv catalyzed cleavage of DNA using modified oligodeoxynucleotides. *Nucleic Acids Res.* **16**: 11781–11793.
13. Margulies, C., Kaguni, J.M. (1996) Ordered and sequential binding of DnaA protein to oriC, the chromosomal origin of Escherichia coli. *J Biol Chem.* **271**: 17035–17040.
14. Ng, J.K. (2007) Design, development and application of A spatially addressable protein microarray. PhD Thesis, National University of Singapore, Singapore.
15. Abremski, K., Hoess, R. (1984) Bacteriophage-P1 site-specific recombination – purification and properties of the Cre recombinase protein. *J Biol Chem.* **259**: 1509–1514.
16. Sadowski, P. (1986) Site-specific recombinases – changing partners and doing the twist. *J Bacteriol.* **165**: 341–347.

Chapter 8

Selection of Peptide Ligands for Human Placental Transcytosis Systems Using In Vitro Phage Display

Saleem Basha, Shruthi Vaidhyanathan, and Giovanni M. Pauletti

Abstract

Fetal pharmacotherapy generally relies on nonspecific biodistribution of therapeutic agents to the unborn child following drug administration into the maternal circulation system. Physiologically, transfer of polar, high-molecular weight solutes across the placenta is facilitated by a specialized, vesicular transport mechanism termed transcytosis. To develop biotechnology-based drugs such as proteins, DNA, and siRNA as clinically effective therapeutics, transcytosis systems have been evaluated as a promising strategy to augment drug transfer across endothelial and epithelial barriers. Screening of random peptide libraries using phage display is a powerful technology to identify peptide sequences with high affinity for surface proteins on desired target cells. Here, we describe assembly of a diverse, cyclic heptapeptide library on the icosahedral T7 bacteriophage platform. This phage-displayed library of random peptides was used for functional in vitro screens across BeWo cell monolayers to identify peptide ligands that facilitate placental transcytosis of viral particles across this cell culture model of the human trophoblast barrier.

Key words: BeWo cell monolayers, Cyclic heptapeptide, Functional in vitro screen, Transcytosis ligand, Human placenta, Phage display, T7 bacteriophage

1. Introduction

Physiologically, receptor-mediated transcytosis is a vesicular transport mechanism facilitating transfer of polar macromolecules across biological membranes. With the desire to develop biotechnology-based drug such as proteins, DNA, and siRNA as clinically effective therapeutics, transcytosis has been evaluated as a promising strategy to enhance biodistribution of polar drugs across various endothelial and epithelial barriers (1, 2). To date, a small number of transcytosis receptors have been identified (e.g., transferrin and insulin receptor), and drug delivery systems comprising high affinity ligands for those transcytosis receptors

Seetharama D. Satyanarayanajois (ed.), *Drug Design and Discovery: Methods and Protocols*,
Methods in Molecular Biology, vol. 716, DOI 10.1007/978-1-61779-012-6_8,

(e.g., antibodies) were demonstrated to successfully augment transmembrane transport of polar drugs (3). However, broad expression of those transcytosis systems throughout the organism results in widespread, nonspecific tissue distribution leading to reduced efficacy and/or increased adverse events. The objective of our research is to identify peptide ligands for transcytosis receptors expressed in the human placenta that facilitate efficient transfer of colloidal, drug-loaded nanocarriers such as nanoparticles and liposomes from the mother to the unborn child in utero.

Screening of random peptide libraries displayed on bacteriophages (i.e., phage display) is a powerful biological combinatorial library technology to select peptide sequences with high affinity for surface proteins on desired target cells (4, 5). Recent reports underline that this strategy is also successful in identifying peptide sequences that interact with novel receptors promoting steps of delivery subsequent to surface binding, including transcytosis (6–8). Commercial availability of the T7Select®415-1 bacteriophage vector facilitated assembly of a constrained, cyclic heptapeptide library. Previously, it was demonstrated that random peptides expressed on the lytic T7 bacteriophage platform exhibit less sequence bias than conventionally used, M13 filamentous phage-displayed peptide libraries (9). Ligand peptides for putative placental transcytosis systems were selected using four sequential rounds of functional screens across BeWo cell monolayers, an in vitro cell culture model of the human trophoblast barrier.

2. Materials

2.1. Amplification and Cloning of Template DNA

1. Synthesize oligonucleotides for generation of template DNA to assemble diverse heptapeptide library (Fig. 1): 5′-CGG GGATCCGAATTCAGGGGGGGGG TGC(NNK)$_7$ TGCG GGTAAGCTTGCGGC-3′. Store in freezer at −20°C.
2. Synthesize oligonucleotides as primers for polymerase chain reaction (PCR). Store in freezer at −20°C:

   Forward primer: 5′-CGGGGATCCGAATTCAG-3′

   Reverse primer: 3′-CGGCGTTCGAATGGGTA-5′.
3. 2 mM $MgCl_2$ in DNAse-free, double-distilled water (dd H_2O).
4. 10 mM dNTPs represent equal mixture of natural 2′-deoxynucleoside-5′-triphosphates dATP, dGTP, dCTP, and dTTP in DNAse-free dd H_2O; pH = 7.5. Store in freezer at −20°C.
5. Platinum® *Taq* PCR_x DNA Polymerase, 5 U/μL (Invitrogen Corp., Carlsbad, CA) supplied with 10× PCR_x Enhancer

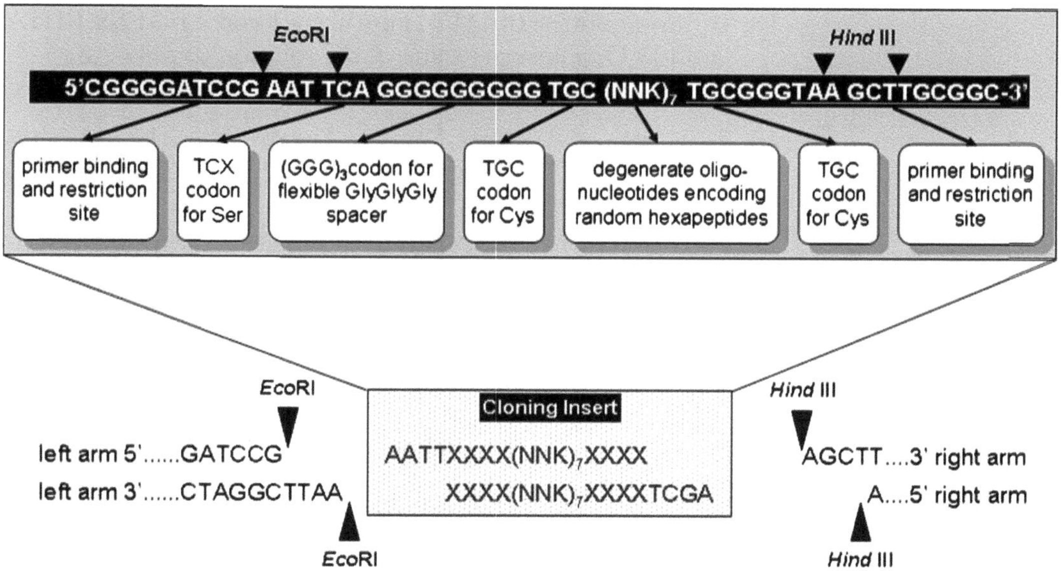

Fig. 1. Rational design of degenerate oligonucleotides to assemble random library of cyclic heptapeptides using the T7Select®415-1b bacteriophage vector. Both the 5′- and 3′-ends of the oligonucleotide strand are flanked by a codon for a Cys residue to facilitate formation of disulfide-cyclized heptapeptides. In addition, the design includes constant regions on both ends that serve as primer binding sites for PCR amplification and restriction sites for *Eco*RI and *Hind*III digestion required for cloning of template DNA into the commercial T7Select®415-1b vector. The 5′-end of the synthetic strand also contains codons for three Gly residues that act as a flexible spacer for the phage-displayed peptide inserts. *Eco*RI cleavage of designed oligonucleotide insert places C in second position resulting in a TCX codon for the amino acid Ser.

Solution, 50 mM $MgSO_4$ in DNAse-free dd H_2O, 10× PCR_x Amplification Buffer, 50 mM $MgCl_2$ in DNAse-free dd H_2O, and 10× PCR Buffer, minus Mg^{2+}. Store in freezer at −20°C.

6. 40% (w/v) acrylamide/bisacrylamide (19:1) solution in double-distilled (dd) H_2O.
7. 10× TAE buffer: 400 mM Tris–OH, 200 mM acetic acid, and 10 mM EDTA in double-distilled H_2O. Adjust pH value of the buffer to pH = 8.3.
8. 10% (w/v) Ammonium persulfate freshly prepared in dd H_2O.
9. 0.77 mg/mL *N*,*N*,*N*′,*N*′-Tetramethylethylenediamine (TEMED) stock solution in dd H_2O.
10. Running buffer (5×): 125 mM Tris–OH and 960 mM glycine in dd H_2O. Adjust pH value to pH = 8.7.
11. Prestained molecular weight markers, 50–10,000 bp (Hi-Lo™ DNA Marker, Minnesota Molecular, Minneapolis, MN). Store refrigerated at 4°C.
12. Ethidium bromide solution: dilute 1% (w/v) stock solution in dd H_2O to 0.5 μg/mL.

13. Diffusion buffer: 0.3 M sodium acetate and 2 mM Na_2EDTA in dd H_2O; adjust pH value of the solution to pH = 7.8.
14. 70–95% (v/v) ethanol in doubled-distilled H_2O.
15. 20 U/μL *Eco*RI (New England Biolabs, Ipswich, MA) supplied with 10× NEBuffer 1 and 100× NEB BSA (10 mg/mL). Store in freezer at −20°C.
16. 20 U/μL *Hind*III (New England Biolabs, Ipswich, MA) supplied with 10× NEBuffer 2 and 100× NEB BSA (10 mg/mL). Store in freezer at −20°C.
17. 1 mg/mL BSA solution: dilute 100× NEB BSA 1:10 using DNAse-free dd H_2O.
18. 1.5% (w/v) Agarose ME gel (Acros Organics, Geel, Belgium, melting point: 86.5–89.5°C).
19. QIAEX II Gel Extraction Kit (Qiagen Inc., Valencia, CA) supplied with QIAEX II Suspension, Buffer QX1 (with pH indicator), and buffer PE.
20. 10 U/μL T4 DNA Polynucleotide Kinase (New England Biolabs, Ipswich, MA) supplied with 10× Kinase Reaction Buffer. Store in freezer at −20°C.
21. 1 mM Adenosine triphosphate (ATP) in DNAse-free dd H_2O.
22. 1 mM EDTA in DNAse-free dd H_2O; pH value adjusted to pH = 8.0.
23. TE buffer: 10 mM Tris–HCl and 1 mM EDTA in dd H_2O, pH value adjusted to pH = 8.0.
24. 3 M Sodium acetate in dd H_2O; pH value adjusted to pH = 5.8.
25. T7Select®415-1b Cloning Kit (EMD Biosciences, Madison, WI) comprised of T7Select® *Eco*RI/*Hind*III Vector Arms, T7Select® Control Insert, T7Select® Packaging Extract, T7Select® Packaging Control DNA, BL21 glycerol stock, T7SelectUP primer, and T7SelectDOWN primer.
26. 20 U/μL T4 DNA ligase (New England Biolabs, Ipswich, MA) supplied with 10× T4 DNA ligase reaction buffer.
27. 100 mM Dithiothreitol in DNAse-free dd H_2O.
28. Luria–Bertani (LB) medium: 10 g of Bacto®Tryptone, 5 g of yeast extract, and 10 g of NaCl dissolved in 1,000 mL of dd H_2O. Adjust pH value to pH = 7.5, and autoclave at 121°C for 20 min.

2.2. Propagation and Characterization of T7 Bacteriophages

1. Top agarose: 3 g of agarose, 3 g of NaCl, 3 g of yeast extract, and 5 g of Bacto®Tryptone in 500 mL of dd H_2O; autoclave at 121°C for 20 min.

2. LB agar plate: 7.5 g of agar in 500 mL of LB medium; heat to boil under stirring for 1 min. Adjust volume to 500 mL of dd H_2O and autoclave at 121°C for 20 min. Let agar cool to ~55°C. Pour 10 mL of LB agar into a sterile Petri dish (100×15 mm), swirl plate in circular motion, and let cool until solid. Store upside down at 4°C.
3. 10 mM EDTA in dd H_2O; adjust pH value to pH = 8.0.
4. QIAquick PCR Purification Kit (Qiagen Inc., Valencia, CA) supplied with QIAquick Spin Columns, buffer PB, buffer PE, buffer EB, pH Indicator *I*, collection tube (2 mL), and loading dye.

2.3. BeWo Cell Culture and Functional Screen of Peptide Library

1. Human choriocarcinoma BeWo cell line (Cat. No. CCL-98, American Type Culture Collection, Manassas, VA). Store in liquid nitrogen at −196°C.
2. Complete Hams F-12 medium consists of Ham's F-12 medium (HyClone Laboratories, Logan) supplemented with 10% (v/v) head-inactivated, sterile-filtered fetal bovine serum, 100 U/mL penicillin, 100 µg/mL streptomycin, 0.1 mM nonessential amino acids, and 2 mM L-glutamine. Store refrigerated at 4°C.
3. PBS/EDTA solution: 0.02% (w/v) EDTA-Na dissolved in phosphate buffered saline (PBS). Adjust pH value to pH = 7.4 and sterilize by filtration using 0.2-µm pore size. Store refrigerated at 4°C.
4. Trypsin/EDTA solution: 0.25% (w/v) porcine trypsin and 0.05% (w/v) EDTA-Na dissolved in Hanks' Balanced Salt Solution without Ca^{2+} and Mg^{2+}. Adjust pH value to pH = 7.4 and sterilize by filtration using 0.2 µm pore size. Store refrigerated at 4°C.
5. Transwell® system with 12 mm diameter polyester membrane, 0.4 µm pore size (Cat. No. 3460, Corning Inc., Acton, MA).
6. Rat Tail Collage solution: dilute 95% (v/v) ethanol with dd H_2O to 60% (v/v), sterilize by filtration using 0.2-µm pore size, and mix three volumes of sterile 60% (v/v) ethanol with one volume of rat tail collagen type I supplied in 0.02 N acetic acid (Cat. No. 354236, BD Biosciences, Bedford, MA). Store refrigerated at 4°C.
7. HBSS: 13.1 g of Hanks' Balanced Salts (Sigma-Aldrich, St. Louis, MO), 0.4 g of $NaHCO_3$, 3.5 g of d-glucose, and 2.9 g of HEPES in 1,000 mL of dd H_2O. Adjust pH value to pH = 7.4 and sterilize by filtration using 0.2 µm pore size. Store refrigerated at 4°C.

3. Methods

Phage-displayed libraries of random peptides are assembled as fusion with viral capsid proteins. Various research groups successfully applied this biological combinatorial library tool to identify peptide ligands exhibiting significant affinity for cell surface receptors (4, 5). Binding of ligands to surface-exposed transcytosis receptors is also required, but must be followed by internalization of the ligand–receptor complex, movement of endocytosed vesicle through the cytosol, and release of the ligand from the receptor into the receiver compartment at the abluminal membrane. As a consequence of this mandatory endocytosis step, physical dimensions of the bacteriophage platform used to display the peptide library are highly relevant to successfully identify transcytosis ligands. The T7 bacteriophage vector was selected for assembly of the cyclic heptapeptide library due to its spherical, icosahedral procapsid structure. The estimated diameter of the viral head of this bacteriophage is between 50 and 80 nm, which appears sufficiently small to fit within endocytic vesicles following internalization (10). In addition, the dimensions of the T7 bacteriophage coincide with the preferred size range of pharmaceutically used, commercial nanocarriers (11, 12).

Identification of viable peptide ligands for human placental transcytosis systems critically depends on the ability to experimentally collect phage clones after successful transfer across the trophoblast barrier. Previously, it was demonstrated that the BeWo cell line, which was isolated from a human choriocarcinoma specimen, expresses many physiological features of human trophoblast cells (13). When cultured in the two-chamber Transwell® system, polarized cell monolayers are obtained mimicking the placental barrier in vivo (14). Sampling from the apical and basolateral compartment, respectively, facilitates experimental access to the "maternal" and "fetal" compartments separated by the trophoblast-like BeWo cell monolayer. Using this arrangement, phage clones successfully traversing the trophoblast barrier via transcytosis can be conveniently collected from the basolateral compartment by liquid sampling. Since the predicted diameter of the T7 procapsid is at least tenfold larger than the estimated paracellular pore radius of BeWo cell monolayers, it is reasonable to assume that in vitro transport of T7 bacteriophages collected from the "fetal" compartment predominantly occurs via transcellular transcytosis.

3.1. Preparation and Amplification of Template DNA

1. Synthesize 67 bp single-stranded, degenerate oligonucleotides using conventional solid-phase DNA synthesis protocols (15). The generic sequence of desired template DNA is 5′-CGGGGATCCGAATTCAGGGGGGGGGTGC(NNK)$_7$

TGCGGGTAAGCTTGC GGC-3′ (see Fig. 1), where N = equal mixture of A, G, C, and T, and K = equal mixture of G and T. (see Note 1). Store purified, degenerate oligonucleotides in DNAse-free dd H_2O (50–100 μM) at 4°C.

2. Prepare template DNA for a diverse peptide library on the T7 bacteriophage platform by amplifying 67 bp degenerate oligonucleotide strands using PCR. Transfer ~100 ng of single-stranded oligonucleotide into a 200 μL thin-wall PCR tube, add 10 pmoles of each forward and reverse primer, 1 μL of 2 mM $MgCl_2$ solution, 1 μL of 10 mM dNTPs, and 2.5 U of Platinum® Taq PCR_x DNA Polymerase.
3. Adjust the final volume to 50 μL with DNAse-free dd H_2O and incubate tube in a thermal cycler at 95°C for 2.5 min to completely denature the template and activate the enzyme. Perform 30 consecutive PCR amplifications using the following reaction conditions: denature at 90°C for 30 s, anneal at 50°C for 30 s, and extend at 72°C for 2 min. Hold PCR mixture after completion at 4°C until purification.
4. Purify amplified DNA by nondenaturing polyacrylamide gel electrophoresis using a protocol described earlier by Sambrook and colleagues (16). All glass plates for gels and the combs are scrubbed clean, rinsed extensively with dd H_2O, and air-dried. To prepare a 0.75-mm thick, 6% polyacrylamide gel, mix 5.25 mL 40% acrylamide:bisacrylamide (19:1) solution, 2 mL of 10× TAE buffer, and 27.75 mL of dd H_2O.
5. Add 100 μL of ammonium persulfate solution and 25 μL of TEMED stock as polymerization catalyst and pour the gel immediately onto the glass plate. Insert a square tooth comb into the gel and wait about 30 min until polymerization is completed before removing the comb.
6. Dilute 100 mL of 5× Running buffer with 400 mL of dd H_2O using a 1,000 mL Erlenmeyer flask and fill upper and lower chamber of gel unit. Load 50 μL of PCR sample in each well. Dedicate one well for molecular weight markers. Assemble the gel unit, connect to the power supply, and run gel for 4 h at 40 mA.
7. Remove gel from glass plates, wash with dd H_2O, and stain DNA bands by submerging gel under gentle rocking for 15 min in ethidium bromide solution (see Note 2). Visualize gel under UV light ($\lambda = 365$ nm) and cut gel slices containing 67 bp DNA bands using a scalpel.
8. Transfer gel slice into sterile 1.5-mL microcentrifuge tube, add 1.0 mL of Diffusion buffer, incubate for 30 min at 50°C using a shaking water bath, and clear mixture by centrifugation (10 min at 11,200 × *g*). Quantitatively transfer supernatant

into a fresh, sterile microcentrifuge tube and allow cooling to room temperature. Discard pellet.

9. Add 1 mL of ice-cold 95% ethanol, incubate mixture for 60 min at −20°C, and clear by centrifugation (10 min at 11,200 × *g*). Carefully aspirate supernatant, wash pellet once with 950 μL of 70% ethanol, chill the tube in a dry ice/ethanol mixture for 10 min followed by centrifugation at 11,200 × *g* for 10 min. Discard supernatant and resuspend pellet in 10 μL of DNAse-free dd H_2O. Estimate DNA concentration spectrophotometrically at λ = 260 nm using dd H_2O as blank (see Note 3).

3.2. Cloning of Template DNA into T7Select® EcoRI/HindIII Vector Arms

1. Digest purified template DNA with restriction enzymes *Eco*RI and *Hind*III for 90 min at 37°C. Combine ~100 ng of DNA with 2.0 μL of NEBuffer 2, 10 U of *Eco*RI, 10 U of *Hind*III, 2.0 μL of BSA solution, and adjust volume to 20 μL using DNAse-free dd H_2O.
2. Prepare a 10-mm thick, 1% (w/v) agarose gel by dissolving under heating 0.3 g agarose in a mixture of 3 mL of 10× TAE buffer and 27 mL of dd H_2O using a 125 mL Erlenmeyer flask. Adjust volume to 30 mL with dd H_2O, pour melted agarose onto gel casting deck, and insert comb. After gel solidifies, remove comb and load 20 μL samples, including DNA ladder, into wells. Run gel at 5 V/cm for 90 min.
3. Identify double-digested, 67 bp DNA band under UV light (λ = 365 nm), cut gel slice carefully around the DNA band, and collect it in a 1.5 mL sterile microcentrifuge tube for extraction using the QIAEX II Gel Extraction Kit.
4. Weigh gel slice in tube and add 600 μL of Buffer QX1 to each 100 mg of gel. Include 10 μL of resuspended QIAEX II silica particles and incubate mixture for 10 min at 50°C using a heatblock. Separate silica-adsorbed DNA from dissolved gel components by a 30 s spin at 11,200 × *g*, carefully remove supernatant, and wash pellet first with 500 μL of Buffer QX1 followed by two washes with 500 μL of Buffer PE. Dissolve air-dried pellet in 20 μL of DNAse-free dd H_2O and estimate concentration of purified template DNA spectrophotometrically at λ = 260 nm (see Note 3).
5. Phosphorylate the two 5′-ends of purified template DNA using T4 DNA Polynucleotide Kinase. Combine ~100 ng of DNA with 1 μL of 1 mM ATP, 2 μL of 10× Kinase Reaction Buffer, and 5 U of T4 DNA Polynucleotide Kinase in a sterile 500-μL microcentrifuge tube. Adjust volume to 20 μL with DNAse-free dd H_2O and incubate this mixture for 20 min at 37°C. Stop phosphorylation by adding 10 μL of 1 mM EDTA and inactive enzyme at 75°C for 10 min.

6. After dilution with 100 μL of DNAse-free dd H_2O, purify DNA by phenol/chloroform extraction. Combine sample with 250 μL of TE buffer-saturated phenol and 250 μL of $CHCl_3$, mix biphasic system efficiently by vortex for 10 s, and separate the layers by centrifugation at 11,200 × *g* for 5 min. Carefully transfer the top, aqueous phase into a fresh tube, add an equal volume of $CHCl_3$, and repeat procedure until interface is no longer visible. Dilute the final aqueous phase with 20 μL of 3 M sodium acetate and 400 μL of ice-cold 95% ethanol, and incubate mixture at −20°C for 1 h. Collect precipitated DNA by centrifugation (11,000 × *g* for 10 min) and discard supernatant. Dissolve air-dried pellet in 10 μL of DNAse-free dd H_2O and estimate concentration of purified, phosphorylated template DNA spectrophotometrically at $\lambda = 260$ nm (see Note 3).
7. Ligate purified, phosphorylated template DNA into the cloning site of the T7Select® *Eco*RI/*Hind*III Vector Arms (see Note 4). Combine in a sterile 1.5-mL microcentrifuge tube ~1.3 ng of purified, phosphorylated template DNA, 0.5 μg of T7Select® *Eco*RI/*Hind*III Vector Arms, 1 μL of 10× T4 DNA ligase reaction buffer, 0.5 μL of 1 mM ATP, 0.5 μL of 100 mM DTT, and 10 U of T4 DNA Ligase; adjust volume to 10 μL with DNAse-free dd H_2O, and incubate reaction mixture at 16°C for 15 h.
8. Thaw a 25 μL aliquot of T7 Packaging Extract on ice, add 5 μL of completed ligation mixture, mix gently with a pipet tip, and incubate packaging mixture at room temperature (20–25°C) for 2 h (see Note 5). Stop packaging reaction by adding 270 μL of LB medium and amplify entire packaged phage library in a single round using liquid culture method described in Subheading 3.3.

3.3. Phage Amplification and Plaque Assay

1. Dilute a fresh, overnight-grown culture of competent *E. coli* BL21 strain in 200 volumes of LB medium and incubate at 37°C for 3–4 h in a bacterial shaker to prepare logarithmically grown bacteria (log phase culture, see Note 6).
2. Infect log phase culture with phage sample and incubate at 37°C under shaking until complete lysis occurs (see Note 7).
3. Prepare serial dilutions of phage lysate from $1{:}10^2$ to $1{:}10^{10}$ in LB medium (see Note 8) and combine 100 μL of each dilution with 250 μL of log phase BL21 culture in a sterile, 5 mL polystyrene tube. After 5 min incubation at room temperature (20–25°C), mix by vortex, add 5 mL of warm (45–50°C) liquid Top agarose, and pour entire content of the tube onto a LB agar plate.

4. Spread top agarose layer evenly by gently swirling the LB agar plate and incubate at 37°C for 3–4 h until clear areas in bacterial lawn (plaques) appear on LB agar plate. Count number of plaques at a dilution that results in maximal 100–200 clearly separated plaques per plate (see Note 9). The phage titer expressed as plaque-forming units (pfu) equals number of plaques counted on LB agar plate × dilution factor × 10 (to account for the 100 μL plated). Total number of phages per unit volume is determined by multiplying the titer by the total sample volume (e.g., packaging reaction: 0.3 mL).

3.4. Sequence Analysis of Phage Recombinants

1. Scrape a plaque of interest, which is clearly separated from neighboring plaques, from top agar layer using a sterile loop or pipet tip and disperse in 100 μL of 10 mM EDTA inside a sterile 1.5 mL microcentrifuge tube. Vortex briefly and place for 10 min on a heating block set at 65°C. After cooling to room temperature, centrifuged for 5 min at 11,200 × *g*. Use supernatant that contains phage DNA for subsequent PCR amplification.
2. Prepare PCR reaction mixture in a thin-walled 200 μL PCR tube using 1 μL of phage DNA, 5 μL of 10× PCR Buffer, minus Mg^{2+}, 0.5 μL of PCR_x 50 mM $MgCl_2$, 0.5 μL of each T7SelectUP Primer and T7SelectDOWN Primer, 1 μL of 10 mM dNTPs, and 2.5 U of Platinum® *Taq* PCR_x DNA Polymerase.
3. Adjust final volume to 50 μL with DNAse-free dd H_2O and incubate tube in a thermal cycler at 95°C for 2.5 min to completely denature the template and activate the enzyme. Perform 30 consecutive PCR amplifications using the following reaction conditions: denature at 90°C for 30 s, anneal at 50°C for 30 s, and extend at 72°C for 2 min. Hold PCR mixture after completion at 4°C until purification.
4. Dilute PCR mixture with 250 μL of QIAquick Buffer PB, load onto QIAquick Spin Column assembly, and centrifuge at 11,200 × *g* for 60 s. Discard filtrate and wash filter-bound DNA with 750 μL of QIA quick Buffer PE using the same centrifugation protocol. Transfer filter unit into new collection tube, and elute DNA from filter by centrifugation using 50 μL of DNAse-free dd H_2O.
5. Confirm expected size of PCR amplification product by agarose gel electrophoresis as described in Subheading 3.2. Submit purified PCR product for DNA sequencing following conventional cycle sequencing protocols (17) with the T7SelectDOWN Primer.
6. Decode primary sequence of peptide insert using standard genetic code (18). To estimate the diversity of an assembled

phage display library sequence, ~30% of all plaques recovered on an LB agar plate that was prepared from a dilution of the assembled library (at least 30–50 plaques). Divide the number of different peptide sequences decoded from sequencing results by the total number of DNA samples submitted, correct for the fraction of total plaques submitted (i.e., 30%), and multiply this diversity with the titer dilution.

3.5. BeWo Cell Culture

1. Maintain BeWo cell line in a humidified atmosphere of 5% (v/v) CO_2 at 37°C using Complete Ham's F-12 medium. Grow cell stock in 75 cm^2 cell culture flasks and replace medium every other day. Subculture cells when approximately 80% confluent.
2. Remove culture medium and wash cells with 6 mL of prewarmed (37°C) PBS/EDTA Solution. Aspirate excess solution and incubate cells at room temperature (20–25°C) for 2 min. Slowly expose cells to 2 mL of prewarmed (37°C) Trypsin/EDTA solution. Remove excess solution and incubate cells at 37°C for 5 min. Collect dissociated cells in 6 mL of prewarmed (37°C) Complete Ham's F-12 medium (see Note 10).
3. Passage cells at 1:5 (v/v) split ratio, and transfer 2 mL of dissociated cell suspension into new 75 cm^2 culture flask filled with 12 mL of prewarmed (37°C) Complete Ham's F-12 medium.

3.6. BeWo Cell Monolayers on Transwells®

1. Coat each Transwell® insert with rat tail collage type I by adding 66 μL of Rat Tail Collagen solution into the center of the filter. Swirl carefully in a circular motion to distribute the viscous solution throughout the entire filter. Dry under UV light ($\lambda = 254$ nm) overnight.
2. Fill receiver (basolateral) compartment of Transwell® system with 1.5 mL of prewarmed (37°C) Complete Ham's F-12 medium. Incubate for at least 2 h in humidified atmosphere of 5% (v/v) CO_2 at 37° before seeding BeWo cells onto collagen-coated insert.
3. Dissociate ~80% confluent BeWo cell culture as described in Subheading 3.4. Dilute 0.5 mL of cell suspension in 1.5 mL of prewarmed (37°C) Complete Ham's F-12 medium and determine cell concentration under an inverted microscope using a hemocytometer. Estimate cells per mL by multiplying the average count per square by 4 (dilution correction) and 10^4 (hemocytometer volume correction).
4. Adjust cell suspension to 2×10^5 cells/mL using prewarmed (37°C) Complete Ham's F-12 medium. Remove Transwell® from cell culture incubator and add 0.5 mL of adjusted BeWo

cell suspension (1×10^5 cells) into the top (apical) compartment (see Note 11).

5. Return Transwell® into cell culture incubator for development of confluent BeWo cell monolayers. Change cell culture medium every other day starting 24 h postseeding. First, carefully aspirate volume from the basolateral compartment before removing culture medium from the apical compartment. Refill in the same order with prewarmed (37°C) Complete Ham's F-12 medium using 1.5 mL for the basolateral and 0.5 mL for the apical compartment, respectively (see Note 12).

3.7. Functional Screen of Phage-Displayed Peptide Library

1. Use confluent BeWo cell monolayers maintained for 5–8 days on Transwells® for functional screen of phage-displayed peptide library assembled on T7 bacteriophage. Figure 2 summarizes most relevant steps of this protocol.
2. Determine phage titer of naïve, phage-displayed library of random heptapeptides using plaque assay as described in Subheading 3.3. Remove aliquot of this library and dilute in prewarmed (37°C) HBSS to 2×10^{10} pfu/mL.
3. Aspirate cell culture medium from basolateral and apical compartments of the Transwell® system and wash BeWo cell monolayer three times with prewarmed (37°C) HBSS (1.5 mL basolateral; 0.5 mL apical).
4. Move filter inserts into a new cluster plate and fill 1.5 mL of prewarmed (37°C) HBSS into the basolateral compartment. Initiate functional screen by adding 0.5 mL (~10^{10} pfu) of naïve, phage-displayed peptide library in prewarmed (37°C) HBSS to the apical donor compartment. Each round of screening is performed in triplicate using three different BeWo cell monolayers. Return Transwell® for 60 min to humidified atmosphere of 5% (v/v) CO_2 at 37°C.
5. Collect phage population in apical and basolateral compartments in separate, sterile 1.5 mL microcentrifuge tubes. Determine phage titer in donor and receiver solutions after each round of screening using 10 μL aliquot (see Subheading 3.3).
6. Amplify entire phage population collected from receiver compartment in competent BL21 strain and titer sublibrary of phage-displayed peptides for the next round of functional screen as outlined in Subheading 3.3. Repeat steps 3–6 described in this section for additional three rounds to select phage clones traversing this in vitro model of the human trophoblast barrier predominantly via transcellular transcytosis.
7. Calculate enrichment factor of transcytosed phage clones by dividing phage titer in receiver compartment from *n*th round

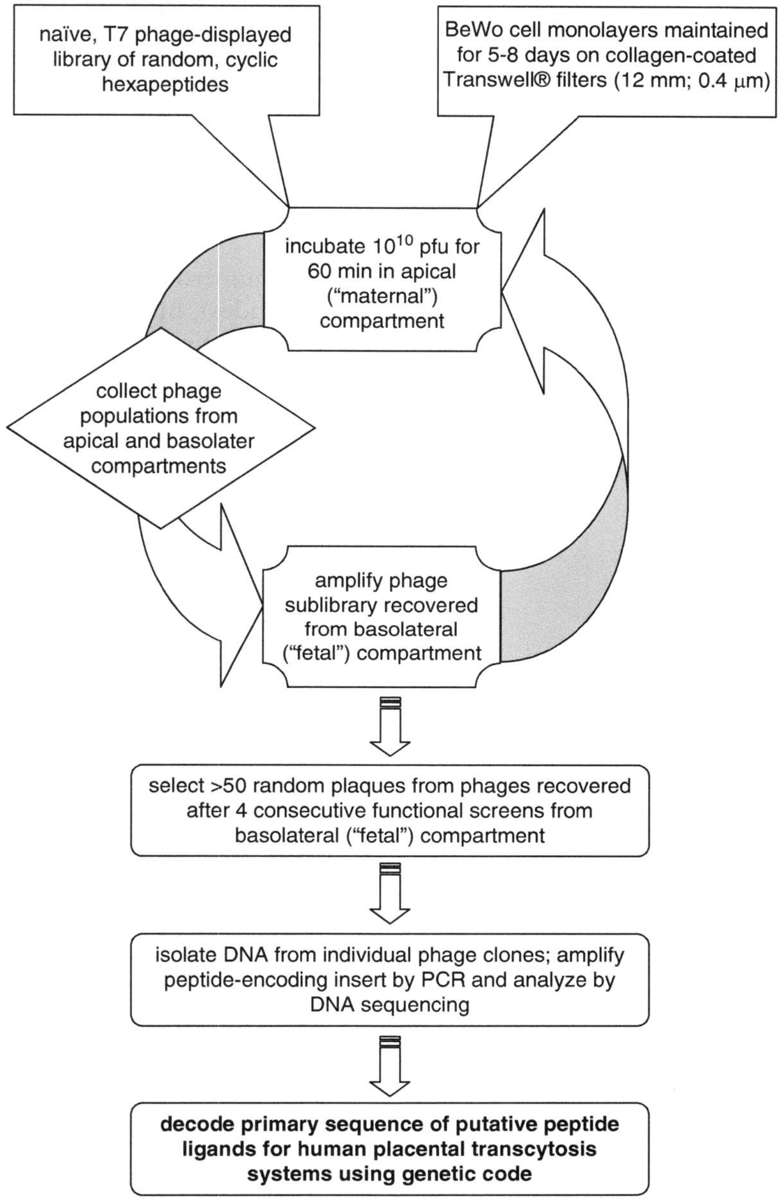

Fig. 2. Schematic overview of functional in vitro screen used to select phage clones expressing putative peptide ligands for human placental transcytosis systems.

by the corresponding number determined for the previous (n–1)th round times 100%.

8. Select >50 random plaques after the fourth round of functional screens from an appropriate dilution of phage population recovered from the receiver compartment. Isolate phage DNA from individual clones and PCR amplify DNA region encoding for the peptide insert. Decode primary sequence of

the peptide inserts using standard genetic code (18) to identify putative peptide ligands for human placental transcytosis systems.

4. Notes

1. To introduce numerous mutations in a small DNA region (20–80 nucleotides), mutant oligonucleotides are generated during organic synthesis by modulating relative molarities of nucleotide precursors at each step of the synthesis. This results in a complex mixture of related molecules called *degenerate oligonucleotide*.
2. Ethidium bromide is a potential mutagen. Always use personal protection equipment such as gloves when working with this chemical.
3. Use 1:100–1:1000 dilutions in DNAse-free dd H_2O to measure absorbance in a clean quartz cuvette (conventional polystyrene cuvettes significantly absorb at $\lambda = 260$ nm!). The average extinction coefficient of double-stranded DNA at $\lambda = 260$ nm is 0.020/(μg/mL) cm. According to the Beer–Lambert Law, 50 μg/mL DNA results in an absorbance or optical density (OD) of 1.0 at this wavelength.
4. For maximal cloning efficiency, use molar DNA insert/phage vector ratio of 3:1. The 37 kb T7Select® *Eco*RI/*Hind*III Vector Arms corresponds to approximately 0.04 pmol/μg. Assuming an average molecular weight of 330 Da for each base in the oligonucleotide, 1 ng of purified 67 bp template DNA equals approximately 0.05 pmoles.
5. T7Select®415-1b Cloning Kit is supplied with 25 μL single reaction volumes of T7Select® Packaging Extract. Each aliquot will package up to 1 μg of vector DNA without loss of efficiency. To test packaging efficiency independently, add 0.5 μg of T7Select® Packaging Control DNA to 25 μL of T7Select® Packaging Extract.
6. Monitor bacterial growth spectrophotometrically at $\lambda = 600$ nm. Log phase culture of *E. coli* results in absorbance at this wavelength between 0.6 and 0.8 ($OD_{600} = 0.6–0.8$).
7. Amplification of T7 bacteriophages in *E. coli* BL21 strain using shaking flask method typically yields 10^{10}–10^{11} phage/mL. As phage titer is proportional to aeration of the culture, use culture volume <20% of flask volume.
8. Initial phage concentration used to inoculate log phase host bacteria is not too critical as T7 phages grow rapidly in competent BL21 strain. Adding a single plaque or phage lysate at

a volume ratio between 1:100 and 1:1000 usually results in good amplification.

9. Recommended dilutions depend on the source of phage sample. To determine packaging efficiency or number of primary recombinants in newly assembled library, use dilution ranges from $1:10^4$ to $1:10^7$. To determine titer of amplified lysate, use dilution ranges from $1:10^7$ to $1:10^{10}$. To monitor enrichment of phages during screening, use dilution ranges from $1:10^2$ to $1:10^5$.
10. Assess status of cell dissociation by gently hitting upright flask against palm of hand. Cells sliding down on plastic support indicate sufficient detachment. Proceed with collection in Complete Ham's F-12 medium to avoid further enzymatic digestion by trypsin.
11. Gently invert stock cell suspension before removing aliquot for seeding onto collagen-coated filter insert. Move quickly from filter to filter to avoid variable seeding densities due to cell sedimentation in pipet.
12. Slowly add new culture medium at the side of the insert to limit removal of BeWo cells from filter support.

Acknowledgments

The authors are grateful to Drs. Anil G. Menon and Vasily V. Ivanenkov from the University of Cincinnati, College of Medicine, for their advice and encouragement. This work was supported in part by a grant from the National Institutes of Child Health & Human Development (HD048512).

References

1. Simionescu, M., Popov, D., and Sima, A. (2009) Endothelial transcytosis in health and disease. *Cell Tissue Res.* **335**: 27–40.
2. Swaan, P. W. (1998) Recent advances in intestinal macromolecular drug delivery via receptor-mediated transport pathways. *Pharm Res.* **15**: 826–834.
3. Jones, A. R., and Shusta, E. V. (2007) Blood-brain barrier transport of therapeutics via receptor-mediation. *Pharm Res.* **24**: 1759–1771.
4. Barry, M. A., Dower, W. J., and Johnston, S. A. (1996) Toward cell-targeting gene therapy vectors: selection of cell-binding peptides from random peptide-presenting phage libraries. *Nature Med.* **2**: 299–305.
5. Pasqualini, R., and Ruoslahti, E. (1996) Organ targeting in vivo using phage display peptide libraries. *Nature* **380**: 364–366.
6. Ivanenkov, V., Felici, F., and Menon, A. G. (1999) Uptake and intracellular fate of phage display vectors in mammalian cells. *Biochim Biophys Acta.* **1448**: 450–462.
7. Ivanenkov, V. V., Felici, F., and Menon, A. G. (1999) Targeted delivery of multivalent phage display vectors into mammalian cells. *Biochim Biophys Acta.* **1448**: 463–472.
8. Morpurgo, M., Kirschner, M., and Radu, A. (2002) An approach to increased polyplex gene delivery by peptides selected from a phage display library. *J Biochem Biophy Methods* **52**: 31–43.

9. Krumpe, L. R., Atkinson, A. J., Smythers, G. W., Kandel, A., Schumacher, K. M., McMahon, J. B., Makowski, L., and Mori, T. (2006) T7 lytic phage-displayed peptide libraries exhibit less sequence bias than M13 filamentous phage-displayed peptide libraries. *Proteomics* **6**: 4210–4222.
10. Lamaze, C., and Schmid, S. L. (1995) The emergence of clathrin-independent pinocytic pathways. *Curr Opin Cell Biol.* 7: 573–580.
11. Debbage, P. (2009) Targeted drugs and nanomedicine: present and future. *Curr Pharm Design* **15**: 153–172.
12. Stroud, R. M., Serwer, P., and Ross, M. J. (1981) Assembly of bacteriophage T7. Dimensions of the bacteriophage and its capsids. *Biophys J.* **36**: 743–757.
13. Sastry, B. V. (1999) Techniques to study human placental transport. *Adv Drug Delivery Rev.* **38**: 17–39.
14. Liu, F., Soares, M. J., and Audus, K. L. (1997) Permeability properties of monolayers of the human trophoblast cell line BeWo. *Am J Physiol.* **273**: C1596–C1604.
15. Gait, M. J. (1991) DNA/RNA synthesis and labelling. *Curr Opin Biotech.* **2**: 61–68.
16. Sambrook, J., Fritsch, E. F., and Maniatis, T. (2001) Gel Electrophoresis of DNA and Pulsed-field Agarose Gel Electrophoresis. In: Sambrook J and Russell D (eds) Molecular Cloning: A Laboratory Manual (s.). Cold Spring Harbor Laboratory Press, Cold Spring Harbor, NY pp 5.1–5.86.
17. Shendure, J. A., Porreca, G. J., and Church, G. M. (2008) Overview of DNA sequencing strategies. *Curr Protoc Mol Biol.* **81**: 7.1.1.–7.1.11.
18. Hartwell, L., Goldberg, M., and Hood, H. (eds.) (2008) Genetics: From Genes to Genomes. McGraw-Hill, Boston, MA.

Chapter 9

Optimization of the Tetrazolium Dye (MTT) Colorimetric Assay for Cellular Growth and Viability

Paul W. Sylvester

Abstract

The MTT colorimetric assay is an established method of determining viable cell number in proliferation and cytotoxicity studies. This assay is based on the cleavage of the yellow tetrazolium salt, MTT, to form a soluble blue formazan product by mitochondrial enzymes, and the amount of formazan produced is directly proportional to the number of living, not dead cells, present during MTT exposure. Since the MTT assay is rapid, convenient, and economical, it has become a very popular technique for quantification of viable cells in culture. However, various parameters have been identified that can affect cellular metabolism and other factors, which significantly modify MTT-specific activity and can result in calculated false high or false low cell counts. Therefore, it is essential to establish assay parameters with the proper controls for each cell line and/or drug treatment in order to optimize assay conditions and minimize confounding effects. These parameters should include determining appropriate cell densities, culture medium, optimal concentrations and exposure times for MTT, fresh culture medium at the time of assay to avoid nutrient depletion, and controlling for drug treatment effects that may influence cellular metabolism. By controlling these important parameters, the MTT colorimetric assay provides accurate and reliable quantification of viable cell number.

Key words: Cell growth assay, Cell viability assay, Colorimetric assay, MTT, Tetrazolium dye

1. Introduction

The discovery and development of novel drug therapies for the treatment of cancer involves the intensive research efforts of investigators in academia, the pharmaceutical industry, as well as governmental agencies. Initially, disease-oriented preclinical drug discovery includes the rapid in vitro screening of candidate drugs against a panel of human tumor cell lines. In general, tumor cells are exposed to various antitumor agents for a fixed duration of time and, afterwards, cell number and/or viability is determined.

Seetharama D. Satyanarayanajois (ed.), *Drug Design and Discovery: Methods and Protocols*,
Methods in Molecular Biology, vol. 716, DOI 10.1007/978-1-61779-012-6_9,

Many methodologies exist that can perform such a function and include techniques as simple as manually counting cells or cell nuclei, to much more elaborate efforts such as measuring ^{3}H-thymidine incorporation, fluorometric DNA assay, and flow cytometry. However, the majority of these techniques are labor intensive, time consuming, produce difficult to handle waste products that are toxic or radioactive, and are expensive to perform. However, one of the most popular and convenient ways to determine viable cell number in 24- or 96-well microtiter plates is the rapid colorimetric tetrazolium dye procedure commonly referred to as the MTT assay developed by Mosmann (1).

As initially described, the MTT assay is based on the cleavage of the yellow-colored tetrazolium salt, 3-(4,5-dimethylthiazol-2-yl)-2,5-diphenyl tetrazolium bromide, into a blue-colored formazan by the mitochondrial enzyme succinate-dehydrogenase (2). The assumed advantage of this cell assay system is that this reaction can only take place in living cells with functional mitochondria. It was also assumed that the amount of formazan formed during a given exposure period is directly proportional to the number of viable cells per well. Therefore, the MTT assay system is widely viewed as a convenient, reliable, and quantitative method for measuring cell proliferation and viability (3). However, many of these early assumptions were overly optimistic regarding the specificity of this assay system. Over time, it became clearly evident that nonmitochondrial enzymes can also specifically reduce tetrazolium salts at various cellular locations outside the mitochondria, and that the level of MTT reduction varies greatly between different cell types (4, 5). Furthermore, MTT-specific activity in nearly all cell lines significantly decreased with increased cell culture duration (3). Over time, other critical conditions became evident that were required for accurate assay performance.

Information presented in this review will summarize the various metabolic and chemical factors that can alter MTT-specific activity and thereby significantly affect quantification of cell number. Although the MTT colorimetric assay is a convenient and reliable method for measuring cell proliferation and viability, these characteristics absolutely depend on the establishment of assay conditions that optimize accuracy and eliminate confounding factors that affect MTT-specific activity (see Note 1).

2. Materials

2.1. Cell Culture and Harvesting

1. Control media: Dulbecco's Modified Eagles's Medium (DMEM)/Ham's F12 Medium (F12) at a ratio of 1:1 (Sigma Chemical Co, St. Louis, MO), supplemented with 10 μg/mL

insulin, 100 U/mL penicillin, 100 μg/mL streptomycin, and 10% bovine calf serum (BCS, Hyclone, Logan, UT).

2. Phosphate-buffered saline (PBS): sterile Ca^{2+}- and Mg^{2+}-free phosphate-buffered saline.
3. Harvesting medium: 0.05% trypsin containing 0.025% EDTA in PBS.
4. Bovine calf serum.
5. 2,4-Dinitrophenol.
6. Crystal violet/citric acid cell lysis solution: 2.1 g citric acid (Sigma) and 0.1 g crystal violet dye dissolved in 100 mL water and filtered with #2 Whatman paper.
7. Teflon cell scraper.
8. Hemocytometer
9. 2 mM D-glucose (dissolved in PBS or nutrient-depleted culture medium and then sterilized by filtration through a 0.2-μm filter).

2.2. MTT Preparation

1. MTT assay solution: 2–5 mg/mL MTT (thiazolyl blue tetrazolium bromide) in PBS (see Note 2).
2. Isopropanol or DMSO.

3. Methods

Viable cell number can be determined most easily in 24- or 96-well culture plates using the MTT colorimetric assay. The number of cells/well is calculated against a standard curve prepared at the start of each experiment, so that the same cell and MTT preparations are used for both the standard curve and the experiment. Standard curves are prepared by plating various concentrations of isolated cells (10^4–10^6), as previously determined by hemocytometer, in triplicate in the culture plates. Depending on the type of cell to be counted, standard curves are prepared so that MTT absorbance readings of experimental samples are obtained in the linear part of the curve. Sample absorbance readings that near the minimal or maximal detection levels will not provide accurate viable cell number counts.

3.1. Isolation of Cells

1. Many cell lines, such as the highly malignant +SA mammary epithelial cells (6–8), attach and grow on the surface of plastic culture plates. The MTT assay method is best suited for monolayer culture, but can also be used in 3-dimensional cell cultures using collagen or matrigel. Isolation of cells prior to experimentation can be routinely accomplished with a

trypsin-EDTA solution. Feed-stock cells can be grown in 100 mm culture plates and maintained on culture medium for a period of time until they reach 80% confluence (still in log phase of growth). In order to harvest cell for experimentation, medium is removed and cells are then rinsed in sterile PBS or just base medium that is free of serum or bovine serum albumin, in order to remove any remaining protein. After rinsing, PBS is removed, and trypsin-EDTA solution is added to cells. The amount of trypsin added depends on size of cell culture plate or flask. For example, the amount of trypsin to harvest cells grown in 100 mm plates is usually 2 mL, while 1 mL of trypsin would be used to harvest cells grown in a T-25 culture flask. Once cells are exposed to trypsin, culture plates or flasks are then returned to the incubator for 5 min. Time of exposure to trypsin is very critical. If exposure time is too short, isolation and harvest efficiency is poor, whereas if exposure time is too long, trypsin will induce cell lysis and death. After the 5 min incubation period, an equal amount of BCS as the amount of trypsin solution used (1–2 mL) is added to each plate in order to stop (quench) the trypsin digestion. Cells can then be isolated using a teflon cell scraper or rubber policeman and by using a pipette to flush the bottom of the plate.

2. The cell suspension is then collected from all plates or flasks, placed in a sterile conical tube, and centrifuged at 300 × *g* for 5–10 min to pellet the cells. Digestion medium is then removed, and cells are resuspended in 5–20 mL of culture medium (depending on the number of cells isolated). A 100 μL of this cell suspension is then placed in a 12 × 75 mm test tube (sterility of tube is not required) and 900 μL of crystal violet/citric acid solution is added to the tube to bring total volume to 1 mL. The tube is then vigorously vortexed for 2 min. This procedure will cause cell lysis, but leave nuclei intact. Since cell size and shape display a wide range of variance, it is much simpler and more accurate to count the darkly crystal violet-stained round nuclei of each cell instead of the irregularly shaped intact cells.
3. Add 10 μL of the lysed cell mixture to each side of a hemocytometer and count the cells, remembering that the cells have been diluted tenfold in order to determine the number of cells/mL in the harvested cell suspension.

3.2. Preparation and Construction of MTT Standard Curve

1. Once cells are counted, cells can be diluted to a concentration that allows easy preparation of the MTT standard curve. For example, if the isolated +SA cell concentration is 5×10^6 cells/mL, then cells, medium, and MTT can be pipetted into the wells

Table 1
Typical cellular dilutions and media volumes used to construct a MTT standard curve (density of isolated cells in suspension is 5×10^6 cells/mL)

Group number	Cell number (1×10^5)	Volume of cell suspension (μL)	Volume of medium (μL)
1	0	0	1,000
2	0.5	10	990
3	1.0	20	980
4	1.5	30	970
5	2.0	40	960
6	2.5	50	950
7	3.0	60	940
8	4.0	80	920
9	5.0	100	900
10	6.0	120	880
11	8.0	160	840
12	10.0	200	800

of a 24-well culture plate in triplicate (appropriate adjustment can be made when using 96-well plates): Table 1 shows an example of cell and medium dilution that would be typical for preparation of a MTT standard curve at the start of a given experiment. After completing the standard curve and plating cells at the appropriate concentration (5×10^4 per well in 24-well plates for neoplastic +SA mammary epithelial cells), cells are returned to the incubator for a 24 h period to allow for suspended cells to reattach to the surface of the plastic culture plate.

2. The next day, medium is removed from the wells of the standard curve and experimental groups that will be counted (Day 0), and fresh medium is added to these wells. As discussed later in this chapter, the refeeding of cells fresh medium prior to MTT exposure is an absolute requirement in order to obtain accurate viable cell number. Afterwards, 200 μL of the sterile MTT stock solution (2 mg/mL in PBS) is then added to each well of the standard curve and each well of the experimental groups to be counted that day. If the stock MTT

solution used in the above example is 2 mg/mL, the final MTT concentration in medium is 0.83 mg/mL. The concentration of the stock MTT solution can be modified (2–5 mg/mL) depending on the type of cell that is being used and culture plate (24- or 96-well) in order to optimize MTT-specific activity.

3. The standard curve and experimental cell culture plate containing cells exposed to MTT are returned to the incubator at 37°C for a 4 h period. This incubation period was determined to be optimal for +SA mammary tumor cells to produce the greatest amount of formazan reduction in the least amount of time. Different cell types with higher or lower metabolic rates may require adjustment in length of the incubation period in order to optimize the MTT assay for that particular type of cell.
4. Afterwards, the MTT containing medium is removed from all wells and the remaining cells containing formazan crystals are dissolved in 1 mL of isopropanol. Again, this volume of isopropanol can be adjusted depending on the type of culture plate being used (200 μL for 96-well plates) in order to optimized absorbance intensity.
5. Optical density of each well can then be determined with a microplate reader using an absorption spectrum that can range between 565 and 630 nm against the blank wells in the standard curve. For +SA mammary tumor cells, maximum absorbance was observed using a 570 nm filter.
6. The MTT standard curve is constructed by plotting the dependent variable (number of cells) on the *x*-axis against the independent variable (optical density) on the *y*-axis using linear/linear or log/log regression analysis, depending on what type of regression provides the best fit for a particular cell line and range of the standard curve.
7. The number of viable cells in experimental treatment groups can then be determined by reading absorbance values from individual wells in control and treatment groups against the standard curve. If treatment effects on the growth of cells are to be monitored over a period of days, then each day another set of wells (multiple treatment group plated at the start of the experiment) can be exposed to MTT and cell number in each group can be calculated from the original standard curve prepared at the start of the experiment. Again, it is essential that the same preparation of cells and MTT are used for both the standard curve and the experiment, and fresh standard curves must be prepared at the start of each subsequent experiment. An example of a MTT standard curve similar to one described above is shown in Fig. 1.

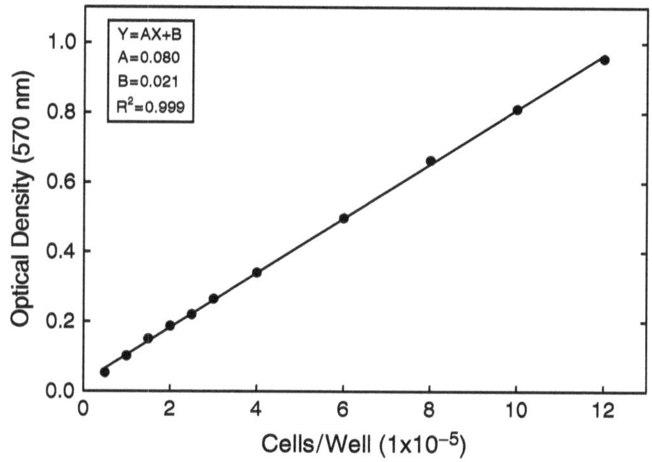

Fig. 1. A representative MTT standard curve for neoplastic +SA mouse mammary epithelial cells (8). Isolated cells were counted manually with a hemocytometer, and then various concentrations (5×10^4 to 1×10^6) were plated in triplicate into 24-well culture plates, fed 1 mL of control culture media, and returned to the incubator for a 24 h period to allow for cell to reattach to the plastic culture plates. The next day, media was removed and cells were fed 1 mL fresh media, and then 200 μL of 5 mg/mL MTT was added to each well so that final concentration was 0.83 mg/mL MTT. Plates were returned to the incubator (37°C) for a 4 h incubation period. Afterward, media was removed and 1 mL of isopropanol was added to each well to dissolve the formazan crystals. Optical density was measured at 570 nm zeroed against the blank wells (0 cells/well) for each well and a linear/linear plot created showing the relationship of the concentration of formazan produced vs. number of cells per well.

3.3. Parameters Determining Optimal MTT Assay Performance

3.3.1. Optimal MTT Concentration

Initial studies conducted by Mosmann (1) and Denizot and Lang (9) compared the use of MTT concentration between 0 and 4 mg/mL with a constant number of cells per well and found that the amount of formazan produced showed a steep increase between 0 and 1 mg/mL, then reached a plateau between 1 and 2 mg/mL. Both investigators concluded that standardizing the MTT concentration to 1 mg/mL for cell viability and proliferation assays was an acceptable compromise because this concentration produced excellent results and was cost-effective. Using various cell lines, it was determined that a concentration of 0.83 mg/mL MTT produced essentially the same results as 1 mg/mL (data not shown) and was selected for use in studies with +SA mammary tumor cells as described in this chapter.

3.3.2. Optimal Incubation Time

1. Neoplastic +SA mouse mammary epithelial cells were initially plated at density of 5×10^5 cell/well in 24-well culture plates and maintained on 1 mL/well control media as described above and then returned to the incubator for a 24 h period to allow cells to reattach to the plastic culture plate.

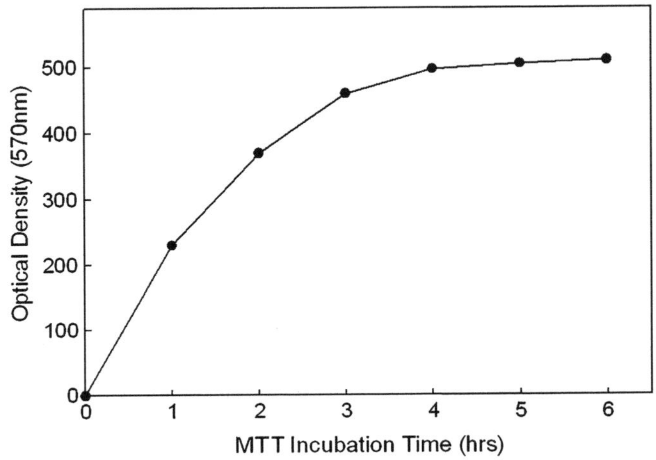

Fig. 2. Time-course relationship of formazan production after +SA cells was exposed to 0.83 mg/mL MTT. +SA mouse tumor cells were initially plated at a density of 5×10^5 cells/well in 24-well culture plates, fed 1 mL control media, and then returned to the incubator for a 24 h period to allow cells to reattach to the plastic culture plates. The next day, cell were divided into different groups with the same number of cells/well in each group, media was removed and replaced with 1 mL fresh control media, and then 200 μL of 2 mg/mL MTT was added to each well. Cells were returned to the incubator and MTT-specific activity was determine at 0, 1, 2, 3, 4, 5, and 6 h following MTT exposure (6 wells/group).

2. The next day, medium was removed and replaced with 1 mL fresh control media and 200 μL of 2 mg/mL MTT in sterile PBS was added to each well. Cells were returned to the incubator and MTT-specific activity was determined at 0, 1, 2, 3, 4, 5, and 6 h following MTT exposure (6 wells/group).
3. Figure 2 shows that there is a continuous increase in MTT-specific activity between 0 and 3 h, which then reached a plateau between 3 and 4 h after treatment exposure.
4. It was concluded from these results that a standardized incubation time of 4 h following MTT exposure was an acceptable compromise for further studies because it produced the optimal specific activity in the least amount of time (Fig. 2) (see Note 3).

3.3.3. Glucose Depletion in Culture Medium Significantly Reduces MTT-Specific Activity

1. Nutrient-depleted control medium was collected after 4 days in culture from 100 mm culture plates containing near confluent cultures of neoplastic +SA mouse mammary epithelial cells. Cells were initially plated at a density of 1×10^6 cells/culture plate and then maintained in the same 10 mL control medium for a 4-day incubation period. Afterwards, media from these culture plates was collected for use in subsequent experiments (see Note 4).

2. In other studies, +SA mammary tumor cells were initially plated at density of 5×10^5 cells/well in 24-well culture plates and maintained on 1 mL control media. Cells were returned to the incubator for 24 h in order to allow cells to reattach to the plastic culture plates.
3. The next day, media was removed and cells were divided into different treatment groups and fed the following treatment media: (1) fresh control media; (2) PBS; (3) PBS supplemented with 2 mM D-glucose; (4) nutrient-depleted media; and (5) nutrient-depleted media supplemented with 2 mM D-glucose. Afterwards, 200 μL of 2 mg/mL MTT in sterile PBS was added to each well, and cells were returned to the incubator. MTT-specific activity was determined after a 4 h incubation period.
4. The results in Fig. 3 show that equal number of cells produced the highest MTT-specific activity when given fresh media prior to MTT exposure. In contrast, formazan production by an equal number of cells maintained in glucose-free PBS showed a large reduction in MTT-specific activity, and this effect was partly reversed by supplementation with 2 mM

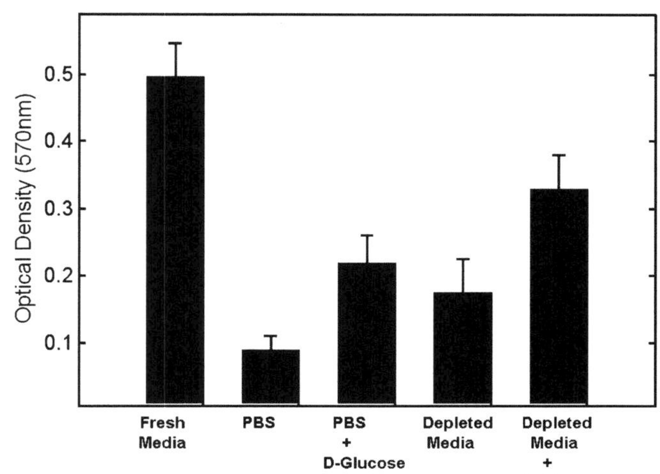

Fig. 3. Effects of glucose on MTT-specific activity. +SA mammary tumor cells were initially plated at density of 5×10^5 cell/well in 24-well culture plates, fed 1 mL control media, and then returned to the incubator for 24 h to allow cells to reattach to the plastic culture plates. The next day, media was removed and cells were divided into the following treatment groups containing the same number of cells/cell in all groups, and fed the following treatment media: (1) Fresh media, control; (2) PBS, glucose-free buffered saline; (3) PBS + D-glucose, PBS supplemented with 2 mM D-glucose; (4) depleted Media, nutrient-depleted media; and (5) depleted media + D-glucose, nutrient-depleted media freshly supplemented with 2 mM D-glucose. Afterwards, 200 μL of 2 mg/mL MTT in sterile PBS was added to each well (6 wells/group), and cells were returned to the incubator, and MTT-specific activity was determine after a 4 h incubation period.

D-glucose. Likewise, cells exposed to nutrient-depleted media showed a large reduction in formazan production as compared to an equal number of cells given fresh media, and supplementation with 2 mM D-glucose greatly increases MTT-specific activity in these cells.

5. These results demonstrate that it is essential that the MTT assay is performed in the presence of fresh media given to cells immediately prior to MTT exposure in order to obtain optimal formazan production. MTT-specific activity is greatly reduced in cells maintained in glucose-free media or nutrient-depleted media (Fig. 3).

3.3.4. Metabolic Uncouplers Greatly Enhance MTT-Specific Activity

1. Neoplastic +SA mouse mammary epithelial cells were plated at various densities (1, 2, 3, 4, and 5×10^5) cells/well in 24-well culture plates and fed 1 mL control media, then returned to the incubator for a 24 h period in order to allow cells to reattach to the plastic culture plates.
2. The next day, media was removed and replaced with 1 mL fresh control media containing 0 or 1 μM 2,4-dinitrophenol. Afterwards, 200 μL of 2 mg/mL MTT in sterile PBS was added to each well. Cells were returned to the incubator and MTT-specific activity was determined in each treatment group (6 wells/group) after a 4 h exposure to MTT.

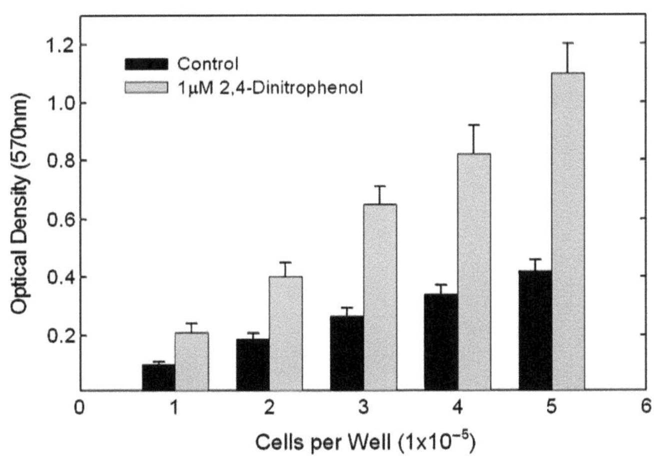

Fig. 4. Effect of the metabolic uncoupler, 2,4-dinitrophenol, on MTT-specific activity. +SA mammary tumor cells were plated at various densities (1, 2, 3, 4, and 5×10^5) cells/well in 24-well culture plates, fed 1 mL control media, and returned to the incubator for a 24 h period to allow cells to reattach to the plastic culture plates. The next day, media was removed and replaced with 1 mL fresh control media containing 0 or 1 μM 2,4-dinitrophenol. Afterwards, 200 μL of 2 mg/mL MTT was added to each well. Cells were returned to the incubator for a 4 h period and then MTT-specific activity was determined in each treatment group (6 wells/group).

3. Results in Fig. 4 show that cells exposed to 1 μM 2,4-dinitrophenol, an established metabolic uncoupler, display an increase in MTT-specific activity as compared to the same number of cells maintained in control media.
4. These results demonstrate that great care must be taken in establishing the proper controls and parameters when using the MTT assay to count cells treated with drugs that alter respiration and metabolism. Cells exposed to uncouplers, such as 2,4-dinitrophenol, displayed a very large "false high" in cell number as compared to the same number of cells from the vehicle-treated control group (see Note 5).

4. Notes

1. The MTT assay is an excellent method for quantification of viable cells in culture. The metabolic activity between different cell lines shows great variability and therefore the MTT standard curve needs to be characterized and optimized for each new cell line. It is also important when testing drug effects on proliferation and viability to include the proper controls for drug effects on cellular metabolism during treatment. By establishing proper assay conditions and controls, the MTT assay is an accurate and reliable method for counting viable cells.
2. MTT dissolves very slowly, so MTT and PBS can be placed on stirring plate and mixed vigorously for 10–20 min, and then filtered through a 0.2-μm filter to sterilize the solution and remove any insoluble particles remaining. This solution can be stored for up to a month at 4°C protected from light.
3. Other parameters have also been identified that play a critical role in modulating MTT-specific activity. Optimization of MTT concentration and exposure time is very important because different cell types display a wide variability in dose- and time-response in maximal formazan production (4, 5).
4. One of the most critical conditions that need to be accounted for when performing the MTT assay is glucose depletion in the culture medium. Previous studies have shown that cells with the highest glucose metabolism display the greatest reduction in MTT-specific activity over time in culture (3). These studies also showed that transfer of cells to a glucose-free medium was associated with an immediate decrease in tetrazolium salt reduction that was pH-independent, indicating that cellular transport and constant metabolism of glucose are required for optimal formazan production (3).

5. Phenol red, the red-colored pH indicator commonly present in many culture media, has an absorbance that overlaps with formazan and its presence in the assay can significantly affect sample absorbance and produce a high background in the blank samples and false highs in treatment cell samples (9). This problem can be eliminated with the use of phenol red-free media. Drugs and chemical agents can also significantly modify MTT-specific activity if these treatments increase or decrease mitochondrial respiration or cause metabolic uncoupling. Drug-induced respiratory uncoupling will produce a large false high, whereas agents that decrease metabolic respiration and electron transport will produce a false low in MTT-specific activity as compared to vehicle-treated controls containing identical cell numbers (3, 10).

Acknowledgments

The author would like to thank Dr. Margot M. Ip for her technical advice during the characterization of the MTT assay and Dr. Howard L. Hosick for generously providing the highly malignant +SA mouse mammary epithelial cell line for use in these studies. This work was supported in part by a grant from the National Institutes of Health (Grant CA 86833).

References

1. Mosmann, T. (1983) Rapid colorimetric assay for cellular growth and survival: application to proliferation and cytotoxicity assays. *J Immunol Methods* **65**: 55–63.
2. Slater, T.F., Sawyer, B., Straeuli, U. (1963) Studies on succinate-tetrazolium reductase systems. I ii. Points of coupling of four different tetrazolium salts. *Biochim Biophys Acta* 77: 383–393.
3. Vistica, D.T., Skehan, P., Scudiero, D., Monks, A., Pittman, A., Boyd, M.R. (1991) Tetrazolium-based assays for cellular viability: a critical examination of selected parameters affecting formazan production. *Cancer Res* **51**: 2515–2520.
4. Sylvester, P.W., Birkenfeld, H.P., Hosick, H.L., Briski, K.P. (1994) Fatty acid modulation of epidermal growth factor-induced mouse mammary epithelial cell proliferation in vitro. *Exp Cell Res* **214**: 145–153.
5. Carmichael, J., DeGraff, W.G., Gazdar, A.F., Minna, J.D., Mitchell, J.B. (1987) Evaluation of a tetrazolium-based semiautomated colorimetric assay: assessment of chemosensitivity testing. *Cancer Res* **47**: 936–942.
6. Anderson, L.W., Danielson, K.G., Hosick, H.L. (1979) New cell line. Epithelial cell line and subline established from premalignant mouse mammary tissue. *In Vitro* **15**: 841–843.
7. McIntyre, B.S., Briski, K.P., Gapor, A., Sylvester, P.W. (2000) Antiproliferative and apoptotic effects of tocopherols and tocotrienols on preneoplastic and neoplastic mouse mammary epithelial cells. *Proc Soc Exp Biol Med* **224**: 292–301.
8. Anderson, L.W., Danielson, K.G., Hosick, H.L. (1981) Metastatic potential of hyperplastic alveolar nodule derived mouse mammary tumor cells following intravenous inoculation. *Eur J Cancer Clin Oncol* **17**: 1001–1008.
9. Denizot, F., Lang, R. (1986) Rapid colorimetric assay for cell growth and survival. Modifications to the tetrazolium dye procedure giving improved sensitivity and reliability. *J Immunol Methods* **89**: 271–277.
10. Maioli, E., Torricelli, C., Fortino, V., Carlucci, F., Tommassini, V., Pacini, A. (2009) Critical appraisal of the MTT assay in the presence of Rottlerin and uncouplers. *Biol Proced Online* **11**: 227–240.

Chapter 10

Imaging NF-κB Signaling in Mice for Screening Anticancer Drugs

Delira Robbins and Yunfeng Zhao

Abstract

The activation of NF-κB has been implicated in various forms of cancer. Thereafter, targeting NF-κB has been suggested for cancer therapy. Instant and accurate tools to monitor NF-κB activation are necessary for such drug screening. Currently, there are various assays available to study NF-κB activation in vitro, however, techniques involving the imaging of NF-κB in vivo models remains limited. Male *NF-κB-RE-luc* (Oslo) mice from Xenogen Corporation (Alameda, California) provide a great model for studying and imaging anticancer drugs that target NF-κB signaling. In addition, the bioluminescent (LPTA) animal model DBA/1, BALB/C-Tg (*NF-κB-RE-luc* (Oslo)), carries a transgene containing three NF-κB response element sites from the Igk light chain promoter and modified firefly luciferase cDNA (Promega pGL-3). The reporter is inducible during inflammatory processes triggered by LPS and TNF-α. This model provides for the rapid study of transcriptional regulation of the NF-κB gene and the treatment of inflammatory diseases and cancer. Therefore, in this chapter, we will provide step-by-step methods on utilizing the *NF-κB-RE-luc* animal model. In addition, we will provide notes on effective compound administration and imaging strategies that have been proven effective in previous studies.

Key words: Anticancer drugs, Bioluminescence imaging, Bioluminescence, Luciferase, NF-κB

1. Introduction

Cancer can be described as the deregulation of control growth that can lead to tumorigenesis at distant sites. This process can be characterized by epigenetic changes, somatic mutations, and progressive cellular differentiation. On the micro level, there are several methods used to investigate the various mechanisms of cancer. Traditionally, investigators use immunoblotting, electrophoretic mobility-shift assay, and light microscopy to give insight to the changes that occur in the various stages of carcinogenesis. Immunoblotting is advantageous, in that it allows the investigator

Seetharama D. Satyanarayanajois (ed.), *Drug Design and Discovery: Methods and Protocols*,
Methods in Molecular Biology, vol. 716, DOI 10.1007/978-1-61779-012-6_10,

to observe changes that occur at the transcriptional, translational, and even posttranslational level. In addition, this technique is highly specific with the use of antibodies that can identify specific genetic sequences within the protein of interest. For example, Western blot analysis is often used to detect protein expression in various cellular fractions. This methodology is also useful in detecting posttranslational modifications such as phosphorylation. As a result, this technique can also give insight to the activation of signal transduction pathways that are present during cancer development. In addition, it shows how phosphorylated proteins may play a role in tumorigenesis. On the other hand, Northern and Southern blotting can be used to detect RNA and DNA expression, respectively. These techniques can reveal how gene activation and transcription can contribute to carcinogenesis as well.

Electrophoretic mobility-shift assay is another technique used to detect genetic changes that may contribute to carcinogenesis. This assay allows the investigator to monitor the DNA binding of transcription factors. In this assay, the sample is coincubated with DNA and separated electrophoretically. Radio-labeled hybridization allows for the detection of DNA binding of various transcription factors. Therefore, if the transcription factor binds, a shift occurs. The shift corresponds to the increased molecular weight of the DNA:protein complex, which in turn retards movement through the gel. Overall, these techniques can lead to the discovery of novel targets for cancer prevention.

On the whole body level, several modalities such as fluorescence imaging, computerized tomography (CT), magnetic resonance imaging (MRI), single photon emission computed tomography (SPECT), and positron emission tomography (PET) have been employed to monitor tumor progression (1). However, each method possesses both strengths and weaknesses. MRI and CT are more anatomical in the analysis of images of various organ structures within the body; whereas PET and SPECT image the physiological processes, therefore producing functional images (2). Nevertheless, many of these effective imaging strategies are not well-suited for small animals (1). In addition, these methods can be encumbering by both time and expense (2).

Nevertheless, bioluminescence is one of the most novel but effective approaches in the scientific world. Bioluminescence imaging is based on the sensitive detection of visible light produced during enzyme-mediated oxidation of a molecular substrate when the enzyme is expressed in vivo as a molecular reporter (3). Bioluminescence can be defined as the natural enzymatic ability to generate the release of photons of light. There are many species that produce enzymes that catalyze the oxidation of a substrate in order to emit photons. These enzymes are known as luciferases. There are various species that contain luciferases such as various strains of *Salmonella*, the Jack-O-Lantern mushroom (*Omphalotus olearius*), dinoflagellates, sea pansy (*Renilla reniformis*), and marine creatures such as Squid. The most popular species currently used is the firefly. Firefly luciferase has been shown in previous studies to limit fluctuations in imaging by remaining stable for the duration of the study. The strong signal emitted from luciferase is able to penetrate several millimeters to centimeters of tissue (4). One of the most common substrates used for bioluminescence is luciferin. One advantage of luciferin is that no toxicity has been shown to occur in previous studies following repeated administration. Substrates like luciferin are usually administered intraperitoneally or intravascularly depending on the research conducted. Luciferase converts luciferine into oxyluciferin in an ATP-dependent manner. As a result, only viable cancer cells contribute ATP to this process. Therefore, only metabolically active cells contribute to the bioluminescence measurements, increasing the selectivity of bioluminescence (2).

There are several advantages of using luciferase detection. This assay allows for the continuous study of disease progression from early (nonpalpable tumors) to the later stages of tumor metastasis (1). Therefore, this reporter gene system is advantageous in that, it allows the investigator to evaluate numerous drug therapies directed at various stages in the disease course (1). Several studies have proven that bioluminescence imaging is powerful and is a quantitative tool for the analysis of a broad range of cancer prevention therapies in living animals. This method of imaging is useful because it reduces equipment cost and scanning time. In addition, it allows for the scanning of multiple animals in a single image acquisition.

Bioluminescence is a very sensitive method. It allows the investigator to study a myriad of molecular interactions from host–pathogen interactions, to tumor models focusing on growth, metastasis, and therapeutic efficacy. In addition, previous studies have shown that bioluminescence imaging has high correlation with in vitro and in vivo studies (5). On the contrary, bioluminescence also gave insight into the presence of mutant genes, their function, and how these genes can potentially contribute to various diseases such as cancer. Bioluminescence is high-throughput (6). This method can also be used to assess real-time gene expression. To evaluate real-time gene expression, mice are engineered to express luciferase under the transcriptional control of promoters from the gene of interest. Therefore, compounds that can interfere with genomic binding may decrease the intensity of the bioluminescence, whereas other pharmacological agents that induce gene expression may increase intensity and give insight into other potential therapeutic targets. In addition, bioluminescence provides the advantage of imaging gene activation in multiple organ systems (5). Zangani et al. found that bioluminescence imaging provided signals from diseased organs several weeks before the clinical manifestations of symptoms occurred. In addition, they were able to analyze NF-κB activation in lymphoid organs, the large intestine, as well as from the kidney (5).

NF-κB is a transcription factor that has a unique role in carcinogenesis being that it is interwoven with inflammation as well. However, the molecular mechanism that contributes to this unique ability is often undefined (7). It has been suggested that the mRNA expression of cytokines that influence tumor growth may be modulated by transcriptional activation (7). NF-κB is a heterodimeric transcription factor composed of members of the Rel family of proteins, including p65 (Rel A), p50 (NF-κB1), p52 (NF-κB2), RelB, and c-Rel (8). NF-κB can be activated by various stimuli such as the binding of epidermal growth factor receptor, or via the Ras signaling transduction pathway. These pathways are constitutively active in various cancers including epidermal carcinomas, often causing these pathways to become pharmacological targets for novel therapies (9, 10). Oftentimes, assays such as electrophoretic mobility-shift assay and reporter-gene assays are used to examine the activation and function of various transcription factors, however these processes cannot be examined in vivo, and thus limit the understanding of protein function, composition, and activation throughout the various stages of carcinogenesis. Herein, we will provide step-by-step instructions on how to utilize bioluminescence imaging as a tool for detecting NF-κB expression in the selection of anti-NF-κB drug candidates.

2. Materials

2.1. Animal Model

1. Male *NF-κB-RE-luc* (Oslo) mice (Xenogen Corporation; Alameda, CA) (see Notes 1 and 2).

2.2. Reagents

1. Lipopolysaccharide (LPS): 2.7 mg/kg dose (see Note 3).
2. Ethanol Extraction of drug candidates: 15 mg/mL stock in 95% ethanol (for ethanol extractions only).
3. Ketamine: 3 mL. Store at room temperature.
4. Xylazine: 0.5 mL. Store at room temperature.
5. Normal Saline: 26.5 mL. Store at room temperature.
6. Luciferin: 150 mg.

2.3. Equipment

1. IVIS^{100} Series Imaging System (Caliper Life Sciences, Hopkinton, MA).

3. Methods

3.1. NF-κB Activation

1. Lipopolysaccharide (LPS): 2.7 mg/kg to activate NF-κB.
2. Inject *NF-κB-RE-luc* (Oslo) mice intraperitoneally every other day with vehicle or the compound of interest for 1 week.
3. The mice should be imaged on the IVIS[100] series imaging system at 3 and 24 h after LPS injection (see Note 4).

3.2. Compound (Drug Candidate) Preparation

1. Ethanol Extraction: prepare 15 mg/mL stock in 95% ethanol (see Note 5).
2. Determine the concentration of the extract and dilute 1:20 in sterile PBS.
3. Prepare the dose based on a 0.1 mL/25 g dosing chart (see Note 6).
4. Inject the mice intraperitoneally with 0.1 mL/25 g body weight with vehicle or the compound of interest.
5. Administer the vehicle/drug every other day for 1 week prior to LPS injection.
6. The last dose should be given within 30 min prior to the LPS injection.
7. Initially, noninvasive imaging of NF-κB activity should be taken at 3 and 24 h following LPS injection (see Note 7).

3.3. Imaging

3.3.1. Anesthesia

1. Ketamine: 3 mL. Store at room temperature.
2. Xylazine: 0.5 mL. Store at room temperature.
3. Normal Saline: 16.5 mL. Store at room temperature.
4. Dose 0.1 mL/10 g body weight.

3.3.2. Luciferase

1. 150 mg of luciferin.
2. 10 mL of Normal Saline.
3. Dose: 0.3 mL of luciferin per 30 g body weight.

3.3.3. Imaging Using the IVIS[100] Imaging System

1. Launch Living Image Software and initialize the IVIS[100] Imaging System.
2. Sanitize work area, as well as, the inside chamber of the IVIS[100] Imaging System with Clidox.
3. Anesthetize the mouse (ketamine/xylazine cocktail).
4. Inject luciferase intraperitoneally approximately 0.1 mL/10 g of mouse's body mass.
5. Allow for an uptake period of 3–5 min and begin scanning the mouse/mice. Be sure to position the mouse/mice in the

chamber to allow for maximum data collection. Image for 60 s using the bioluminescence option (see Note 8).

6. Label and save data to an appropriate folder. Once all data is collected, quantify the data using Living Image Software.
7. Place mice on heating pad under a light source. The animals should be monitored until the mice regain consciousness.
8. Once consciousness is regained, return mice to their home cage.

3.3.4. Quantitation of Bioluminescence Imaging

1. Click on Living Image Software icon on the desktop screen.
2. Click on Living Image within the toolbar, and select Load LI Data (Ctrl+2). This will allow the user to upload the bioluminescence data to Living Image Software. Select the specific image that will be quantitated.
3. The uploaded image will be accompanied by various parameters (i.e., max bar, min bar, overlay, etc.)
4. *Max Bar/Min Bar.* Changes in the values of the Max/Min Bar will allow the user to modulate the imaging and background intensities. Decreasing the Max Bar lowers the threshold for maximum intensity. Conversely, increasing the Max Bar increases the threshold for maximum intensity. However, the value obtained for counts/photons does not change. Decreasing the Min Bar lowers the threshold for minimum intensity. This causes an increase in background noise that may become problematic when obtaining a region of interest (ROI) measurement. Therefore, to decrease background noise, the minimum intensity should be increased.
5. *Creating a ROI.* There are four shapes that can be used to create a ROI circle, square, contour, and grid. Once chosen, these shapes can be modified to encompass the specific region of choice. Previous experiments have shown that the square option is beneficial in analyzing imaging of the lungs; whereas the circle has been proven to be advantageous in analysis of the thoracic cavity. However, these options are dependent on the interest of the investigator. Once the shape has been chosen, the user has the option of creating either one ROI at a time or multiple ROIs at once. Under the Create tab, there is a menu that allows the user to create 1–10 ROIs or the user has the option of Auto1 or Auto All. Once the correct ROI parameters have been selected, click on the Create tab and the ROI(s) will appear. As mentioned before, the user can modify the shape and even the location of the ROI according to the investigator's interest. Once the proper ROIs have been selected and located, click on the Measure tab. Once the ROI has been measured, a value will appear.

6. *Removal of created ROI.* The user has the option of removing a previously created ROI. Under the Remove tab, there is an option to remove All, All Meas, All Auto, All Bkg, All Subj, ROI 1-the maximum number of ROIs that exist. After this option has been selected, click on the Remove tab, to remove the created ROI(s).
7. *Quantitation of data.* Once the measurement has been made the values will appear. The user has the option of expressing the data in units of counts or photons. Counts are used as a measurement of radiating photons represented in pixels from the raw data of the image. The units for counts are expressed as photons/s (11). On the other hand, the data can be expressed in units of photons. Photons are used as a calibrated measurement of the actual photons being emitted from the source sample (i.e., animal, cells within the petri dish, etc.) The units for photons are expressed as photons/s/cm^2/sr (11). Once these values have been obtained, the data can be exported into Microsoft Excel for further analysis.
8. *Data exportation.* Data can be exported to an analysis software such as Microsoft Excel. To export the imaging data, select the Measurement window. Once select, the user can click the configure tab. The Configure option allows the user to select the measurement parameters to be exported. Select the specific parameters, measurement type, and ROI dimensions. Once selected, this window can be closed. Next click the Export tab, and save the file to the proper drive. Once saved, the user can open the data in the analysis software of choice.
9. *Data analysis.* Analysis software such as Microsoft Excel presents a Text ImportWizard that allows the user to choose how the imaging data will be displayed. Once this has been performed, the data can be presented as units (photons/s, if using counts; or photons/s/cm^2/sr if using photons) on the ordinate vs. the various treatment groups on the abscissa. Statistical analysis can be performed using Prism 3.0 software, or a statistical analysis software of choice.

4. Notes

1. *Standard conditions for animal model.* Mice should be housed in a temperature- and humidity-controlled AAALAC facility with a 12-h light/dark cycle. Mice should be allowed access to food and water ad libitum. All procedures should be approved by the Institutional Animal Care and Use Committee in accordance with NIH guidelines.

2. *Nonresponders.* Nonresponders can occur; therefore animals should be genotyped to determine the transgenicity.
3. *LPS induction of NF-κB.* LPS (2.7 mg/kg body weight) given intraperitoneally has been used to induce NF-κB activity.
4. *Determining how long after drug administration should LPS be administered.* We have found that 10–20 min after drug treatment, LPS should be administered intraperitoneally.
5. *Drug administration.* Dietary administration, so far, has been the ideal route of administration. This route of administration provides constant drug exposure and provides more dramatic effects on NF-κB activity. We have found that giving similar doses by oral gavage resulted in a high incidence of mortality before the animals could be imaged.
6. *Pretreatment body weight.* Animals should be weighed daily and on the day of imaging.
7. *Using multiple time points to image mice.* This may become problematic if not given the adequate recovery time. Imaging time intervals should be greater than 2 h in between imaging. It has been found in previous experiments that repeated dosing and imaging at 2 h or less decreases the chances of recovery from sequential dosing of anesthesia.
8. *Animal model usage.* This animal model can be used repeatedly for various experiments. However, each animal should be imaged prior to drug treatment to establish the proper baseline level of NF-κB activity. Also, allow a 5–7 day "washout" period to allow for proper drug excretion. This time may vary depending on the pharmacokinetics of the drug. In addition, animals should be imaged between experiments to provide a background control. It is important to note that in this animal model, previous studies have shown higher levels of intensity in the lymph nodes around the neck region, thymus, and Peyer's patches (4).

Acknowledgments

The authors would like to acknowledge Tracee Terry, Heather Kleiner-Hancock, Ph.D., Michael Mathis, Ph.D., and the LSU Health Sciences Center Animal Facility in Shreveport, LA for their support.

References

1. Contag, C.H., Jenkins, D.,Contag P.R., and Negrin, R.S. (2000) Use of reporter genes for optical measurements of neoplastic diseases In vivo. *Neoplasia* **2**: 41–52.
2. Klerk, C.P., Overmeer, R.M., Niers, T.M.H., Versteeg, H.H., Richel, D.J., Buckle, T., et al. (2007) Validity of bioluminescence measurements for noninvasive in vivo imaging of tumor load in small animals. *Biotechniques* **43**: 7–13.
3. Sadikot, R.T. and Blackwell, T.S. (2005) Bioluminescence imaging. *Proc Am Thorac Soc* **2**: 537–540.
4. Sato, A., Klaunberg, B., and Tolwani, R. (2004) In vivo bioluminescence imaging. *Comp Med* **54**: 631–634.
5. Zangani, M., Carlsen, H., Kielland, A., Os, A., Hauglin, H., Blomhoff, R., et al. (2009) Tracking early autoimmune disease by bioluminescent imaging of NF-κB activation reveals pathology in multiple organ systems. *Am J Pathol* **174**: 1358–1367.
6. Kim, S.B., Ozawa, T., Walanabe, S., and Umezawa, Y. (2004) High-throughput sensing and noninvasive imaging of protein nuclear transport by using reconstitution of split *Renilla* luciferase. *Proc Natl Acad Sci USA* **101**: 11542–11547.
7. Ondrey, F., Dong, G., Sunwoo, J., Chen, Z., Wolf, J.S., Crowl-Bancroft, C.V., et al. (1999) Constitutive activation of transcription factors NF-κB, AP-1 and NF-IL6 in human head and neck squamous cell carcinoma cell lines that express proinflammatory and proangiogenic cytokines. *Mol Carcinog* **26**: 119–129.
8. Baldwin, A.S. (1996) The NF-κB and IκB proteins: New discoveries and insights. *Annu Rev Immunol* **14**: 649–683.
9. He, Y., Zeng, Q., Drenning, S.D., Melhem, M.F., Tweardy, D.J., Huang, L., et al. (1998) Inhibition of human squamous cell carcinoma growth in vivo by epidermal growth factor receptor antisense RNA transcribed from the U6 promoter. *J Natl Cancer Inst* **90**: 1080–1087.
10. Sun, L. and Carpenter, G. (1998) Epidermal growth factor activation of NF-κB is mediated through IκBα degradation and intracellular free calcium. *Oncogene* **16**: 2095–2102.
11. Xenogen Corporation. (2006) Xenogen Living Image Software Manual **2.6**. Xenogen Corporation, San Francisco, CA.

Chapter 11

Evaluation of Anticancer Agents Using Flow Cytometry Analysis of Cancer Stem Cells

Vineet Gupta, Qian-Jin Zhang, and Yong-Yu Liu

Abstract

Flow cytometry can sensitively detect and efficiently sort cells based on fluorescent signals integrated into cellular markers of proteins or DNA. It has been broadly applied to assess cell division, apoptosis and to isolate cells including stem cells. As the seeds for tumorigenesis and metastasis, cancer stem cells (CSCs) are often more resistant to cytotoxins and anticancer agents than other heterogeneous cells in tumors. Analyzing CSCs under treatments is an effective way to evaluate new therapeutic agents for cancers. We introduce a method using flow cytometry to assess breast CSCs ($CD44^{+}/CD24^{-/low}$) in human MCF-7/Dox breast cancer cells, after the treatment of mixed-backbone oligonucleotide against glucosylceramide synthase. Flow cytometry analysis of CSCs is a reliable, effective, and easy-handling approach to screen agents targeting CSCs.

Key words: Cancer stem cells, CD44, CD2, Flow cytometry, Glucosylceramide synthase, Mixed-backbone oligonucleotide

1. Introduction

Tumorigenesis and cancer progression depend on a small subset of cancer cells known as cancer stem cells (CSCs). In addition to initiating primary tumors, CSCs are the seeds of tumor metastasis and relapse after clinical remission (1, 2). Besides sharing the same properties of normal adult stem cells in self-renewal and generation of diverse cells, CSCs display cancerous characteristics and are resistant to cytotoxins (3). In human breast cancer, the cells with $CD44^{+}/CD24^{-/low}$ markers are identified as breast cancer stem cells (BCSCs) (4). These cells are more resistant to anticancer agents and radiation than other heterogeneous cells in tumors (5, 6). Thus, the significant drug resistance with cancerous stemness earmarks CSCs as novel targets for cancer treatments (7, 8).

Seetharama D. Satyanarayanajois (ed.), *Drug Design and Discovery: Methods and Protocols*,
Methods in Molecular Biology, vol. 716, DOI 10.1007/978-1-61779-012-6_11,

Analysis of CSCs under treatments becomes a more effective way to evaluate new therapeutic agents for cancers. Here, we describe a method using flow cytometry to assess BCSCs in an established cell line after the treatment of mixed-backbone oligonucleotide (MBO-asGCS) against glucosylceramide synthase (GCS) (9). Based on specific stem cell markers, such as $CD44^{+}/CD24^{-/low}$, flow cytometry can quantitatively determine the alterations of BCSCs after treatments (4, 5, 10). Established cancer cell lines that are enriched with CSCs have been broadly used as sources to study the properties of stem cells (5, 11). Human MCF-7/Dox breast cancer cell line has greater than 20% of side-population cells or $CD44^{+}/CD24^{-/low}$ cells as we assessed. MCF-7/Dox cells grow well in standard culture condition. The use of MCF-7/Dox cells, rather than the isolated BCSCs, allows directly assessing the effects of agents on BCSCs in a simple procedure.

We use MBO-asGCS as an example of agents that disrupt CSCs. GCS catalyzes the first glycosylation of ceramide in glycosphingolipid synthesis and has a vital role in mouse embryo development (12, 13). Enhanced capacity of ceramide glycosylation allows human embryonic stem cells growth (14). Our works suggest that MBO-asGCS can effectively disrupt BCSCs (unpublished data). MBO-asGCS treatment significantly decreases BCSCs (13.84 vs. 20.59) detected by flow cytometry analysis and immunostaining of CD44/CD24.

Taken together, the flow cytometry analysis of CSCs presented is a reliable, effective, and easy-handling approach to screen new agent to target CSCs.

2. Materials

1. Drug-resistant MCF-7/Dox human breast cancer cells (University of Texas, M.D. Anderson Cancer Center, Houston, TX). MCF-7/Dox cells were derived from the parental drug-sensitive MCF-7 human breast cancer cells by stepwise selection with doxorubicin (15).
2. RPMI-1640 medium (Invitrogen, Carlsbad, CA): supplemented with 10% fetus bovine serum (FBS) (Hyclone, Logan UT), 100 U/mL penicillin, 100 μg/mL streptomycin, and 584 mg/L l-glutamine.
3. Phosphate-Buffered Saline (PBS): pH 7.4 prepared by 10 times dilution of PBS (10×) with distilled water following autoclave sterilization.
4. 0.25% Trypsin with EDTA·4Na (Invitrogen).
5. Lipofectamine™2000 (Invitrogen).

6. Opti-MEM I reduced-serum medium (Invitrogen).
7. An MBO was designed to target the ORF 18–37 of human GCS and designated as MBO-asGCS. A scrambled control had the same chemical components as MBO-asGCS, but no sequence specificity designated as MBO-SC. MBOs were purified by reverse-phase HPLC and desalting after synthesis (Integrated DNA Technologies, Inc., Coralville, IA) (9, 16). MBOs were dissolved in sterile water in 150 μM and stored at −80°C after aliquot.
8. Blocking buffer: 5% goat serum in PBS.
9. FITC anti-human CD44 antibody (BioLegend, San Diego, CA) (25 μg in 100 μL); Alexa Fluor® 647 anti-mouse CD24 antibody (Cat. 101817, BioLegend) (25 μg in 100 μL).
10. Polystyrene round bottom test tubes (5 mL, 12×75 mm) (BD Bioscience, San Jose, CA) are used as the flow-cytometer tube.
11. Sheath Fluid (BD Bioscience).
12. BD FACSCalibur™ Flow Cytometer equipped with lasers argon (L1) and red diode (L2) (BD Bioscience).
13. Software in BD FACSCalibur: BD CellQuest Pro (BD Bioscience).
14. BD Falcon 4-well CultureSlide (BD Bioscience).
15. Mouse anti-human CD44 monoclonal antibody (Cat. C7923, Sigma-Aldrich) (200 μg/mL).
16. Rabbit anti-human CD24 polyclonal antibody (FL-80) (Cat. SC-11406, Santa Cruz Biotechnology, Santa Cruz, CA) (200 μg/mL).
17. Alexa Fluor®488 goat anti-rabbit IgG (H+L) (2 mg/mL in 0.5 mL) (Cat. A-11008, Invitrogen).
18. Alexa Fluor®555 goat anti-mouse IgG (H+L) (2 mg/mL in 0.5 mL) (Cat. A-21422, Invitrogen).
19. VECTASHIELD Mounting Medium with DAPI (4′, 6-diamidino-2-phenylindole) (Vector Laboratories Inc., Burlingame, CA).

3. Methods

3.1. Cells Treated with MBO-asGCS

1. Seed MCF-7/Dox cells (~2×10^6 cells) in 100 mm tissue culture dishes and add 10 mL of 10% FBS RPMI 1640 medium per dish.
2. Culture the cells at 37°C in a CO_2 incubator until the cells achieve 70–80% confluence. This usually takes 18–24 h.

3. Prepare transfection solution in two 15-mL sterile test tubes:

   Solution A: add 8 μL of MBO-asGCS stock solution (150 μM) into 3 mL Opti-MEM I medium, to prepare 3 mL of 200 nM MBO-asGCS solution per dish.

   Solution B: add 20 μL of Lipofectamine 2000 into 3 mL Opti-MEM I medium to prepare 3 mL liposome solution per dish.
4. Gently shake the Solutions A and Solution B and stand them still at room temperature (~26°C) for 5 min.
5. Gently mix Solution A and B together in one tube and stand it still at room temperature for 20 min to form MBO-liposome complex. For Vehicle control, Solution B is mixed with additional 3 mL Opti-MEM I medium.
6. During this period (see step 5 above), remove the medium from the cell dishes (see step 2 in the Subheading 3.1) and rinse the cells once with 10 mL of sterile PBS.
7. Slowly drop the transfection solutions (see step 5 in Subheading 3.1) into cell dishes with gently shaking. Experimental dishes are transfected with MBO-asGCS/ Lipofectamine, and the Vehicle dish is mock-transfected with Lipofectamine only.
8. Incubate the cells in dishes at 37°C for 5 h in a CO_2 incubator.
9. Add 20% FBS RPMI 1640 medium, 6 mL per dish. The final concentration of FBS will be 10% in medium with 100 U/ mL penicillin, 100-μg/mL streptomycin, and 584 mg/L l-glutamine.
10. Continuously culture cells for an additional 48 h, and then analyze the cells using flow cytometry and immunostaining.

3.2. Sample Preparation

1. Remove medium from the cell dishes (see step 10 in Subheading 3.1), and detach cells by spreading 500 μL of 0.25% trypsin-EDTA to the dishes.
2. Add 10 mL PBS to collect all cells from each dish and spin down cells in 15-mL tubes, 720 rcf, and at room temperature for 5 min.
3. Resuspend the cell pellets in PBS at a density of 10^6 cells/100 μL. Prepare two vials (10^6 cells/100 μL in 1.5-mL Eppendorf tube) for each sample.
4. Add 5 μL of FITC-CD44 and 5 μL of Alexa647-CD24 antibodies into each cell tube marked the Stained. Add 10 μL of PBS into the Unstained tubes.
5. Incubate the cells with the fluorescent antibodies for 30 min at 4°C in refrigerator. Cells are covered with aluminum foil to prevent fluorescence quenching (see Note 1).

6. Spin down the cells at 720 rcf, room temperature for 10 min. Resuspend the cell pellets in 1 mL of PBS and spin down the cells.
7. Resuspend the cell pellets in 1 mL of PBS and transfer into the flow-cytometer tubes on ice and cover with aluminum foil. These samples including the Unstained Vehicle, Vehicle, Unstained MBO-SC, MBO-SC, Unstained MBO-asGCS, and MBO-asGCS are ready for flow cytometer analysis (see Note 2).

3.3. Analysis of BCSCs by Flow Cytometer

3.3.1. Start-Up Flow Cytometer

1. Open the front lid of the flow cytometer (BD FACSCalibur), fill the sheath fluid, and empty the waste tank.
2. Turn on the cytometer, and then turn on the computer.
3. In the front lid of cytometer, turn switch from the Change Tank position to the Pressurize position.

3.3.2. Create Experimental Windows

1. Open the CellQuest Pro program from the computer. An untitled document with Tool Palette will automatically appear. The following steps will create an experimental window (Fig. 1).
2. Click Acquire from the Menu bar, select Connect to Cytometer. A Browser Window will appear. This step connects cytometer to computer.

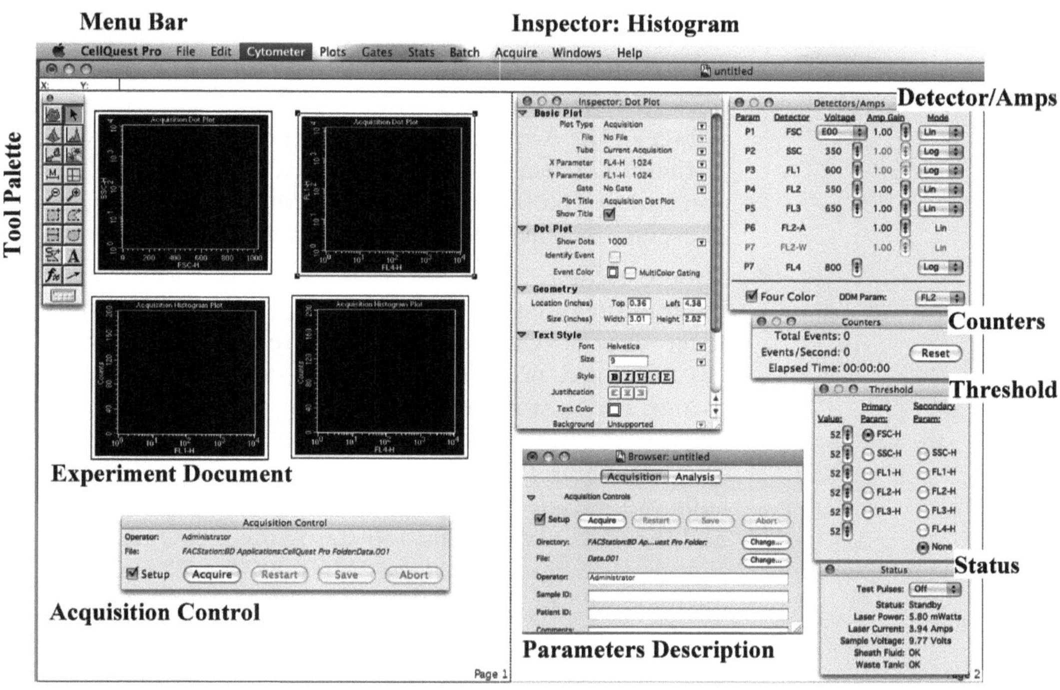

Fig. 1. Analysis parameters in the CellQuest program. A typical experiment of flow cytometry assay in the dot and contour plots is settled with parameters in the detector/amps, threshold, counters, and acquisition control windows.

3. Click Cytometer followed by selecting Detector/Amps from the Menu bar. In the Detector/Amps window, check Four Color and select FL2 for DDM Param. This step will allow FL4 Detector showing in the Detectors/Amps window.
4. Click the Dot Plot icon from the Tool Palette or click Plots followed by selecting Dot Plot from the Menu bar. Customize the plot size in the untitled document. In this step, an Inspector:Dot Plot window will automatically appear. In this window, change Analysis to Acquisition position. Select FSC-H 1024 and Lin for X Parameter and SSC-H 1024 and Log for Y Parameter in the Inspector:Dot Plot window. Thus, the FSC on *X*-axis and SSC on *Y*-axis (FSC vs. SSC) will be shown in the dot plot window. This dot plot will be used to detect all cells.
5. Repeat step 4 to establish second dot plot for detecting two colors of fluorescence (green and red). Select FL1 1024 for green color (FITC) and FL4 1024 for red color (Alexa Fluor® 647) in the Inspector:Dot Plot window. The dot plot window will show the Alexa Fluor® 647-CD24 on *X*-axis and FITC-CD44 on *Y*-axis (FL4 vs. FL1).
6. Click Cytometer from the Menu bar, and select Detector/Amps, Threshold, Status, and Counters separately. This will allow appearing four different windows. These parameters include detector/amps need to be adjusted while analyzing the samples. Keep all these windows aside the experiment document.
7. Click Acquire from the Menu bar and select Acquisition. The storage of the Acquisition and storage dialog box will appear. In the box, select acquisition gate accept, all events, collection criteria 10,000 of all events are counted and storage gate all events, and then click on OK (Fig. 1).
8. Choose Acquire from the Menu bar and select Parameter Description and a new window will appear. In the window, select change Directory button, create a new folder as "BCSC," and provide the location for this folder. Select change File, a window of File Name Editor will appear. In Custom Prefix, provide the file name as "MCF-7/DOX." The File Name Prefix will be Custom Prefix and File Name Suffix will be File Count. In the File Count put "1" and click on OK. Once data acquisition starts, the CellQuest Pro will automatically save the data as "MCF-7/Dox 1" (FCS file) in the folder of "BCSC."

3.3.3. Data Acquisition

1. From the Tool Palette, select the quadrant marker and divide the second dot plot (FL4 vs. FL1) in four quadrants (Fig. 2).

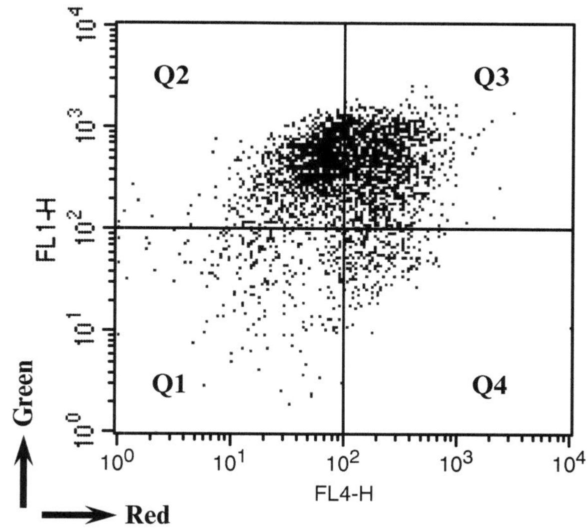

Fig. 2. A dot plot for double-fluorescence cell assay. In the dot plot, the *X*-axis and the *Y*-axis represent the FL4 (red, Alexa647) and the FL1 (green, FITC), respectively. The dot plot is divided into four quadrants (Q1, Q2, Q3, and Q4). The quadrant Q1 will have the green-negative and red-negative cells, Q3 will have the green-positive and red-positive cells. The Q2, the green-positive and red-negative cells; the Q4, the green-negative and red-positive cells.

Q1. Lower left quadrant (LL), showing both negative cells

Q2. Upper left quadrant (UL), showing green-positive cells

Q3. Upper right quadrant (UR), showing both positive cells

Q4. Lower right quadrant (LR), showing red-positive cells

2. Adjust the parameters (Voltage and Amp Gain in the Detector/Amps window) while analyzing the Unstained cells. The same parameters should be used for the stained cells. These parameters should be adjusted every time when analyzing different types of cells or cells treaded in different conditions (see Notes 3 & 4).
3. Put the unstained sample, "unstained vehicle" (see step 7 in Subheading 3.2) in the Sample port of the cytometer (see Note 3).
4. Change the cytometer in Run mode, and Speed Low.
5. Go into the Acquisition Control window and check for the Setup box.
6. Click on the Acquire now. This will allow us to view samples in all the plots and adjust the instrument settings.
7. While looking at the sample in the first dot plot (FSC vs. SSC), adjust the Voltage and Amp Gain in the Detector/ Amps window to make sure all events are in this plot. Then, looking at the second dot plot (FL4 vs. FL1), adjust the

Voltage and the Amp Gain from the Detector/Amps window, until entire events in the first quadrant Q1 (Fig. 2).

8. Look in the contour plots, and make sure that peak in the contour plots with the filter FL1 and the FL4 in the left. Otherwise, adjust the Voltage in the Detector/Amps to position the peak in the left side of the contour plots.
9. After necessary changes in the instrument settings, click on the Pause and then the Abort in the Acquisition Control window.
10. Uncheck the Setup box, file name "MCF-7/Dox 1" will appear in the Acquisition Control window. Click on the Acquire button in the Acquisition Control.
11. Once cytometer finishes counting of the 10,000 events, the CellQuest Pro will automatically save the counting data of "unstained vehicle" in the file "MCF-7/Dox 1" and the "BCSC" folder. For the Unstained samples, these cells should be in the lower left quadrant, Q1.
12. The file named "MCF-7/Dox 2" for next sample will automatically appear in the Acquisition Control window, once cytometer finishes last counting. It is necessary to analyze the stained sample using the same instrument settings as unstained one. Put the Stained sample, "vehicle" in the Sample port (see step 7 in Subheading 3.2) and repeat the steps 10 and 11 in Subheading 3.3.3 to acquire the data for the Vehicle. The counting data for the "vehicle" will be automatically saved as "MCF-7/Dox 2" (see Notes 5 & 6).
13. Repeat the steps 3–11 in Subheading 3.3.3 with the sample of "unstained MBO-SC" to acquire the data for the "unstained MBO-SC." The counting data for the "unstained MBO-SC" will be automatically saved as "MCF-7/Dox 3."
14. Repeat the steps 3–11 in Subheading 3.3.3 to acquire the data for the "MBO-SC." The counting data for the "MBO-SC" will be automatically saved as "MCF-7/Dox 4."
15. Repeat the steps 3–11 in Subheading 3.3.3 with the sample of "unstained MBO-SC" to acquire the data for the "unstained MBO-SC." The counting data for the "unstained MBO-SC" will be automatically saved as "MCF-7/Dox 5."
16. Repeat the steps 3–11 in Subheading 3.3.3 to acquire the data for the "MBO-SC." The counting data for the "MBO-SC" will be automatically saved as "MCF-7/Dox 6" (see Note 7).

3.3.4. Data Analysis

1. Choose plot from the Menu and select Dot Plot. This will open the Plot Inspector window. In the Plot Inspector window, click on the Select File and choose the file name (MCF-7/Dox 1) for analysis.
2. Once the data appear on the dot plot, select the FL4 on *X*-axis and the FL1 on *Y*-axis.

3. From the Tool Palette, select the Quadrant icon, divide the plot into four quadrants and adjust dividing lines to locate the unstained cell sample in the both negative quadrant (Q1) (Fig. 3a, b).
4. In the Pool Palette, select the Rectangular icon, place the cursor in the desired quadrant, and create a region around that quadrant. To deselect a region, click on the region in the plot and the Delete in the Menu bar.
5. In the Stats, select the Region Stats in the Menu. A Region Stats window will appear, and it will provide us the events in desired region from the total 10,000 events.

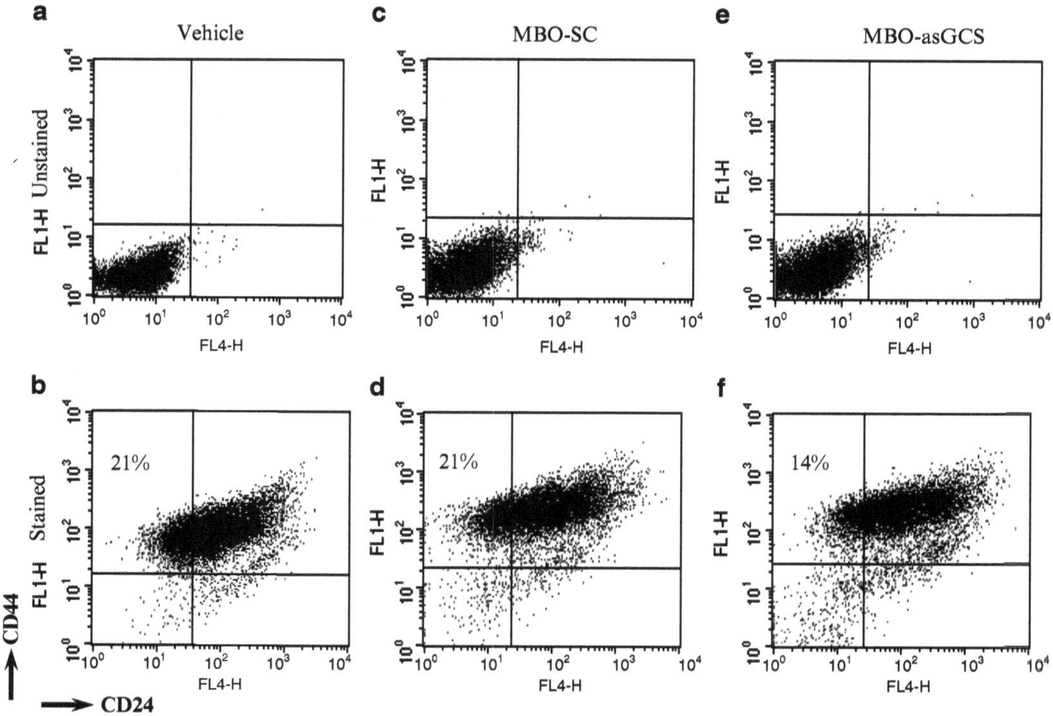

Fig. 3. Effects of MBO-asGCS on BCSCs (CD44+/CD24−/low). MCF-7/Dox cells were exposed to MBO-asGCS or MBO-SC (200 nM) for 48 h and incubated with FITC-CD44 and Alex647-CD24 antibodies. (**a**) Unstained cells for the vehicle. Cells cultured in the absence of MBOs (lipofectamine, vehicle) were used to settle the parameters for cell assay, and all the cells are in the quadrant 1 (Q1). (**b**) Stained vehicle. Cells cultured in the absence of MBOs (lipofectamine, vehicle) were incubated with FITC-CD44 and Alexa647-CD24 antibodies. The BCSC population (Q2) is 20.59 ± 1.92%, from triplicate assay. (**c**) Unstained cells for MBO-SC treatment. Cells treated with MBO-SC were used to settle the parameters, and all the cells are in quadrant 1(Q1). (**d**) Stained cells for MBO-SC treatment. Cells treated with MBO-SC were incubated with FITC-CD24 and Alexa647-CD44 antibodies. The BCSC population in the quadrant 2 (Q2) is 20.69 ± 1.44%, from triplicate assay. (**e**) Unstained cells for MBO-asGCS treatment. Cells treated with MBO-asGCS were used to settle the parameters and all the cells are in the quadrant 1 (Q1). (**f**) Stained cells for MBO-asGCS treatment. Cells treated with MBO-asGCS were incubated with FITC-CD24 and Alexa647-CD44 antibodies. The BCSC population in the quadrant 2 (Q2) is 13.84 ± 0.4%, from triplicate assay; $P < 0.001$ as compared to the vehicle (**b**).

6. Repeat the steps 1–5 in Subheading 3.3.4 with the file of "MCF-7/Dox 2" to generate the dot plot for the "vehicle." The same fashion of quadrants and the desired region generated from the sample of "unstained vehicle" should be used for the "vehicle." The cells in the rectangular region of the Quadrants 2 (Q2) are designated as BCSCs and the percentage of these cells after reduced the Unstained (see step 5 in Subheading 3.3.4) is presented with the dot plot (Fig. 3c).
7. Repeat the steps 1–6 in Subheading 3.3.4 with the files of "MCF-7/Dox 3" and "MCF-7/Dox 4" to create the dot plots for the "unstained MBO-SC" and "MBO-SC" (Figs. 3c, d).
8. Repeat the steps 1–6 in Subheading 3.3.4 with the files of "MCF-7/Dox 5" and "MCF-7/Dox 6" to create the dot plots for the "unstained MBO-asGCS" and "MBO-asGCS" (Fig. 3e, f).

3.4. Analysis of BCSCs by Immunostaining

1. Seed the cells (25,000 cell/chamber) in four-chamber slide and add 0.4 mL of 10% FBS RPMI 1640 medium and culture cells for 24 h.
2. Flip the medium out, and rinse the cells with 400 μL of PBS.
3. After rinsing, fix the cells with 400 μL of ice-cold methanol at 4°C for 5 min.
4. Flip the methanol out and keep the chamber upside down on paper towel and dry it in air for 5 min.
5. Rinse the chambers with 400 μL of PBS, 5 min for 3 times, to rehydrate the cells.
6. Add 400 μL of blocking solution (5% goat serum in PBS) and incubate at room temperature for 30 min.
7. Flip the blocking solution out and add 250 μL of primary antibody solution. Mouse anti-human CD44 and rabbit antihuman CD24 antibodies are diluted with the blocking solution in 1:100.
8. Keep the slide on wet paper towel in plastic box to incubate at 4°C in refrigerator, overnight.
9. Remove the antibody solution and wash the chambers with 400 μL of PBS for 5 min, 3 times.
10. Add 250 μL of the secondary antibody solution into the chamber slides. The Alexa Fluo®488 goat anti-rabbit IgG (H+L) (for CD24) and Alexa Fluor®555 goat anti-mouse IgG (H+L) (for CD44) are diluted with the blocking solution in 1:1,000.
11. Incubate slides covered with aluminum foil at room temperature for 1 h (see Note 1).

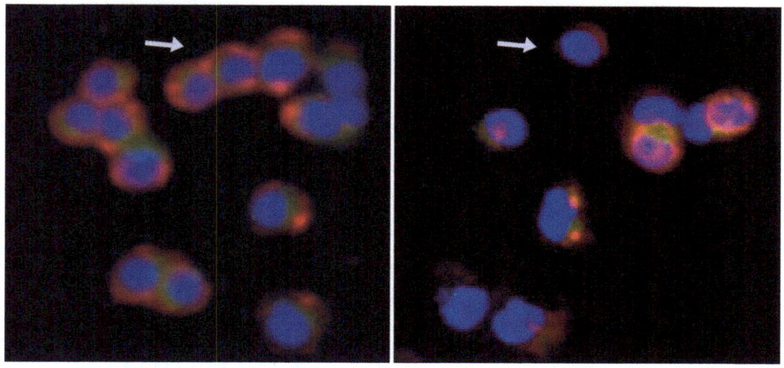

Fig. 4. Fluorescent immunostaining of $CD44^{+}/CD24^{-/low}$ cells. MCF-7/Dox cells were treated with MBO-asGCS (200 nM, 48 h) or vehicle (lipofectamine) and stained with BCSC markers. *Green* represents the Alexa488-CD24; *red*, Alexa555-CD44; *blue*, DAPI. *Arrow heads* indicate the $CD44^{+}/CD24^{-}$ cells of BCSCs.

12. Remove the second antibody solution and wash the slides with 400 μL of PBS for 5 min and 3 times.
13. Remove the chambers from slide with the Remove Tool and observe the slides under fluorescent microscope to visualize the slide background.
14. Drop the VECTASHIELD Mounting Medium to cover cell section. This is for nucleus-counter staining and preventing fluorescence quenching. Use the slips to cover slides.
15. Observe slides under Olympus IX71 microscope coupled with digital camera (DP71). Images are captured using Olympus DP controller software (Fig. 4).

4. Notes

1. Fluorescence antibodies are susceptible to light, it is necessary to avoid the exposure to light. Once the fluorescent antibodies are applied to the cells, use aluminum foil to cover the tubes or slides.
2. Immediately analyze cell samples. Once the antibody incubation is completed, it is always advisable to start the flow cytometer assay.
3. It is necessary to vortex sample just before placing it to the Sample Port. It can decrease cell clumps and avoid block of the Sample Port.
4. Adjust the parameters with unstained cells every time, before you start to acquire data for different cell line or cells treated

with different conditions. Each cell line or treatment has its own cell sizes and internal complexity that determine the cell signals detected by cytometer.

5. It is necessary to measure the BCSCs for each sample in triplicate. For data acquisition, apply the same parameters and the same tube of sample, and repeat the Subheading 3.3.3, step 12 two times to acquire counting data for the stained sample. In data analysis, repeat the Subheading 3.3.4, step 6 two times to generate the data for the Region Stats for the triplet.
6. For many groups of samples, note down the order of data acquisition to prevent confusion. The CellQuest Pro program saves the files under the same name plus counting order, such as "MCF-7/Dox 1," "MCF-7/Dox 2," and "MCF-7/Dox 3" in the recent analysis.
7. Once the sample is analyzed (see step 11 in Subheading 3.3.3), always put the cytometer on the Stand-by mode to save the laser use.

Acknowledgments

This work was supported by United State Public Health Service/NIH grant P20 RR16456 (Y.Y.L) and grant 5G12RR026260-02 (Q.J.Z) from NCRR. We thank Dr. Benny Blaylock and Dr. Sharon Meyer (College of Pharmacy, University of Louisiana at Monroe) for their kind advices on flow cytometer.

References

1. Reya, T., Morrison, S. J., Clarke, M. F., and Weissman, I. L. (2001) Stem cells, cancer, and cancer stem cells. *Nature.* **414**: 105–11.
2. Dalerba, P., Cho, R. W., and Clarke, M. F. (2007) Cancer stem cells: models and concepts. *Annu Rev Med.* **58**: 267–84.
3. Visvader, J. E., and Lindeman, G. J. (2008) Cancer stem cells in solid tumours: accumulating evidence and unresolved questions. *Nat Rev Cancer.* **8**: 755–68.
4. Al-Hajj, M., Wicha, M. S., Benito-Hernandez, A., Morrison, S. J., and Clarke, M. F. (2003) Prospective identification of tumorigenic breast cancer cells. *Proc Natl Acad Sci U S A.* **100**: 3983–8.
5. Fillmore, C. M., and Kuperwasser, C. (2008) Human breast cancer cell lines contain stem-like cells that self-renew, give rise to phenotypically diverse progeny and survive chemotherapy. *Breast Cancer Res.* **10**: R25.
6. Phillips, T. M., McBride, W. H., and Pajonk, F. (2006) The response of CD24(-/low)/CD44+ breast cancer-initiating cells to radiation. *J Natl Cancer Inst.* **98**: 1777–85.
7. Tang, C., Ang, B. T., and Pervaiz, S. (2007) Cancer stem cell: target for anti-cancer therapy. *FASEB J.* **21**: 3777–85.
8. Korkaya, H., and Wicha, M. S. (2009) HER-2, notch, and breast cancer stem cells: targeting an axis of evil. *Clin Cancer Res.* **15**: 1845–7.
9. Patwardhan, G. A., Zhang, Q. J., Yin, D., Gupta, V., Bao, J., Senkal, C. E., Ogretmen, B., Cabot, M. C., Shah, G. V., Sylvester, P. W., Jazwinski, S. M., and Liu, Y. Y. (2009) A new mixed-backbone oligonucleotide

against glucosylceramide synthase Sensitizes multidrug-resistant tumors to apoptosis. *PLoS One*. **4**: e6938.

10. Petriz, J. (2007) Flow cytometry of the side population (SP). *Curr Protoc Cytom*. **Chapter 9**, Unit9 23.
11. Gupta, P. B., Onder, T. T., Jiang, G., Tao, K., Kuperwasser, C., Weinberg, R. A., and Lander, E. S. (2009) Identification of selective inhibitors of cancer stem cells by high-throughput screening. *Cell*. **138**: 645–59.
12. Yamashita, T., Wada, R., Sasaki, T., Deng, C., Bierfreund, U., Sandhoff, K., and Proia, R. L. (1999) A vital role for glycosphingolipid synthesis during development and differentiation. *Proc Natl Acad Sci U S A*. **96**: 9142–7.
13. Liour, S. S., and Yu, R. K. (2002) Differential effects of three inhibitors of glycosphingolipid biosynthesis on neuronal differentiation of embryonal carcinoma stem cells. *Neurochem Res*. **27**: 1507–12.
14. Salli, U., Fox, T. E., Carkaci-Salli, N., Sharma, A., Robertson, G. P., Kester, M., and Vrana, K. (2009) Propagation of undifferentiated human embryonic stem cells with nano-liposomal ceramide. *Stem Cells Dev*. **18**: 55–66.
15. Mehta, K. (1994) High levels of transglutaminase expression in doxorubicin-resistant human breast carcinoma cells. *Int J Cancer*. **58**: 400–6.
16. Liu, Y. Y., Gupta, V., Patwardhan, G. A., Bhinge, K., Zhao, Y., Bao, J., Mehendale, H., Cabot, M. C., Li, Y. T., Jazwinski, S. M. (2010) Glucosylceramide synthase upregulates MDR1 expression in the regulation of cancer drug resistance through cSrc and beta-catenin signaling. *Mol Cancer*. **9**:145.

Chapter 12

Chemical Screening with Zebrafish Embryos

Hanbing Zhong and Shuo Lin

Abstract

Functional chemicals are very useful tools for molecular biology studies. Due to its small size, large progeny clutch, and embryonic transparency, zebrafish serves as a superb in vivo animal model for chemical compound screens and characterization. During zebrafish embryogenesis, multiple developmental phenotypes can be easily examined under the microscope, therefore allowing a more comprehensive evaluation for identifying novel functional chemicals than cell-based assays. Ever since the first zebrafish-based chemical screen was conducted in the year 2000, many functional chemicals have been discovered using this strategy. In this chapter, we describe how to perform a typical zebrafish-based chemical screen and discuss the details of the protocol by using the example of the identification and characterization of two new Smo inhibitors with a *Gli:GFP* transgenic line.

Key words: Chemical library, Fluorescent protein, Screening, Transgenic, Zebrafish

1. Introduction

Genetic loss-of-function and gain-of-function are the most powerful approaches to studying gene function and dissecting signal transduction pathways. Although modern genetics has developed many versatile and easy-to-use tools (1, 2), it is still usually laborious and time-consuming to generate knockout and transgenic organisms. By contrast, chemicals, particularly small molecules, offer easier and more precise temporal control of gene function by allowing addition and removal of a given compound at preselected time points. A chemical capable of specifically modifying a biological process is not only a useful molecular biological tool but also a potential drug candidate. To date, the number of such chemicals is still low compared to the number of functional genes. Whole organism-based chemical screening is an effective way to identify novel functional chemicals, because it represents a forward

Seetharama D. Satyanarayanajois (ed.), *Drug Design and Discovery: Methods and Protocols*,
Methods in Molecular Biology, vol. 716, DOI 10.1007/978-1-61779-012-6_12,

genetics approach allowing systematic identification of modifiers of any biological process without prior knowledge of the targets (3).

Among the established animal models, *C. elegans*, *Drosophila*, and zebrafish (embryo) are all small enough to grow in microformat plates. Among them, zebrafish is the only vertebrate animal that is appropriate for large-scale chemical screening. Zebrafish embryos develop rapidly, and rudiments of most organs are formed by 1 day post fertilization (dpf). By 3 dpf, embryogenesis is largely completed, and the embryos hatch from their chorions with functional circulatory and nervous systems. This rapid embryonic development of zebrafish provides a great deal of morphological information. Multiple traits (body axis, brain, eye, ear, heart, and skin) can be easily examined. Furthermore, by using tissue-specific fluorescent protein transgenic lines, many internal organs (liver, pancreas, intestine, pituitary, blood vessel, etc.) can be conveniently examined. Adult females produce large clutches of embryos (100+) per mating, allowing analysis of a large number of chemicals in a multiwell plate. Thus, zebrafish embryos are very suitable for screening chemical libraries, especially for identifying developmental modifiers.

In 2000, Peterson et al. first demonstrated that small-molecule developmental modifiers can be isolated through chemical screening with zebrafish embryos by visual examination, in which about 1,100 compounds were tested and several molecules were found to regulate the development of the central nervous system, neural crest, ear, and cardiovascular system (4). Since this proof of principle chemical screen in zebrafish (5), a number of additional chemical compound screens using zebrafish have been performed with various designs and readouts, including suppression of genetic mutations (6, 7), expression pattern changes of molecular markers revealed by in situ hybridization (ISH) (8, 9), and fluorescent pattern changes of transgenic reporters (10) (for a review, see ref. (5)). Here, we describe a framework of chemical screening in zebrafish with emphasis on screening with transgenic lines.

2. Materials

2.1. Zebrafish Husbandry

The zebrafish scientific research community essentially adopts the following husbandry condition.

1. Fish water: pH 7.2–7.6, conductivity 500 μS, nitrates <5 ppm.
2. Temperature 28.5°C.
3. Light cycle: 14 h on and 10 h off.

2.2. Chemical Libraries

1. Prestwick Chemical Library (Prestwick Chemical, Illkirch, France), containing 1,120 small molecules. Ninety percent of them are marketed drugs and the remaining 10% are bioactive alkaloids or related substances.
2. DIVERSet™ library (ChemBridge Corporation, San Diego, CA, USA), which is carefully selected to cover the broadest pharmacophore spectrum within a limited number of compounds. The whole library contains 50,000+ compounds (a subset of this library can be purchased).

2.3. Screening with Zebrafish Embryos

1. Petridish.
2. Transfer pipette.
3. U-bottom 96-well plates.
4. Methylene blue.
5. Cellgro Antibiotic-Antimycotic Solution (Mediatech, Manassas, VA). Stock is 100×.
6. 0.3% (w/v) 1-phenyl-2-thiourea (PTU, Sigma-Aldrich) in fish water (100×).

2.4. Generate RNA Probes

1. Nuclease-free water (Applied Biosystems/Ambion, Austin, TX, USA).
2. 5× transcription buffer with polymerase (Promega, Madison, WI, USA).
3. 100 mM DTT.
4. RNA polymerase (Promega, Madison, WI, USA).
5. RNasin RNase Inhibitor (Promega, Madison, WI, USA).
6. NTP labeling mixture (Roche, Indianapolis, IN, USA).
7. RNeasy MinElute Cleanup Kit (Qiagen, Valencia, CA, USA).

2.5. In Situ Hybridization (ISH)

1. 30 mg/mL protease (Protease from *Streptomyces griseus*, type XIV) (Sigma-Aldrich) in 10 mM Tris–HCl, pH 7.0, 10 mM NaCl.
2. 10× PBS buffer: 137 mM NaCl, 2.7 mM KCl, 4.3 mM Na_2HPO_4, 1.4 mM KH_2PO_4 in DEPC treated water. Adjust to pH 7.3, autoclave and store at room temperature (RT).
3. PBST: 1× PBS buffer with 0.2% Tween-20.
4. 4% (w/v) paraformaldehyde in 1× PBS. Dissolve by heating to 65°C and mixing regularly. Aliquot and store at –20°C.
5. 10 μg/mL proteinase K (EMD, Gibbstown, NJ, USA) in PBST.
6. SSC buffer (20×): 3 M NaCl, 0.3 M NaCitrate in DEPC-treated water. Adjust to pH 7.0, autoclave and store at RT.

7. Hybridization buffer: 50% (v/v) ultra pure formamide, 5× SSC, 5 μg/mL heparin, 5 mM EDTA, 0.5 mg/mL ribosomal RNA (Sigma-Aldrich), 0.1% Tween-20. Adjust to pH 6.0. Store at −20°C.
8. Acetone Powder: Freeze zebrafish in liquid nitrogen and grind them under liquid nitrogen in mortar to fine powder. Transfer powder into centrifuge tube, add 0.9% (w/v) NaCl and keep on ice for 5 min. Add 8 mL of chilled acetone per 2 mL of powder suspension. Mix well and incubate on ice for 30 min. Spin at 10,000 ×*g* for 10 min. Discard supernatant. Resuspend the pellet in fresh chilled acetone of same volume used previously, mix, and incubate for 10 min. Repeat centrifugation and resuspend in acetone. Let it sit for several seconds, collect supernatant. Discard the precipitate. Aliquot and store acetone powder at −20°C.
9. Anti-Digoxigenin-AP Fab fragments (Roche, Indianapolis, IN, USA).
10. Lamb serum: Be heated at 57°C for 10 min. Aliquot and store at −20°C.
11. Alkaline phosphatase (AP) buffer: 100 mM NaCl, 50 mM $MgCl_2$, 100 mM Tris–HCl, pH 9.5, 0.1% Tween-20, 1 mM levamisol (option).
12. NBT (Nitro-Blue Tetrazolium Chloride) stock: 50 mg NBT in 0.7 mL of dimethyl formamide anhydride plus 0.3 mL water. BCIP (5-Bromo-4-Chloro-3′-Indolylphosphate *p*-Toluidine Salt) stock: 50 mg of BCIP in 1 mL of dimethyl formamide anhydride. Both NBT and BCIP should be stored at −80°C since their degradation products increase background dramatically.
13. 24-well plate.

2.6. Imaging

1. Dissecting microscope.
2. Inverted compound microscope.

3. Methods

3.1. Design of a Screen

1. Goal and readout of the screen: The goals and readouts of a chemical screen should be considered carefully. When targeting a biological process or a signaling pathway, one should define molecular markers that are reflective of the pathway activity. If possible, one should use transgenic lines with fluorescent protein reporters in live fish embryos. In general, an ideal readout should be accurate, sensitive, rapid, and reliable to detect the modulation of a biological process. Every method

has its pros and cons. Direct visual examination is easy but does not detect minor internal morphological alterations. ISH can reveal the expression of any molecular marker, but it takes at least 3 days to complete the assay. Transgenic lines mimic the endogenous molecular markers with reporter genes, usually fluorescent proteins, allowing sensitive and convenient examination, but it takes usually 6 months or more to generate a stable transgenic line.

2. Choosing a chemical library: A number of commercial chemical libraries are available. How to choose the suitable one is a pivotal and difficult question. Useful introduction and guidance are outlined in a review from Mayer (11). In general, a focused library will facilitate mechanism studies, while a more random library will promote novel discoveries. Two libraries commonly available and useful are Prestwick Chemical Library and DIVERSet™ library. As mentioned above, Prestwick Chemical Library contains 1,120 small-molecules. Ninety percent of them are marketed drugs and the remaining 10% are bioactive alkaloids or related substances. Therefore, it presents a great degree of empirically possible "drug-likeliness." Prestwick library is very good for pilot screening to validate the experimental design. The DIVERSet library is carefully selected to cover the broadest pharmacophore spectrum within a limited number of compounds. The whole library contains 50,000+ compounds. Due to its diverse collection, this library is suitable for identifying new functional chemicals and biological targets.
3. Timing of exposure to chemicals: The time for chemical treatment depends on the goal of the screen and the nature of the chemical libraries. According to published literatures and our own experience, the earlier you add chemicals to embryos, the higher the death rate and side effects, which will obstruct the search for a specific phenotype. For a screen targeting organogenesis, chemicals can be added to embryos at the shield stage (at ~6 h post fertilization (hpf)) to minimize undesirable embryonic death and side effects. It is highly recommended to perform a pilot screen (of ~200 chemicals) at the beginning of the study to estimate the death rate and "hit" rate. One needs to compromise death rate and "hit" rate to find a proper concentration range of a chemical library.
4. Confirm "hits": Once an interesting chemical compound is isolated, it is necessary to repeat the test. Most chemical screening core facilities can offer several microliters of a chemical from the stock plate. If possible, repeat the compound testing at multiple concentrations in at least 1 log dose range – for example, at 1, 5, 10, and 20 μM. A functional compound should modulate biological processes in a dose-dependent manner.

3.2. Setup Mating of Zebrafish

Adult females should be trained to lay eggs weekly. Well-trained females will yield eggs in ~20 min after release from a physical separator that prevents uncontrolled mating of female and male in a mating cage. One pair mating is preferred because usually multipair mating results in a wide range of embryo stages, which impairs the scoring of chemical effects at later time points. Embryos can be raised in fish water. Embryos are staged according to the description by Kimmel et al. (12).

3.3. The Procedure of a Typical Screen (Fig. 1)

1. Day 1 afternoon, place one or two males with one female zebrafish in one mating cage for each breeding pair. Typically, 10–20 pairs are set up to allow adequate supply of eggs.
2. Day 2 morning, release separator.
3. About 20 min later, collect embryos into individual petri dishes, wash with fresh fish water and keep at 28.5°C for 1 h. At this step, collect embryos every 20 min to avoid mixture of different stages, and do not pool embryos from different clutches together before checking their quality.
4. Check embryo quality and only keep healthy embryos (transparent and dividing synchronically). Pool together the healthy embryos in order to decrease the bias of individual disparities. Usually three clutches of the same stage are pooled together.

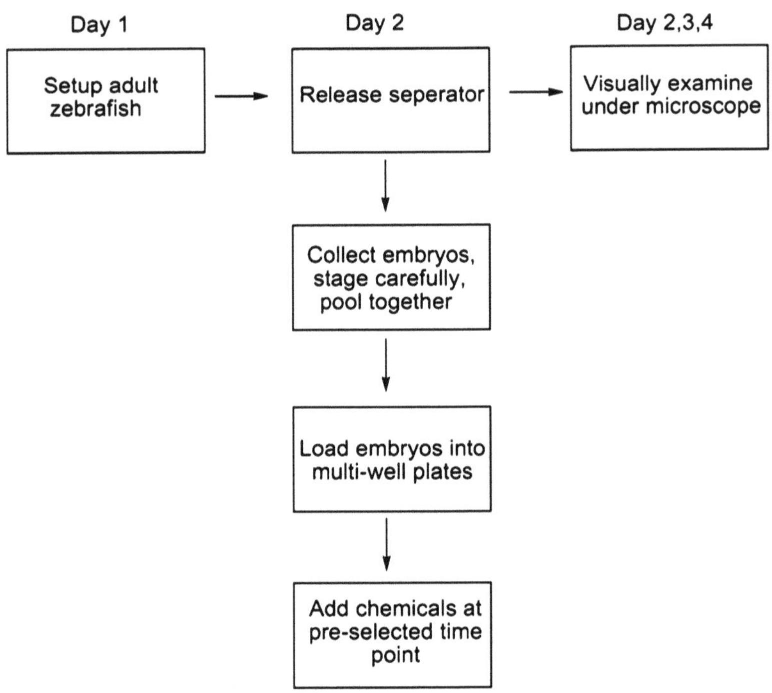

Fig. 1. Flowchart of a chemical screen in zebrafish with readout of direct visual examination.

5. Load embryos into U-bottom 96-well plates, 4–7 embryos per well depending on the amount of embryos harvested on the day. At this step, add a drop of methylene blue into fish water, which will help doing transfer.
6. Gently remove fish water from each well without damaging embryos, then add 200 μL fresh fish water with 1× Antibiotic-Antimycotic.
7. Add chemicals at a preselected time point using an automated microplate pipetting system or by hand. One percent DMSO in fish water serves as a negative control (Notes 1, 2, and 3).
8. If using transgenic reporters, on the succedent days, visually examine and score embryos consecutively under the microscope to identify expected phenotypes (Note 4).
9. If using ISH of molecular markers, embryos will be fixed and performed with ISH, then be examined and scored (Note 5).

3.4. In Situ Hybridization

3.4.1. Generate Dig-Labeled RNA Probe

1. Combine the following reagents in order.

   1.0 μg linearized DNA template.

   4.0 μL 5× transcription buffer.

   2.0 μL DTT.

   2.0 μL NTP labeling mixture.

   1.0 μL RNasin RNase Inhibitor.

   2.0 μL RNA polymerase.

   Add RNase-free water to final volume of 20 μL.

   Incubate at 37°C for 45 min.

   Usually 1 μg DNA template will produce 10 μg RNA probe.
2. Clean up RNA probes with RNeasy MinElute Cleanup Kit.

3.4.2. Fixation and Dehydration of Embryo

1. Pigment appears around 24 hpf. If one wants to do ISH with embryos older than 24 hpf, PTU should be added into fish water to inhibit pigmentation before 24 hpf at a final concentration of 0.003% (w/v).
2. Most embryos will hatch by 3 dpf. If they do not or embryos younger than 3 dpf are needed, one can dechorionate them with protease digestion or forceps.
3. Fix embryos with 4% paraformaldehyde for 2 h at RT or overnight at 4°C. Less than 100 embryos per 1 mL of 4% paraformaldehyde.
4. Wash fixed embryos with PBST for 5 min at RT.
5. Dehydrate fixed embryos, each step 5 min at RT.

   30% ethanol in 1× PBS

   50% ethanol in 1× PBS

70% ethanol in water

100% ethanol

6. Keep dehydrated embryos at −20°C for at least 2 h. For unknown reason, the step helps decrease NBT/BCIP staining background.

3.4.3. Rehydration and Proteinase K Digestion

1. Transfer dehydrated embryos to 2 mL centrifuge tube, less than 40 per tube/sample. If not mentioned otherwise, the volume of solutions is 400 μL.
2. Rehydrate fixed embryos, each step 5 min at RT.

   70% ethanol in water

   50% ethanol in 1× PBS

   30% ethanol in 1× PBS
3. Wash embryos 2 times with PBST for 5 min at RT.
4. Digest embryos with proteinase K at RT. The aim of proteinase K digestion is to make "holes" in fixed embryos to let RNA probes go into every tissue. To digest gently, the final concentration of proteinase K is 10 μg/mL. The time of digestion is stage and/or probe dependent. For most probes, embryos younger than 1 dpf do not need to be digested; embryos of 2 dpf need to be digested for 20 min; embryos of 3 dpf need to be digested for 30 min.
5. Wash embryos with PBST for 5 min.
6. Refix embryos with 4% paraformaldehyde for 20 min at RT.
7. Wash embryos 4 times with PBST for 5 min at RT.

3.4.4. Hybridization

1. Equilibrate embryos in hybridization buffer until they sink.
2. Wash with new hybridization buffer and prehybridize for at least 2 h at 65°C.
3. Use hybridization buffer to dilute RNA probe to 3 ng/mL. Equilibrate probe solution in hybridization buffer to 65°C and add to embryos.
4. Hybridize overnight at 65°C.
5. The temperature of hybridization varies on probe by probe basis. Before doing large scale ISH, one should try several temperatures of hybridization between 60 and 70°C.
6. Remove and save probe solutions. Probe in hybridization buffer may be used for several times until staining signal becomes weak.
7. Wash embryos with the following solutions at 65°C.

   3 volume of hybridization buffer plus 1 volume of 2× SSC for 15 min.

   1 volume of hybridization buffer plus 1 volume 50% 2× SSC for 15 min, 2 times.

2× SSC for 15 min.

0.2× SSC for 30 min, 2 times.

3.4.5. Prepare Anti-Digoxigenin-AP Fab Fragments (Anti-Dig) Solution

1. While doing hybridization, one can prepare Anti-Dig solution.
2. Each sample needs 40 μL of acetone powder. Vortex acetone powder stock and transfer acetone powder needed to a new tube.
3. Centrifuge at 5,000 × *g* for 2 min, discard acetone.
4. Wash pellet with PBST, centrifuge at 5,000 × *g* for 2 min, discard PBST.
5. Add 40 μL of PBST, vortex.
6. Absence of acetone powder dramatically increases staining background. Acetone powder can be replaced by commonly used blocking reagents.
7. Add 0.8 μL of 2% lamb serum.
8. Add 0.1 μL of Anti-Digoxigenin-AP Fab fragments, shake at 4°C for at least 4 h or overnight.
9. Centrifuge at 5,000 × *g* for 2 min, save supernatant (acetone powder absorbed Anti-Dig solution).

3.4.6. Alkaline Phosphatase Staining

1. After hybridization, wash embryos 2 times with PBST for 5 min each.
2. Dilute acetone powder absorbed Anti-Dig with 360 μL of PBST with 2% lamb serum. So the final volume of Anti-Dig solution is 400 μL.
3. Incubate each sample in 400 μL of Anti-Dig solution on a shaker for at least 4 h or overnight at 4°C.
4. Take samples from 4°C, wash 6 times with PBST for 15 min each.
5. Prepare fresh alkaline phosphatase (AP) buffer, because it precipitates over time.
6. Wash 2 times with AP buffer.
7. Prepare developing solution, calculate 400 μL per sample, and keep in dark. For 1 mL AP buffer, add 4.5 μL of 50 mg/mL NBT and 3.5 μL of 50 mg/mL BCIP.
8. Rinse 24-well plate with AP buffer, transfer embryos from centrifuge tube to 24-well plate using AP buffer, remove excess AP buffer from each well.
9. Add 400 μL of developing solution to each well.
10. Incubate in the dark at RT for 2–4 h or until good signal appears. Usually, bluish-purple color develops in 1 h.
11. Stop color developing by washing 2 times with PBST.

12. If one wants to preserve embryos for a long time, dehydrate in
    30% ethanol in 1× PBS for 5 min.
    50% ethanol in 1× PBS for 5 min.
    70% ethanol in water for 5 min.
    100% ethanol for 5 min, then store at –20°C.
13. Rehydrate with PBST and score under microscope. Dehydrating and rehydrating improve the contrast of alkaline phosphatase staining.

3.5. An Example of a Screen: Identification of New Smoothened (Smo) Inhibitors with Gli:GFP Transgenic Embryos

In a previous study, our group identified two potent Smo inhibitors with Gli1-dependent GFP transgenic zebrafish (10). Smo is a seven-pass transmembrane protein and is an important component of the Hedgehog (Hh) signaling pathway. When Hh ligand binds to its membrane receptor Patched1 (Ptch1), Ptch1 relieves its suppression on Smo, leading to the activation of the Gli transcription factors. Gli1 and Gli2 are activators, and Gli3 is a repressor. Hh pathway is one of the fundamental master regulators of animal development, controlling cell fate determination, cell proliferation, and organogenesis. Furthermore, recent studies indicate that the Hh pathway is overactivated in several malignancies and cancers – for example, basal cell carcinoma and deadly brain cancer medulloblastoma (13, 14). Because most abnormal activations of the Hh pathway are caused by Ptch1 or Smo mutations, intense efforts have been invested to search for inhibitors against them. Several compounds inhibiting Smo have been identified, and one of them, GDC-0449, is in clinical trial. GDC-0449 substantially reduces basal cell carcinoma and medulloblastoma. However, one patient with severe medulloblastoma developed resistance to GDC-0449 in 3 months and died soon thereafter (15, 16). Thus, there is a need to search for more compounds that repress the Hh pathway, and a multidrug cocktail may help overcome drug resistance to one particular compound.

Genetic and chemical Hh-deficient zebrafish embryos display the same defective phenotypes, including U-shaped somites, short intersegmental blood vessels (ISVs), and few pancreatic islet cells. To detect Hh activity more directly in real-time, we generated a *Gli:GFP* transgenic line in which GFP was driven by 8× Gli1 binding sites with a minimal promoter. By using this line, we screened a focused library synthesized based on the structure of SAG, a synthetic Hh pathway agonist (17, 18). Cyclopamine was used as a positive control.

Two lead compounds SANT74 and SANT75 were identified (Fig. 2). SANT74 and SANT75 demonstrated similar potencies, so only the results of SANT74 are shown. Embryos treated with SANT74, SANT75, or cyclopamine displayed ventrally curved bodies, U-shaped somites, and abolished GFP expression near the midline, while the negative control group displayed a normal

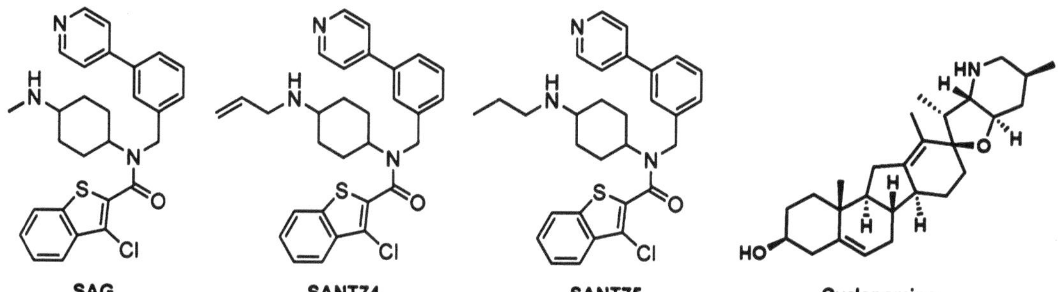

Fig. 2. Molecular structures of SAG, SANT74, SANT75, and cyclopamine. This figure is adapted from the paper published by Yang et al. (10).

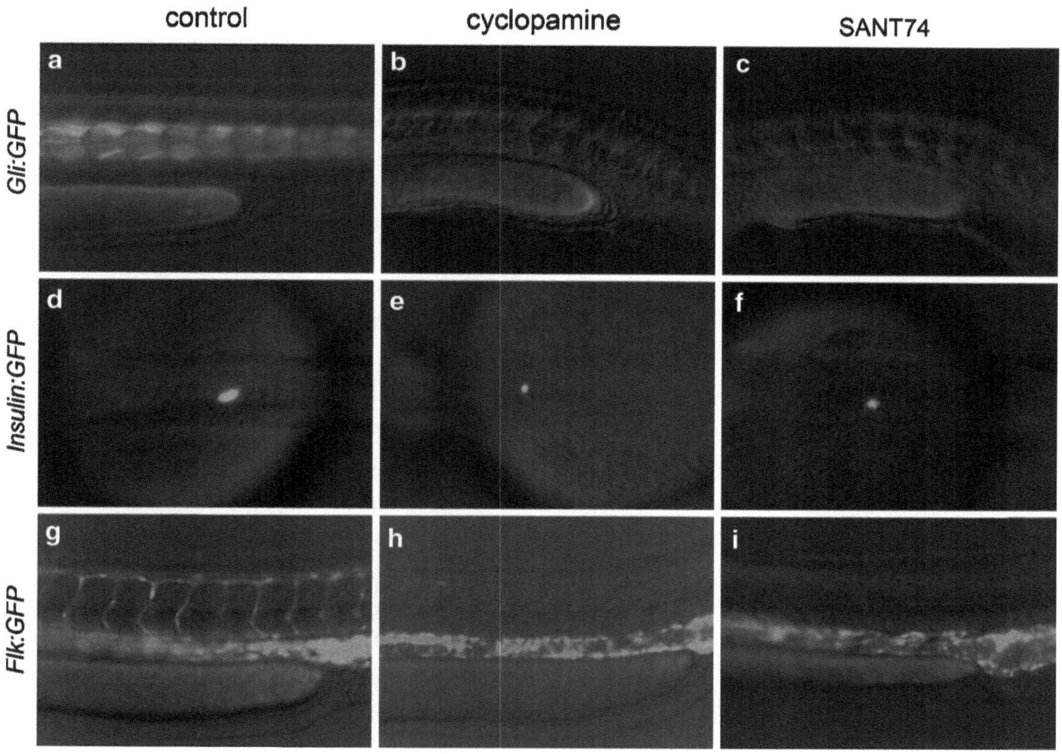

Fig. 3. Identification and characterization of SANT Smo inhibitors in zebrafish. (**a–c**) 36 hpf *Gli:GFP* embryos. (**a**) Control group, the somites near the midline expressed GFP. (**b**, **c**) GFP expression was ablated by 20 μM cyclopamine or SANT74 respectively. (**d–f**) 36 hpf *Insulin:GFP* embryos. (**d**) Control group, the pancreatic islet cells are labeled with GFP. (**e**, **f**) The number of pancreatic islet cells decreased under administration of 20 μM cyclopamine or SANT74 respectively. (**g–i**) 36 hpf *Flk:GFP* embryos. (**g**) Control group, endothelial cells are labeled with GFP. ISVs grow to DLAV (dorsal longitudinal anastomotic vessels). (**h**, **i**) Embryos treated with 40 μM cyclopamine or SANT74 from 17 hpf. They specifically lack ISV but maintain normal V-shaped somites. This figure is adapted from the paper published by Yang et al. (10).

body shape and strong GFP expression in the somite tissue immediately adjacent to the midline (Fig. 3a–c). If SANT74 and SANT75 are specific inhibitors of the Hh pathway, treating zebrafish embryos with them should lead to other well-characterized phenotypes. We then selected pancreatic islet (*Insulin:GFP*) and endothelial cell (*Flk:GFP*) transgenic lines to evaluate SANT74 and SANT75. The results showed that SANT74 and SANT75 dramatically decreased the number of pancreatic islet cells and blocked the growth of ISVs, indicating that they are specific Hh pathway inhibitors.

SANT74 and SANT75 were then tested in the mammalian Shh-LIGHT2 cell line to confirm their inhibitory activities and to calculate IC_{50}. The decreased luciferase readout showed that SANT74 and SANT75 were Hh inhibitors with IC50s in the nanomolar range. Further investigation by the FRET (fluorescence resonance energy transfer) approach indicated that SANT74 and SANT75 were bound to Smo and repressed its activity by regulating Smo conformation.

4. Notes

1. Commercial chemical libraries usually are supplied in 96-well plates in about 5–10 mM solutions in DMSO. In our protocol, 0.5 μL of the DMSO stock is added to embryos in 200 μL fish water. The final concentrations of the chemicals are about 12.5–25 μM.
2. For compounds insoluble in DMSO, ethanol and methanol can be used as alternatives. Zebrafish can tolerate 0.5% ethanol and methanol.
3. Usually with an automated microplate pipetting system, 400–600 chemicals can be screened per week.
4. Automated microscopy readers with image analysis software can offer some help, but improvement of embryo manipulation is needed because zebrafish embryos are mobile after 24 hpf and the tail bends to one side of the body, which can interfere with imaging.
5. Usually ISH is performed with 2 mL centrifuge tube, but ISH with multiwell plate is also doable.

Acknowledgments

We gratefully acknowledge support from the 973 Program of MOST of P. R. China (2009CB941203) and Shenzhen Science and Technology Key Laboratory Promotion Fund. We thank Zahra Tehrani for reading and editing the manuscript.

References

1. Elliott, D.A. and Brand, A.H. (2008) The GAL4 system: a versatile system for the expression of genes. *Methods Mol Biol.* **420**: 79–95.
2. Frese, K.K. and Tuveson, D.A. (2007) Maximizing mouse cancer models. *Nat Rev Cancer.* 7: 645–658.
3. Zhong, H., Liu, N. and Lin, S. (2009) Zebrafish Models for Human Diseases and Drug Discovery. In: Ekins S and Xu JJ (eds) Drug Efficacy, Safety, and Biologics Discovery: Emerging Technologies and Tools. Wiley: Hoboken. p. 115–133.
4. Peterson, R.T., Link, B.A., Dowling, J.E. and Schreiber, S.L. (2000) Small molecule developmental screens reveal the logic and timing of vertebrate development. *Proc Natl Acad Sci U S A.* **97**: 12965–12969.
5. Kaufman, C.K., White, R.M. and Zon, L. (2009) Chemical genetic screening in the zebrafish embryo. *Nat Protoc.* **4**: 1422–1432.
6. Peterson, R.T., Shaw, S.Y., Peterson, T.A., Milan, D.J., Zhong, T.P., Schreiber, S.L., MacRae, C.A. and Fishman, M.C. (2004) Chemical suppression of a genetic mutation in a zebrafish model of aortic coarctation. *Nat Biotechnol.* **22**: 595–599.
7. Stern, H.M., Murphey, R.D., Shepard, J.L., Amatruda, J.F., Straub, C.T., Pfaff, K.L., Weber, G., Tallarico, J.A., King, R.W. and Zon, L.I. (2005) Small molecules that delay S phase suppress a zebrafish bmyb mutant. *Nat Chem Biol.* **1**: 366–370.
8. Goessling, W., North, T.E., Loewer, S., Lord, A.M., Lee, S., Stoick-Cooper, C.L., Weidinger, G., Puder, M., Daley, G.Q., Moon, R.T. and Zon, L.I. (2009) Genetic interaction of PGE2 and Wnt signaling regulates developmental specification of stem cells and regeneration. *Cell.* **136**: 1136–1147.
9. Yeh, J.R., Munson, K.M., Elagib, K.E., Goldfarb, A.N., Sweetser, D.A. and Peterson, R.T. (2009) Discovering chemical modifiers of oncogene-regulated hematopoietic differentiation. *Nat Chem Biol.* **5**: 236–243.
10. Yang, H., Xiang, J., Wang, N., Zhao, Y., Hyman, J., Jiang, J., Chen, J.K., Yang, Z. and Lin, S. (2009) Converse conformational control of smoothened activity by structurally related small molecules. *J Biol Chem.* **284**: 20876–20884.
11. Mayer, T.U. (2003) Chemical genetics: tailoring tools for cell biology. *Trends Cell Biol.* **13**: 270–277.
12. Kimmel, C.B., Ballard, W.W., Kimmel, S.R., Ullmann, B. and Schilling, T.F. (1995) Stages of embryonic development of the zebrafish. *Dev Dyn.* **203**: 253–310.
13. Jacob, L. and Lum, L. (2007) Deconstructing the hedgehog pathway in development and disease. *Science.* **318**: 66–68.
14. Theunissen, J.W. and de Sauvage, F.J. (2009) Paracrine Hedgehog signaling in cancer. *Cancer Res.* **69**: 6007–6010.
15. Von Hoff, D.D., LoRusso, P.M., Rudin, C.M., Reddy, J.C., Yauch, R.L., Tibes, R., Weiss, G.J., Borad, M.J., Hann, C.L., Brahmer, J.R., Mackey, H.M., Lum, B.L., Darbonne, W.C., Marsters, J.C., Jr., de Sauvage, F.J. and Low, J.A. (2009) Inhibition of the hedgehog pathway in advanced basal-cell carcinoma. *N Engl J Med.* **361**: 1164–1172.
16. Yauch, R.L., Dijkgraaf, G.J., Alicke, B., Januario, T., Ahn, C.P., Holcomb, T., Pujara, K., Stinson, J., Callahan, C.A., Tang, T., Bazan, J.F., Kan, Z., Seshagiri, S., Hann, C.L., Gould, S.E., Low, J.A., Rudin, C.M. and de Sauvage, F.J. (2009) Smoothened mutation confers resistance to a hedgehog pathway inhibitor in medulloblastoma. *Science.* **326**: 572–574.
17. Frank-Kamenetsky, M., Zhang, X.M., Bottega, S., Guicherit, O., Wichterle, H., Dudek, H., Bumcrot, D., Wang, F.Y., Jones, S., Shulok, J., Rubin, L.L. and Porter, J.A. (2002) Small-molecule modulators of Hedgehog signaling: identification and characterization of Smoothened agonists and antagonists. *J Biol.* **1**: 10.
18. Chen, J.K., Taipale, J., Young, K.E., Maiti, T. and Beachy, P.A. (2002) Small molecule modulation of Smoothened activity. *Proc Natl Acad Sci U S A.* **99**: 14071–14076.

Chapter 13

iTRAQ™ Labeling Coupled with LC-MALDI Mass Spectrometry for Monitoring Temporal Response of Colorectal Cancer Cells to Butyrate Treatment

Hwee Tong Tan, Teck Kwang Lim, Maxey C.M. Chung, and Qingsong Lin

Abstract

Mass spectrometry (MS)-based quantitative proteomics plays important roles in drug discovery. In this chapter, we describe a stable isotope labeling technique which employs 4-plex iTRAQ™ isobaric reagents coupled with two-dimensional (2-D) liquid chromatography (LC) and MALDI-TOF/TOF MS, for a temporal study of HCT-116 colon carcinoma cells treated with butyrate. Butyrate is a short-chain fatty acid fermentation by-product of fiber that can induce temporal cell maturation, from the early phase of growth arrest, to differentiation, and to the activation of apoptotic cascades. Our quantitative proteomics study uncovered several integrated cellular processes and pathways involved in growth arrest, apoptosis, and metastasis. Selected protein targets are validated by real-time PCR and western blotting.

Key words: Butyrate, 2-D LC, HCT-116 cells, iTRAQ, MALDI-TOF/TOF MS, Temporal study

1. Introduction

Proteomics has been widely applied to drug discovery, such as the identification of drug targets, the study of mechanism of drug action, and the discovery of biomarkers for drug response or drug toxicity (1, 2). iTRAQ™ is one of the most widely used quantitative proteomics technologies which utilizes isobaric reagents with different stable isotope compositions to label the primary amines of peptides including the N-terminal amino and the lysyl ε-amino groups. The relative quantification of proteins from different samples is achieved by mass spectrometry (MS), through the comparison of the reporter ions obtained by MS/MS fragmentation (3). The first generation iTRAQ (4-plex) reagents allow for comparison of up to four different samples, while the second

Seetharama D. Satyanarayanajois (ed.), *Drug Design and Discovery: Methods and Protocols*, Methods in Molecular Biology, vol. 716, DOI 10.1007/978-1-61779-012-6_13,

generation (8-plex iTRAQ) reagents extend the capability to eight samples (4). In this chapter, we showcase this technology by using 4-plex iTRAQ to monitor the temporal response of colon carcinoma cell line HCT-116 to butyrate treatment (5). Due to the high complexity of the iTRAQ-labeled peptide mixture, we utilize two-dimensional liquid chromatography (2-D LC) by coupling strong cation exchange (SCX) with reversed-phase columns to separate the peptide mixtures before MS analyses.

Colorectal cancer is a prevalent disease worldwide, especially in developed countries, with high mortality and morbidity rates (6). High intake of dietary fiber has been shown to reduce the incidence and risk of this neoplasm (7, 8), and butyrate produced from anaerobic fermentation of indigestible carbohydrate is responsible for the chemopreventive properties (9–11). Butyrate not only serves as an energy source for normal colonocytes, but also mediates cell maturation with the promotion of growth arrest followed by differentiation and/or apoptosis of cancer cells (12–16). Since colonic transformation is characterized by multistage alterations of tissue homeostasis, resulting in aberrant cell division and/or cell death (17, 18), these butyrate-caused biological effects are crucial in colorectal cancer therapy. Thus, butyrate has been purported as a potential anticancer agent. In order to systematically elucidate butyrate's mode of actions in an integrated manner, we carried out 4-plex iTRAQ analysis of HCT-116 cells treated with butyrate at three time points (24, 36 and 48 h), spanning from the induction of growth arrest and early phase of apoptosis till the late phase of cell death, with the aim to identify clusters of proteins (and pathways) that showed a consistent trend of differential expression over time (Fig. 1). This study revealed several integrated cellular processes and pathways involved in growth arrest, apoptosis, and metastasis (Fig. 2). We further employed real-time PCR (Fig. 3) and western blotting to validate the molecular responses at both the transcriptional and the translational levels. (5)

2. Materials

2.1. Cell Culture, Butyrate Treatment, and Protein Extraction

1. HCT-116 human colorectal carcinoma cell line (American Type Culture Collection, Rockville, MD).
2. McCoy's 5A medium: 12 g McCoy's medium powder (Sigma, St. Louis, MO), 2.2 g sodium bicarbonate, and 10 mL of 10× antimycotic antibiotics in 890 mL water (see Note 1). This medium is filtered through a 0.22 µm PES filter unit (Nalge Nunc International, Rochester, NY) in a BSL2 laminar hood. 100 mL of heat-inactivated fetal bovine serum (FBS) (Gibco, Green Island, NY) is then added to the medium for use. Store at 4°C.

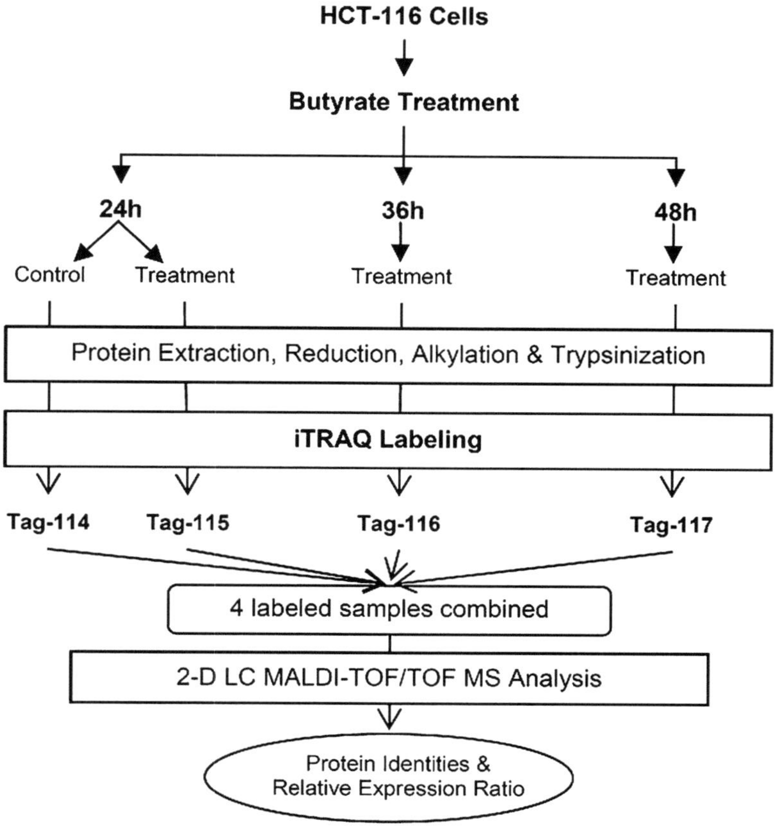

Fig. 1. Workflow outlining the quantitative and temporal proteome analysis of butyrate treatment using iTRAQ labeling. The four iTRAQ tags are used to label proteins extracted from HCT-116 cells treated with butyrate at different time points. iTRAQ labels primary amines of all peptides via the N-termini and ε-amino group of lysine side chain. Following 2-D LC separation of the iTRAQ-labeled peptides, identification and quantitation of iTRAQ-labeled proteins are determined by the amino acid sequence and reporter ions (*m/z* 114–117) generated by MS/MS fragmentation, respectively.

3. Heat-inactivated FBS: heating the FBS at 56°C for 30 min. Store in 50 mL aliquots at −20°C.
4. Sodium butyrate: dissolved at 1 M in sterile water and stored in aliquots at 4°C. Working solutions of 5 mM are prepared by diluting in McCoy's 5A medium, and added into the tissue culture flasks as required.
5. 0.05% (v/v) trypsin – 0.53 mM EDTA solution: diluting with sterile phosphate-buffered saline (PBS). Aliquots are stored at −20°C. The solution is thawed to room temperature prior to use.
6. 500 mM triethylammonium bicarbonate (Sigma) with 1.0% (w/v) SDS: dissolve SDS in 1 M triethylammonium bicarbonate and dilute with water to required concentration.

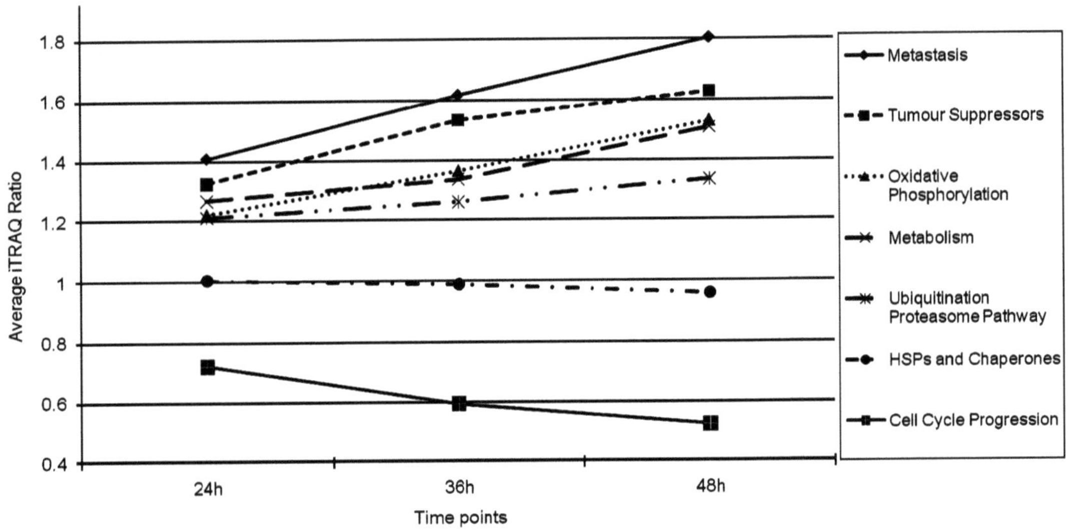

Fig. 2. An overview of the temporal effects of butyrate treatment on the various cellular processes. The differential regulation of the proteins from each cellular process was summarized to illustrate the overall temporal effects of butyrate treatment on HCT-116 cells.

7. Coomassie Plus Protein assay reagent and bovine serum albumin (BSA) standards (Pierce/Thermoscientific, Rockford, IL).
8. PBS (10× PBS): 1.37 M NaCl, 27 mM KCl, and 100 mM phosphate buffer.

2.2. Labeling Protein Samples by 4-Plex iTRAQ Reagents

1. 5 mM Tris-(2-carboxyethyl)phosphine (TCEP) and 10 mM methyl methane-thiosulfonate (MMTS) are supplied with the iTRAQ® Reagents Multiplex Kit (Applied Biosystems, Foster City, ca).
2. Each vial of trypsin with $CaCl_2$, TPCK treated (25 μg) (Applied Biosystems) is dissolved in 25 μL of water prior to use.
3. iTRAQ™ Reagent vials ($Tag_{114-117}$). 70 μL of ethanol is added to each vial prior to labeling samples. Both ethanol and iTRAQ reagents are supplied with the iTRAQ® Reagents Multiplex Kit (Applied Biosystems).
4. ICAT® Cation Exchange Buffer Pack and Cation Exchange Cartridge (Applied Biosystems) (see Note 2). The buffers include cation exchange buffer-load (10 mM potassium phosphate (KH_2PO_4) in 25% acetonitrile (ACN) at pH 3.0), cation exchange buffer-clean (10 mM KH_2PO_4 in 25% ACN/1 M KCl at pH 3.0), cation exchange buffer-elute (10 mM KH_2PO_4 in 25% ACN/350 mM potassium chloride (KCl) at pH 3.0), and cation exchange buffer-storage (10 mM KH_2PO_4 in 25% ACN at pH 3.0, +0.1% sodium azide (NaN_3)).
5. Sep-Pak cartridge (Millipore).

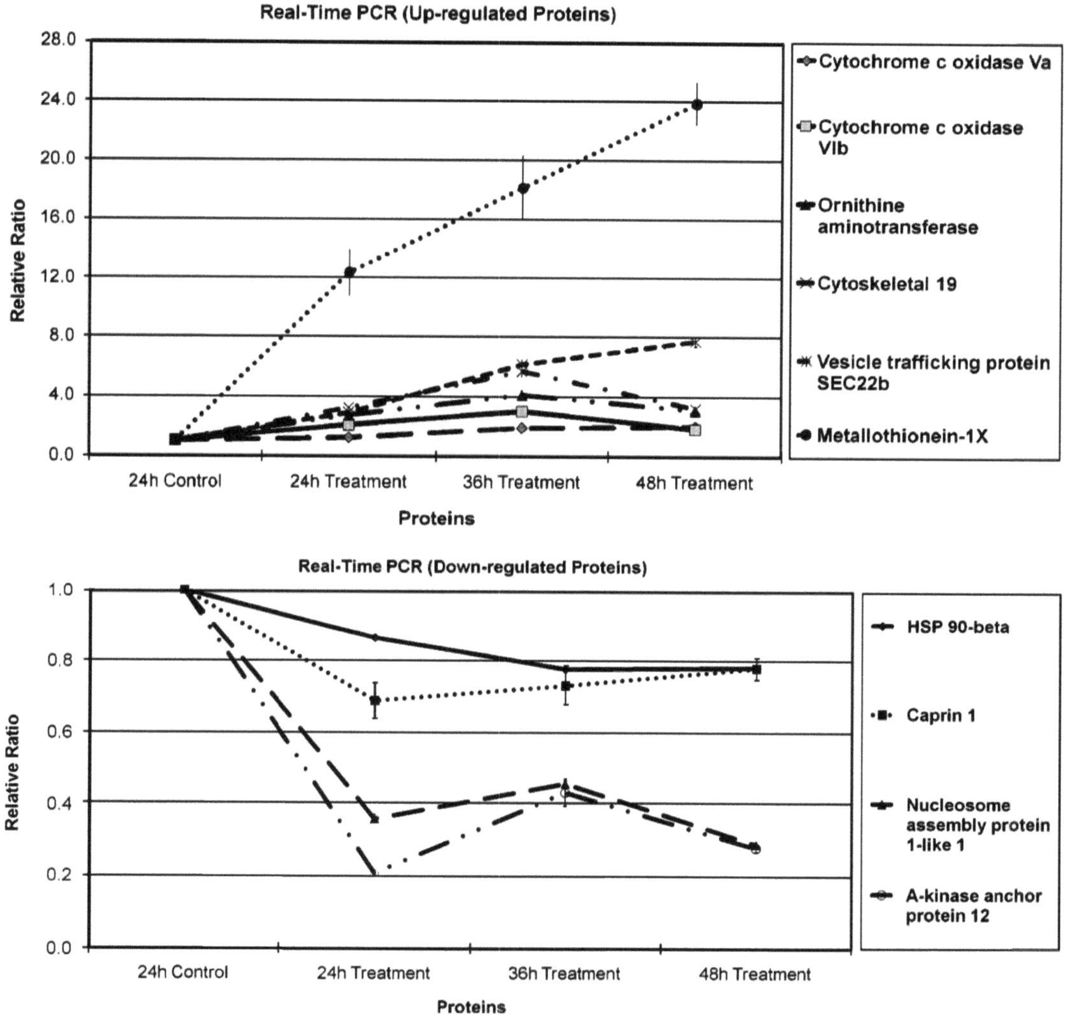

Fig. 3. Validation of the iTRAQ results on selected proteins using real-time PCR. The results verified differential regulation of these proteins upon butyrate treatment. Fold-change ratio assessed by real-time-PCR was expressed as mean values ± standard error (SE) of two batches of cells performed in triplicates.

6. 0.05% Trifluoroacetic acid (TFA).
7. 50% (v/v) ACN and 100% ACN.

2.3. Two-Dimensional Liquid Chromatography Separation of Labeled Peptides

1. Ultimate™ dual-gradient LC system (Dionex-LC Packings, Sunnyvale, CA) equipped with a Probot™ MALDI spotting device.
2. 0.3 × 150-mm SCX column (FUS-15-CP, Poros 10 S) (Dionex-LC Packings).
3. Two 0.3 × 1-mm trap columns (3-µm C_{18} PepMap™, 100 Å) (Dionex-LC Packings).

4. 0.2 × 50-mm reversed-phase column (Monolithic polystyrene-divinylbenzene) (Dionex-LC Packings).
5. Ion-exchange mobile A: 5 mM KH_2PO_4 buffer (pH 3) + 5% ACN.
6. Ion-exchange mobile B: 5 mM KH_2PO_4 buffer (pH 3) + 5% ACN + 500 mM KCl.
7. Reversed-phase mobile A: 2% ACN with 0.05% TFA.
8. Reversed-phase mobile B: 80% ACN with 0.04% TFA. All buffers are filtered through a 0.45 μm PTFE membrane (Sartorius AG, Germany) prior to use (see Note 3).
9. MALDI matrix solution: 7 mg/mL α-cyano-4-hydroxycinnamic acid and 130 μg/mL ammonium citrate dissolved in 75% ACN.
10. 25-nL mixing tee (Upchurch Scientific/IDEX Health & Science, Oak Harbor, WA).

2.4. Mass Spectrometry Analysis of iTRAQ-Labeled Samples

1. 4700 Proteomics Analyzer mass spectrometer (Applied Biosystems).
2. GPS Explorer™ software Version 3.6 (Applied Biosystems).
3. MASCOT search engine (Version 2.1; Matrix Science).
4. International Protein Index (IPI) human database (Version 3.30, 67922 sequences).
5. Six protein mixture supplied with iTRAQ® Reagent Methods Development Kit (Applied Biosystems).
6. A randomized database (67922 sequences) generated using IPI human database Version 3.30 (generated using a Pearl script downloaded from Matrix Science, http://www.matrixscience.com/help/decoy_help.htmL).

2.5. Real-time PCR

1. RNeasy Plus Mini Kit (Qiagen, Chatsworth, CA).
2. 1% (w/v) agarose gel: 1 g agarose in 100 mL of tris-acetate EDTA (TAE) buffer, and mixed with 3 μL of 10 mg/mL ethidium bromide.
3. Nucleic acid loading dye and EZ load 100 bp Molecular Ruler.
4. Primer Express™ software (Applied Biosystems) is used to design primers.
5. Primers are commercially synthesized.
6. MultiScribe™ Reverse Transcriptase and RNase Inhibitor (Applied Biosystems).
7. SYBR Green PCR Master Mix (Applied Biosystems).
8. ABI PRISM 7000 Sequence Detection System instrument (Applied Biosystems).

2.6. Western Blotting

1. 40% Acrylamide/Bis solution (37.5:1) (Bio-Rad) and TEMED (Bio-Rad) stored at 4°C.
2. Separating buffer: 1.5 M Tris–HCl (pH 8.8). Store at 4°C.
3. Stacking buffer: 1.0 M Tris–HCl (pH 6.8). Store at 4°C.
4. Ammonium persulfate (APS): 10% (w/v) solution in water.
5. 10% SDS: 10% (w/v) solution in water.
6. Sample loading buffer (2×): 120 mM Tris, 20% (v/v) glycerol, 4% (w/v) SDS, and 0.2% bromophenol blue. Store in aliquots at −20°C.
7. Water-saturated butanol: shake equal volume of water and sec-butanol in a glass bottle. Allow them to separate, and use the top layer. Store at room temperature.
8. 10× SDS/Tris/glycine running buffer: 250 mM Tris, 1.92 M glycine, and 1% SDS. Store at room temperature. Dilute with water to 1× and store at 4°C before use.
9. Prestained precision plus dual color molecular weight markers (Bio-Rad) are used for western blot. Store in aliquots at −20°C.
10. 0.2 μm Nitrocellulose membranes and 3 MM fiber pad from Bio-Rad, and blotter paper from GE Healthcare.
11. Mini-Protean III and Mini Trans-Blot (Bio-Rad).
12. Towbin transfer buffer: 25 mM Tris, 192 mM glycine, 0.1% SDS, and 20% methanol. The buffer is prepared and prechilled at 4°C prior to use. An ice pack is placed inside the transfer tank, and a magnetic stir bar is stirred continuously to ensure low temperature during the transfer.
13. Tris-buffered saline with Tween 20 (TBS-T) (10× stock): 200 mM Tris–HCl, 1.5 M NaCl, pH 7.5. Dilute to 1× with water, and add Tween 20 to 0.1% for use.
14. Blocking buffer: 5% (w/v) nonfat dry milk in TBS-T.
15. Rabbit anti-GAPDH (1:200) (Santa Cruz, CA), mouse anti-HSP 90-beta (1:1,000) (Stressgen, CA), mouse anti-Gelactin-1 (1:500), mouse anti-SEC22b (1:750), and mouse anti-COX VIb (1:750) (Abnova Corporation, Taiwan). Antibodies are diluted with 1% (w/v) nonfat dry milk in TBS-T.
16. HRP-conjugated antibodies: anti-rabbit IgG (1:2,500) (Santa Cruz), HRP-conjugated anti-mouse IgG (1:5,000) (GE Healthcare), and HRP-conjugated anti-mouse IgM (1:5,000) (Pierce, Rockford, IL). Antibodies are diluted with 1% (w/v) nonfat dry milk in TBS-T.
17. Stripping solution: 100 mM 2-mercaptoethanol, 62.5 mM Tris–HCl (pH 6.8), and 2% (w/v) SDS.
18. Enhanced chemiluminescence (ECL) (GE Healthcare) and Biomax film (Eastman Kodak).

3. Methods

3.1. Cell Culture, Butyrate Treatment, and Protein Extraction

1. HCT-116 human colorectal carcinoma cell line is cultured in 10 mL McCoy's 5A medium in T75 tissue culture flask in a humidified incubator (37°C, 5% CO_2).
2. Upon reaching 60% confluency, the medium is changed to fresh medium or medium containing 5 mM sodium butyrate. All cell culture procedures are performed in a BSL2 laminar hood.
3. After the cells are mock-treated or butyrate-treated for a specific time point (12, 24, 36 and 48 h), they are harvested via trypsinization using 0.05% (v/v) trypsin – 0.53 mM EDTA solution. Firstly, the medium for the cells is removed, and the cells are gently rinsed with 5 mL sterile PBS. 1 mL of trypsin-EDTA is added into the tissue culture flask and incubated for 3–5 min at 37°C. 1 mL of McCoy's medium is then added onto the cells to inactivate the trypsin. The cell suspension is pipetted into a 15 mL tube.
4. The cell suspension is pelleted by centrifugation at 1,000 × *g* for 5 min at 4°C. This step is repeated with washing in 5 mL PBS thrice, followed by a final centrifugation step at 500 × *g* for 3 min at 4°C. The resultant cell pellets are stored at −20°C prior to use for cell lysate preparations.
5. 500 mM triethylammonium bicarbonate/1.0% (w/v) SDS is added into the cell pellet (with a buffer:cell pellet ratio of 4:1) for extraction and denaturation of cellular proteins by boiling at 100°C for 10 min. The cell suspension is vortexed at regular intervals during this period. Subsequently, cellular debris is removed after centrifugation at 18,800 × *g* for 1 h at 23°C.
6. Protein quantitation is performed using the Coomassie Plus Protein Assay reagent. BSA is used at concentration of 0–250 μg/mL range as standard. The samples are diluted to at least 100× to reduce the concentration of SDS to at least 0.01%. 10 μL of each sample is mixed with 150 μL of Coomassie Plus reagent, and absorbance is read at 590 nm using a microplate reader.

3.2. Labeling Protein Samples by 4-Plex iTRAQ Reagents

1. 100 μg protein of each sample is reduced with 5 mM TCEP at 60°C for 1 h, subsequently alkylated with 10 mM MMTS at room temperature for 10 min.
2. After cysteine blocking, each sample is diluted to 0.05% (w/v) SDS with 500 mM triethylammonium bicarbonate prior to trypsinization. Reconstitute each vial of trypsin/$CaCl_2$ with 25 μL of water. To each sample tubes, add 10 μL of the trypsin/$CaCl_2$ solution (see Note 4). Incubate the samples at 37°C for 16 h.

3. In order to maximize labeling efficiency, the volume of the sample digest must be less than 50 μL before labeling. If the volume of the sample digest is greater than 50 μL, dry the sample in a centrifugal vacuum concentrator, and then reconstitute with 30 μL 500 mM triethylammonium bicarbonate (see Note 5).
4. Following trypsinization, each tryptic digest is labeled with one of the four isobaric amine-reactive tags. Add 70 μL of ethanol to each iTRAQ™ Reagent vial. Vortex each vial for 1 min to dissolve the iTRAQ™ Reagent. Transfer the contents of one iTRAQ™ Reagent vial to one sample tube as follows: Tag_{114} – 24 h control; Tag_{115} – 24 h treated; Tag_{116} – 36 h treated; and Tag_{117} – 48 h treated samples. Voltex to mix. Incubate for 1 h at room temperature.
5. These four iTRAQ-derivatized samples are then pooled into a fresh tube and voltexed to mix. Reduce the concentrations of buffer salts and organics by diluting the sample mixture at least tenfold with cation exchange buffer-load. Check that the pH is between 2.5 and 3.3. If not, adjust the pH by adding cation exchange buffer-load and phosphoric acid (see Note 6).
6. To condition the strong cation exchange cartridge, inject 1 mL of the cation exchange buffer-clean. Then inject 2 mL of the cation exchange buffer-load. Slowly inject (~1 drop/second) the diluted sample mixture into the cation exchange cartridge and collect the flow-through in a sample tube (see Note 7). Inject 1 mL of the cation exchange buffer-load to wash the TCEP, SDS, calcium chloride, and excess iTRAQ™ Reagents from the cartridge. Collect the flow-through in the same sample tube.
7. To elute the peptides, slowly inject (~1 drop/second) 500 μL of the cation exchange buffer-elute. Capture the eluate in a fresh 1.5-mL tube.
8. Wash the undigested proteins such as trypsin from the cation exchange cartridge by injecting 1 mL of the cation exchange buffer-clean. After cleaning, inject 2 mL of the cation exchange buffer-storage. Store the cartridge at 4°C.
9. The eluate from the ion-exchange step is then desalted using a Sep-Pak cartridge. Wet the Sep-Pak cartridge with at least 10 mL of 0.05% TFA. Dilute the iTRAQ-labeled sample with 2 mL of 0.05% TFA. Draw the sample with a new syringe and pass through the cartridge. Collect the flow-through. Use the flow-through and run it through the column to enhance the binding efficiency. Inject another 3 mL of Mobile A through the column to remove any salt or contaminant. To elute the peptides, wash with 5 mL of 50% ACN followed by 10 mL of

100% ACN – collect in a 50 mL tube. Dilute the sample with 10 mL of water, mix well, and freeze in −80°C for at least 12 h. Evaporate the sample to dryness in a lyophilizer (see Note 8).

3.3. Two-Dimensional Liquid Chromatography Separation of Labeled Peptides

1. Each of the iTRAQ-labeled peptide mixtures is separated using an Ultimate™ dual-gradient LC system equipped with a Probot™ MALDI spotting device.
2. A 2-D LC separation is performed for each iTRAQ experiment as follows: the labeled peptide mixture is dissolved in ion-exchange mobile A and injected into a 0.3 × 150-mm SCX column (FUS-15-CP, Poros 10 S) for the first dimensional separation. The flow rate is 6 μL/min. Nine fractions are obtained using step gradients of ion-exchange mobile phase B: unbound, 0–5, 5–10, 10–15, 15–20, 20–30, 30–40, 40–50, 50–100% B.
3. The eluting fractions are captured alternatively onto two 0.3 × 1-mm trap columns (3-μm C_{18} PepMap™, 100 Å) and washed with reversed-phase mobile A followed by gradient elution in a 0.2 × 50-mm reverse-phase column (Monolithic polystyrene-divinylbenzene). The gradient elution step is 0–60% reversed-phase mobile B in 15 min at a flow rate of 2.7 μL/min.
4. The LC fractions are mixed directly with MALDI matrix solution at a flow rate of 5.4 μL/min via a 25-nL mixing tee before they were spotted onto a 192-well stainless steel MALDI target plate using a Probot Micro Precision Fraction collector, at a speed of 5 s per well.

3.4. Mass Spectrometry Analysis of iTRAQ-Labeled Samples

1. The samples on the MALDI target plates are analyzed using a 4700 Proteomics Analyzer mass spectrometer. MS/MS analyses are performed using nitrogen at collision energy of 1 kV and a collision gas pressure of 1×10^{-6} Torr.
2. The GPS Explorer™ software Version 3.6 is used to create and search files with the MASCOT search engine for peptide and protein identifications with iTRAQ-labeled samples. The IPI human database (Version 3.30, 67922 sequences) (19) is used for the search, and this is restricted to tryptic peptides.
3. One thousand laser shots are accumulated for each MS spectrum. For MS/MS, 6,000 shots are combined for each precursor ion with a signal-to-noise (S/N) ratio greater or equal to 100. For precursors with S/N ratio between 50 and 100, 10,000 shots are acquired. No smoothing is applied before peak detection for both MS and MS/MS, and the peaks are deisotoped. For MS/MS, only the peaks from 60 to 20 Da below each precursor mass and with S/N ≥10 are selected. Peak density is limited to 30 peaks per 200 Da, and the maximum

number of peaks is set to 125. Cysteine methanethiolation, N-terminal iTRAQ labeling, and iTRAQ-labeled lysine are selected as fixed modifications while methionine oxidation is considered as a variable modification. One missed cleavage is allowed. Precursor error tolerance is set to 100 ppm, while MS/MS fragment error tolerance is set to 0.4 Da (see Note 9). Maximum peptide rank is set to 2. iTRAQ quantification is performed using the GPS Explorer software and normalized among samples (see Note 10). iTRAQ ratios are calculated based on the cluster areas of the iTRAQ reporter fragment peaks (114–117), and the ratios calculation includes only peptides identified with CI % above cutoff thresholds as described below.

4. The average iTRAQ ratio and standard deviation (SD) are determined using the GPS Explorer™ software with the following equations.

$$R = e^{\left(\frac{\sum_{i=1}^{N} X_i}{N}\right)}$$

where R = average iTRAQ ratio

X_i = natural log of iTRAQ ratio of each iTRAQ pair

N = the number of peptides with nonzero iTRAQ ratio.

$$S.D. = e^{(\log R + \log S)} - e^{(\log R)} = e^{(\log R)} \times (e^{(\log S)} - 1)$$

where SD = standard deviation of iTRAQ ratio, and

$$\log R = \frac{\sum_{i=1}^{N} X_i}{N}$$

log S = sd.

R = average iTRAQ ratio.

$$sd = \sqrt{\frac{\sum_{i=1}^{N} (x_i - \log R)^2}{N-1}}$$

where sd = iTRAQ standard deviation.

X_i = natural log of iTRAQ ratio of each peptide.

5. In this work, four biological replicates of iTRAQ-labeled samples are analyzed. Student's *t*-test is performed, and the *p* values based on the iTRAQ ratios of peptides matched to each protein (48 h time point vs. control) are used to assess the significance of temporal differential expression.

Proteins that have p value <0.05 in at least one dataset and shown consistent changes in all datasets are considered as significantly altered in the expression level.

6. To determine the cutoff threshold of fold changes for proteins with single-peptide match, two equal amounts of tryptic digested six protein mixtures are labeled with iTRAQ reagent 114 and 117, respectively, and analyzed with 1-D LC MALDI-TOF/TOF MS (reversed-phase liquid chromatography; similar to abovementioned). The SD based on the ratios of all the identified peptides is 0.15, thus 1.3 (1+2 SD) is determined to be the significant cutoff threshold ($p < 0.05$) for the upregulated proteins, and reciprocally 0.77 is the cutoff threshold for the downregulated proteins. Similar cutoff threshold has been used in other iTRAQ studies (20, 21) (see Note 11).
7. In addition to the IPI human database, a randomized database (67922 sequences) generated using IPI human database Version 3.30 (generated using a Pearl script downloaded from Matrix Science, http://www.matrixscience.com/help/decoy_help.htmL) is also used to search the iTRAQ-labeled samples. The false positive rate is calculated by comparing the peptide hits obtained from these two databases at different ion score CI % (peptide). The minimum ion score CI % is set such that no more than 5% false positive rate is achieved. Based on this cutoff threshold, all the proteins identified from the random database search are single-peptide matched. Hence, proteins identified from the human database that are matched to at least two peptides are statistically confident. For single-peptide-matched proteins, only those with ion score CI % greater than the highest CI % attained from the random database search are selected. With these cutoff thresholds, essentially 0% false positive identification rate at protein level can be achieved.

3.5. Real-Time PCR

1. RNA is isolated from two batches of HCT-116 cells using the RNeasy Plus Mini Kit. First, the harvested cells were disrupted in Buffer RLT and homogenized using syringe and 20-gauge needle. 70% Ethanol is then added to the homogenized lysate and mixed well by pipetting. The samples are then added onto the RNeasy Mini spin column placed in the 2 mL collection tube. Centrifuge at 8,000 × g for 15 s.
2. The spin column membranes are washed once using 700 μL Buffer RW1, centrifuged at 8,000 × g for 15 s. The spin columns are then washed twice with 500 μL Buffer RPE to remove any contaminants from the samples by centrifuging at 8,000 × g for 15 s and 2 min, respectively. The total RNA is then eluted in RNase-free water, centrifuged at 8,000g for 1 min. Purified RNA is quantified by UV spectrophotometry (A_{260} of 1 = 40 μg/mL).

3. RNA purity is assessed by ratio of A_{260}/A_{280} and denaturing agarose gel electrophoresis. 1% (w/v) agarose is prepared by dissolving 1 g agarose in 100 mL TAE buffer and boiled using microwave. After the agarose solution has cooled and poured into the gel casting cassette, 3 μL of 10 mg/mL ethidium bromide is mixed in the agarose solution before the gel polymerise. 2 μg of RNA sample is mixed with nucleic acid loading dye before loading into each well. 5 μL of EZ Load 100 bp Molecular Ruler is loaded in a separate well. Electrophoresis is carried out at constant voltage of 100 V for 30 min. The RNA bands are visualized using the UV detector (see Note 12).
4. MultiScribe™ Reverse Transcriptase is used to reverse transcribe RNA from each sample to cDNA. The RT reaction mix consisted of RNase-free water, TaqMan RT buffer, 5.5 mM $MgCl_2$, 0.8 mM deoxyNTPs mixture, 2.5 μM random hexamers, 0.4 U/μL RNase inhibitors, and 1.25U/μL MultiScribe™ reverse transcriptase. The RT reaction mix is mixed with 2 μg RNA into the wells of a MicroAmp Optical 96-Well Reaction Plate and sealed with MicroAmp Optical Adhesive Cover. Reverse transcription is performed using the ABI PRISM 7000 Sequence Detection System instrument. The thermal cycling parameters are shown in Table 1.
5. Sequences for the primers specific for each gene target are designed using the Primer Express™ software and synthesized. BLAST (NCBI) searches for all primer sequences are performed to confirm gene specificity. PCR is carried out using SYBR Green PCR Master Mix, 10 ng of cDNA template, 300 nM of reverse, and forward primers. For quantification of each gene in the samples, amplification is performed in triplicates using the ABI PRISM 7000 Sequence Detection System instrument.
6. Nontemplate controls are included for each run. Glyceraldehyde-3-phosphate dehydrogenase (GAPDH) is

Table 1
Thermal cycling parameters for reverse transcription reactions

	Incubation	Reverse transcription	Reverse transcriptase inactivation
Step	**Hold**	**Hold**	**Hold**
Time	10 min	30 min	5 min
Temperature	25°C	48°C	95°C

Table 2
Thermal cycling parameters for RT-PCR

		PCR	
		Cycle (40 cycles)	
	AmpliTaq Gold activation	Denature	Anneal/extend
Step	Hold	Cycle	
Temperature	95°C	95°C	60°C
Time	10 min	15 s	1 min

used as the endogenous control reference for normalization. Thermal cycling parameters are as follows: denaturation at 95°C for 10 min followed by 40 cycles at 95°C for 15 s and 60°C for 1 min (Table 2).

3.6. Western Blotting

1. Equal aliquots of proteins extracted from both control and butyrate-treated cells of each time point are resolved in 1-D SDS-PAGE. 5 μg protein of each samples are mixed with equal volume of the 2× Laemmli buffer and boiled at 95°C for 5 min prior to loading into 1.0 mm 12.5% polyacrylamide gels.
2. The glass slides for the gels are cleaned with ethanol before use. The separating polyacrylamide gel (12.5% acrylamide, 0.375 M Tris, pH 8.8, 0.1% SDS, 0.1% APS, and 0.01% TEMED) is prepared by mixing 1.875 mL acrylamide/bis solution, 1.5 mL separating buffer, 60 μL SDS, 60 μL APS, 2.505 mL water, and 6 μL TEMED. Overlay with water-saturated butanol. The separating gel should polymerise within 30 min.
3. The stacking polyacrylamide gel (4% acrylamide, 0.126 M Tris, pH 6.8, 0.1% SDS, 0.1% APS, and 0.01% TEMED) is prepared by mixing 0.15 mL acrylamide/bis solution, 0.189 mL separating buffer, 15 μL SDS, 15 μL APS, 1.131 mL water, and 1.5 μL TEMED. The butanol is poured away. The stacking solution is then added and the comb inserted immediately. The stacking gel should polymerise within 30 min.
4. The running buffer is prepared by diluting the 10× stock with water.
5. After the stacking gel is ready, remove the comb. Add the running buffer into the upper chamber of gel unit and load the sample into the wells. Load the molecular weight marker

in one well. Electrophoresis is performed using the Mini-Protean III gel system at a constant current of 15 mA per gel till the dye front reached the end of gel.

6. Upon completion of electrophoresis, the SDS-PAGE gels are rinsed in prechilled Towbin transfer buffer. The blotting papers, nitrocellulose membranes, and fiber pads are also wet with the transfer buffer before use. Proteins were then blotted onto nitrocellulose membranes using the Mini Trans-Blot system in the Towbin transfer buffer. The transfer setup arrangement is as follows: 1 fiber pad, 2 blotting papers, gel, 1 nitrocellulose membrane, 2 blotting papers, and 1 fiber pad in the transfer cassette. No bubbles are ensured to be present in the sandwich. The transfer cassette is placed in the transfer tank so that the membrane is between the gel and anode. An ice pack is placed inside the transfer tank, and a magnetic stir bar is stirred during the transfer. The transfer is performed at a constant voltage of 100 V.
7. After the transfer is completed, the blots are taken out of the sandwich. The colored molecular weight markers should be visible on the membranes. The membranes are then rinsed with 10 mL PBS and blocked using 10 mL of 5% (w/v) non-fat dry milk in TBS-T overnight prior to immunoprobing with 5 mL antibodies for 1 h each at room temperature on a rocking platform. The membranes are incubated with rabbit anti-GAPDH (1:200), mouse anti-HSP 90-beta (1:1,000), mouse anti-Gelactin-1 (1:500), mouse anti-SEC22b (1:750), or mouse anti-COX VIb (1:750). HRP-conjugated anti-rabbit IgG (1:2,500), HRP-conjugated anti-mouse IgG (1:5,000), or HRP-conjugated anti-mouse IgM (1:5,000) are used as secondary antibodies. Three washes in 10 mL of TBS-T for 15 min each are carried out between each antibody incubation.
8. Subsequent visualization is performed using ECL and Biomax X-ray film in a dark room under safe light conditions. The ECL reagents are mixed and evenly spread onto the membranes. Excess ECL reagents are removed from the blots. The blots are then placed in a plastic protector and placed in the x-ray film cassette. An x-ray film of appropriate size is placed onto the blots for a suitable exposure time in the cassette.
9. For reprobing of the membrane with another antibody, the membrane is incubated with a 30 mL stripping solution for 45 min at 50–60°C, with periodical shaking. After this, the membrane is washed with 30 mL TBS-T for 15 min thrice. Subsequently, the membrane is blocked with blocking buffer prior to incubation with the new primary antibody and secondary antibody for ECL detection as abovementioned.

4. Notes

1. "Water" in this context refers to deionized water that has a resistance of 18.2 mΩ-cm.
2. The cation exchange buffers and cartridge are also supplied with the iTRAQ® Reagent Methods Development Kit (first order only) (Applied Biosystems). We have compared these two products and found that they are the same.
3. It is very critical to filter all the solutions used for liquid chromatography. Particles in the unfiltered solutions may cause the clogging of the columns. It is also crucial to check the compatibility of the filter membranes with the solvents. For example, nitrocellulose membrane will be dissolved in high concentration of ACN.
4. The sample becomes cloudy after adding trypsin/$CaCl_2$ solution. This is due to the formation of calcium carbonate. It does not affect tryptic digestion and iTRAQ labeling. There is no need to separate phases. The cloudiness should disappear after iTRAQ-labeling reaction and the sample is diluted with the cation exchange buffer-load and the pH is adjusted to 2.5–3.3. If cloudiness still exists, centrifugation or filtering should be performed to prevent clogging of the cation-exchange column in the following step.
5. It is crucial to minimize the sample volume at this step. This will facilitate the efficient iTRAQ labeling reaction, which requires greater than 70% organic solvent to be present.
6. Adjusting pH to 2.5–3.3 is critical to ensure efficient binding of iTRAQ-labeled peptides to the cation-exchange cartridge. pH of the diluted sample can be tested by pipetting 1 μL of sample onto a pH paper. Quite often, it is insufficient to adjust pH by adding more cation exchange buffer-load. 1% phosphoric acid is needed to titrate the sample to the desired pH.
7. To ensure efficient binding of the iTRAQ-labeled peptides, the flow-through can also be passed through the column once again.
8. Care should be taken to avoid introducing air bubble into the Sep-Pak cartridge during the desalting steps.
9. MS calibration should be performed right before the MS analysis to ensure the mass accuracy is within 50 ppm across the sample plate. The room temperature should be kept constant. The mass accuracy will be affected if the temperature fluctuates too much (a few degrees). For long MS/MS analysis, the MS instrument should be calibrated daily.

10. In the GPS Explorer software, normalization is done by adjusting the median ratio to 1. This is based on the assumption that the majority of proteins do not change in abundance between the two samples. However, this assumption may not apply to all kinds of studies. Care should be taken not to misinterpret the data. Internal protein standards can be spiked into different samples before iTRAQ labeling and used for normalization instead.
11. The cutoff ratio is determined by data variation, thus it is MS instrument-dependant. Thus, it is suggested that a similar test be done with your own MS system.
12. The A_{260}:A_{280} value should be in the range of 1.7–2.1 to ensure that the RNA sample is free of contaminating proteins, DNA, and reagents such as phenol, ethanol, and salts. The RNA integrity is checked by performing denaturing agarose gel electrophoresis. Good quality RNA samples will show discrete 18 and 28 S ribosomal RNA bands, and the 28 S rRNA band is approximately twice as intense as the 18 S rRNA band.

Acknowledgment

The authors would like to acknowledge National University of Singapore's support for a research scholarship to Hwee Tong Tan. They also thank Singapore Cancer Syndicate for financial assistance (Grant no. MU003).

References

1. Sleno, L., Emili, A. (2008) Proteomic methods for drug target discovery. *Curr Opin Chem Biol.* **12**: 46–54.
2. Hu, S., Yen, Y., Ann, D., Wong, D.T. (2007) Implications of salivary proteomics in drug discovery and development: a focus on cancer drug discovery. *Drug Discov Today* **12**: 911–6.
3. Ross, P.L., Huang, Y.N., Marchese, J.N., Williamson, B., Parker, K., Hattan, S., Khainovski, N., Pillai, S., Dey, S., Daniels, S., Purkayastha, S., Juhasz, P., Martin, S., Bartlet-Jones, M., He, F., Jacobson, A., and Pappin, D.J. (2004) Multiplexed protein quantitation in *Saccharomyces cerevisiae* using amine-reactive isobaric tagging reagents. *Mol Cell Proteomics* **3**: 1154–69.
4. Choe, L., D'Ascenzo, M., Relkin, N.R., Pappin, D., Ross, P., Williamson, B., Guertin, S., Pribil, P., Lee, K.H. (2007) 8-Plex quantitation of changes in cerebrospinal fluid protein expression in subjects undergoing intravenous immunoglobulin treatment for Alzheimer's disease. *Proteomics* 7: 3651–660.
5. Tan, H.T., Tan, S., Lin, Q., Lim, T.K., Hew, C.L., Chung, M.C. (2008) Quantitative and temporal proteome analysis of butyrate-treated colorectal cancer cells. *Mol Cell Proteomics* 7: 1174–85.
6. Jemal, A., Siegel, R., Ward, E., Murray, T., Xu, J., Smigal, C., and Thun, M,J. (2006) Cancer statistics, 2006. *CA Cancer J Clin.* **56**:106–30.
7. Howe, G.R., Benito, E., Castelleto, R., Cornee, J., Esteve, J., Gallagher, R.P., Iscovich, J.M., Deng-ao, J., Kaaks, R., Kune, G.A. et al. (1992) Dietary intake of fiber and

decreased risk of cancers of the colon and rectum: evidence from the combined analysis of 13 case-control studies. *J Natl Cancer Inst.* **84**: 1887–96.

8. Bingham, S.A., Day, N.E., Luben, R., Ferrari, P., Slimani, N., Norat, T., Clavel-Chapelon, F., Kesse, E., Nieters, A., Boeing, H., Tjonneland, A., Overvad, K., Martinez, C., Dorronsoro, M., Gonzalez, C.A., Key, T.J., Trichopoulou, A., Naska, A., Vineis, P., Tumino, R., Krogh, V., Bueno-de-Mesquita, H.B., Peeters, P.H., Berglund, G., Hallmans, G., Lund, E., Skeie, G., Kaaks, R., and Riboli, E. (2003) Dietary fibre in food and protection against colorectal cancer in the European Prospective Investigation into Cancer and Nutrition (EPIC): an observational study. *Lancet* **361**: 1496–501.
9. Cummings, J.H. (1981) Short chain fatty acids in the human colon. *Gut* **22**: 763–79.
10. Cummings, J.H., and Macfarlane, G.T. (1991) The control and consequences of bacterial fermentation in the human colon. *J Appl Bacteriol.* **70**: 443–59.
11. Perrin, P., Pierre, F., Patry, Y., Champ, M., Berreur, M., Pradal, G., Bornet, F., Meflah, K., and Menanteau, J. (2001) Only fibres promoting a stable butyrate producing colonic ecosystem decrease the rate of aberrant crypt foci in rats. *Gut* **48**: 53–61.
12. Heerdt, B., Houston, M.A., and Augenlicht, L.H. (1994) Potentiation by specific short-chain fatty acids of differentiation and apoptosis in human colonic carcinoma cells. *Cancer Res.* **54**: 3288–93.
13. Barnard, J.A., and Warwick, G. (1993) Butyrate rapidly induces growth inhibition and differentiation in HT-29 cells. *Cell Growth Differ.* **4**: 495 – 501.
14. Hague, A., Elder, D.J., Hicks, D.J., and Paraskeva, C. (1995) Apoptosis in colorectal tumour cells: Induction by the short chain fatty acids butyrate, propionate and acetate and by the bile salt deoxycholate. *Int J Cancer* **60**: 400–6.
15. Scheppach, W., Bartram, H.P., and Richter, F. (1995) Role of short-chain fatty acids in the prevention of colorectal cancer. *Eur J Cancer* **31A**: 1077–80.
16. McIntyre, A., Gibson, P.R., and Young, G.P. (1993) Butyrate production from dietary fibre and protection against large bowel cancer in a rat model. *Gut* **34**: 386–91.
17. Fearon, E.R., and Vogelstein, B. (1990) A genetic model for colorectal tumorigenesis. *Cell* **61**: 759–67.
18. Bedi, A., Pasricha, P.J., Alchtar, A.J., Barber, J.P., Bedi, G.C., Giairdiello, F.M., Zehnbauer, B.A., Hamilton, S.R., and Jones, R.J. (1995) Inhibition of apoptosis during development of colorectal cancer. *Cancer Res.* **55**: 1811–6.
19. Kersey, P. J., Duarte, J., Williams, A., Karavidopoulou, Y., Birney, E., and Apweiler, R. (2004) The International Protein Index: An integrated database for proteomics experiments. *Proteomics* **4**: 1985–8.
20. Guo, Y., Singleton, P.A., Rowshan A, Gucek, M., Cole, R.N., Graham D.R., Van Eyk, J.E., and Garcia, J.G., (2007) Quantitative proteomics analysis of human endothelial cell membrane rafts: evidence of MARCKS and MRP regulation in the sphingosine 1-phosphate-induced barrier enhancement. *Mol Cell Proteomics* **6**: 689–96.
21. Pierce, A., Unwin, R.D., Evans, C.A., Griffiths, S., Carney, L., Zhang, L., Jaworska, E., Lee, C.F., Blinco, D., Okoniewski, M.J., Miller, C.J., Bitton, D.A., Spooncer, E., and Whetton, A.D. (2007) Eight-channel iTRAQ enables comparison of the activity of 6 leukaemogenic tyrosine kinases. *Mol Cell Proteomics* **7**: 853–63.

Chapter 14

Heterotypic Cell Adhesion Assay for the Study of Cell Adhesion Inhibition

Seetharama D. Satyanarayanajois, Sharon Ronald, and Jining Liu

Abstract

CD2 is a cell adhesion molecule that mediates T-cell activation by binding to its ligand CD58 on antigen-presenting cells. Interaction between CD2 and CD58 or leukocyte function-associated antigen-3 (LFA-3) helps to optimize immune recognition facilitating contact between T lymphocytes and antigen-presenting cells. Modulation or inhibition of this interaction has been shown to be therapeutically useful in the treatment of autoimmune diseases. Antibodies and small molecules including peptides have been designed to modulate or disrupt the cell adhesion interactions due to CD2 and CD58. E-rosetting assay is a widely used method applied in the study of the modulation of CD2–CD58 interaction, which is either labor-intensive or radio-hazardous. In this chapter, we describe two methods that are used to study cell adhesion inhibition: (a) E-rosetting Assay and (b) Lymphocyte-epithelial assay. The second method, lymphocyte-epithelial assay, is a rapid and sensitive heterotypic cell adhesion assay for studying cell adhesion inhibition. The method relies on the CD2 expression on the surface of Jurkat cells and the CD58 expression on the surface of Caco-2 cells, which were confirmed by flow cytometry and ELISA studies respectively. This heterotypic cell adhesion assay described typically takes less than 4 h to perform, allows the evaluation of inhibitory activity of peptides/small molecules to modulate CD2–CD58 interaction in real cell system.

Key words: Caco-2 cells, CD2, CD58, Cell adhesion inhibition, E-rosetting, Jurkat cells

1. Introduction

A key feature for the recognition of antigen-presenting cells (APCs) by T-cells in the immune response is the interaction of cell surface proteins, including the T-lymphocyte adhesion receptor CD2 with its ligands, CD58 in humans, and CD48 in rodents (1). The interaction between CD2 on T-cells and CD58 on APCs is believed to augment the adhesion between T-cells and APCs (1, 2). In particular, this heterotypic cell adhesion facilitates initial

Seetharama D. Satyanarayanajois (ed.), *Drug Design and Discovery: Methods and Protocols*,
Methods in Molecular Biology, vol. 716, DOI 10.1007/978-1-61779-012-6_14,

cell–cell contact before specific antigen recognition and also enhances T-cell receptor (TCR) affinity by fostering interaction with pMHC (peptide-class II MHC complex). It is documented that the TCR-MHC complex stabilizes in the presence of CD2–CD58 interaction with a 50- to 100-fold greater efficiency than in its absence (3). Although the TCR-pMHC interaction is important for the recognition of antigen to generate T-cell activation for immune response, the affinity of TCR for pMHC is very low – on the order of 10^{-4} to 10^{-6} M. With this low affinity and limited number of antigenic complexes on the surface of APC, the interaction of TCR with antigen seems unlikely to drive the formation of a tight contact. Costimulatory molecules such as CD2 and CD58 help to tighten the gap between the T-cells and APC interface. Furthermore, endothelial cells (EC) in rheumatoid arthritis (RA) have been shown to express elevated levels of CD58. RA-synovial fluid lymphocytes (SFL) that consist mostly of T-cells showed higher expression of CD2 and CD58 relative to normal peripheral blood lymphocytes (4, 5). CD58 is widely distributed among cell types of the synovial microenvironment and provides numerous cell types with which lymphocytes can interact via CD2–CD58 and ICAM-1–LFA-1 adhesion pathways during the course of inflammatory synovitis (6). RA-SFL that consist mostly of T-cells showed higher expression of CD2 and CD58. It is postulated that the onset of autoimmunity may be associated with CD58 upregulation and ligation of CD2 on dendritic cells, and subsequent autocrine release of IL-1β that increases the release of IL-12 which, in turn, activates T-cells. These findings make CD2 and CD58 molecules attractive targets for understanding the mechanism of autoimmune diseases, in particular, RA.

Modulation of T-cell responses in vivo after blockade of the interaction between CD58 and CD2 can potentially be applied in the treatment of autoimmune diseases and transplantation. It has been shown that blockade of the CD2–CD58 interaction (7–9) and/or modulation of the CD2 costimulatory pathway (10) can result in prolonged tolerance toward allografts. The soluble CD58-Ig fusion protein Amevive (LFA3TIP) has been employed in the treatment of psoriasis (11). The humanized versions of antibodies BTI-322 (12) and MEDI-507 (13) have been tested for the treatment of acute organ rejection and graft-versus-host disease. These findings make CD2 and CD58 molecules attractive targets for drug design for autoimmune diseases. To discover and develop inhibitory ligands to modulate CD2–CD58 interaction, it is important to have cellular assays that can monitor CD2–CD58 interaction and its interruption in a model cellular system.

In previous reports related to the study of CD2–CD58 cell adhesion and its inhibition, the modulation of CD2–CD58 interaction was mainly investigated by E-rosetting, by either counting bound cells visually under a microscope or radiolabeling cells with ^{125}I and measuring the residual radioactivity after separating non-E-rosette-forming cells (14). The first method is less expensive and simple, but very labor-intensive. Although the second method is sensitive, rapid, and easier than counting, it requires the use of hazardous radiochemicals. E-rosetting assay has the disadvantage that the results reported the inhibition of adhesion interaction of CD2 protein with sheep CD58 protein (using sheep blood cells), which is different from the interaction with human CD58 protein. In this chapter, we describe two methods that are used to study cell adhesion inhibition: (a) E-rosetting assay and (b) lymphocyte-epithelial assay. E-rosetting is the most widely used method to identify T-cells by CD2–CD58 interaction (15). Sheep red blood cells (SRBCs) express CD58 protein, while Jurkat leukemic T-cells express CD2 protein on their surface. The ability of Jurkat cells to express CD2 was measured by flow-cytometry assay. Binding of Jurkat cells to SRBCs due to CD2 and CD58 interaction results in the formation of E-rosettes. These E-rosettes can be observed under a microscope for the assessment of adhesion of cells. Inhibition of adhesion between the cells by peptides or antibodies to CD2 or CD58 results in the loss of E-rosette formation. Hence, the E-rosetting assay can be used as a method to evaluate the ability of peptides or other small molecules to inhibit cell–cell adhesion.

In the E-rosetting assay mentioned above, the adhesion between cells that express CD2 and CD58 can be monitored by counting the number of cells that form E-rosettes. Although the method has been in use for several years, it is very tedious. Cells that form E-rosettes and cells that do not must be counted under a microscope. At least 200 cells from different samples have to be counted, which leads to variations in the results obtained. Lymphocyte-epithelial assay, a new method to evaluate the cell adhesion ability of peptides, was developed in our laboratory using T-cells and Caco-2 cells. Caco-2 cells express CD58 while Jurkat cells express CD2 protein. The inhibitory activity observed between Caco-2 cells and Jurkat cells provides evidence that the peptides designed from CD2 can inhibit the adhesion between the heterotypic cells. The inhibitory activities of designed CD2 peptides were measured by using fluorescently labeled Jurkat cells and a microplate fluorescence analyzer. The schematic diagram (Fig. 1) gives the overall assay design (16). We have demonstrated that both methods can be successfully applied to evaluate the inhibitory activities of peptides to CD2–CD58 interaction.

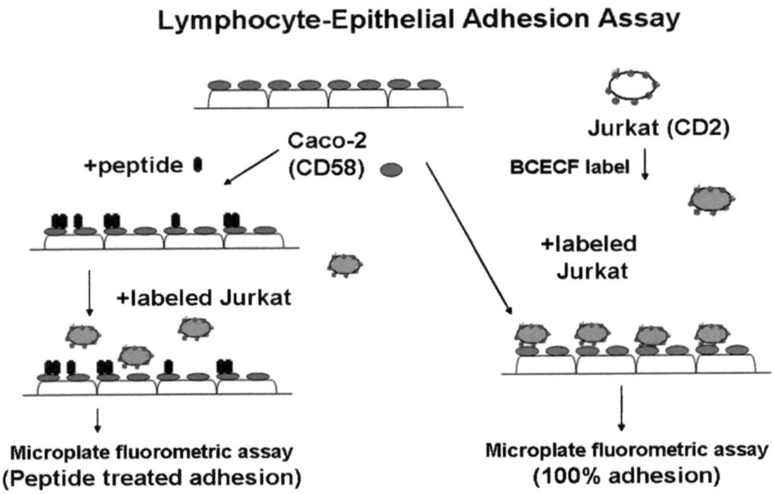

Fig. 1. Schematic diagram of lymphocyte-epithelial adhesion assay.

2. Materials

2.1. Cell Culture

1. Trypsinizing medium: 0.25% Trypsin EDTA, 200 mM L-glutamine, 100 mg/L penicillin/streptomycin, nonessential amino acids, and 100 mM sodium pyruvate (Gibco/BRL, Bethesda, MD).
2. Fetal bovine serum: stored in single use aliquots at –20°C, and then added to tissue culture as required.
3. Cell lines: The human colon adenocarcinoma (Caco-2) cell line and the T-leukemia Jurkat cell line (American Type Culture Collection, Rockville, MD).
4. RPMI1640: (Gibco/BRL, Bethesda, MD) supplemented with 10% FBS, 2 mM L-glutamine, 100 mg/L of penicillin/streptomycin, and 5 mg of bovine insulin in 500 mL medium.
5. Minimum essential medium-α (MEM-α): supplemented with 10% FBS, 1% nonessential amino acids, 1 mM sodium pyruvate, 1% L-glutamine, and 100 mg/L of penicillin/streptomycin.
6. Hemocytometer.
7. 2.2×2.2 cm^2 Coverslips.
8. 25 and 75 cm^2 Tissue culture flasks.
9. 15-mL Conical tubes (Falcon).
10. Brightfield microscope.

2.2. CD58 Expression Examined by ELISA

1. Blocking buffer: 0.3% (w/v) BSA in PBS and stored in single use aliquots at −80°C.
2. Fixing buffer: Paraformaldehyde (PFM): 0.3% (w/v) solution in PBS. The solution needs to be carefully heated (using a stirring hot-plate in a fume hood) to approximately 80°C and dissolve. Cool and store at a 4°C refrigerator.
3. Washing buffer: 0.05 M Tris–HCl (pH 7.4).
4. Mouse anti-human CD58 monoclonal antibody (mAb) clone 1C3 (AICD58.6) (IgG2a) (BD Biosciences, San Jose CA).
5. ELISA kit: with anti-mouse Ig-horseradish peroxidase (HRP) conjugate (1:1,000) and substrate solution (ABTS) (BD Biosciences, San Jose CA).
6. Microplate reader.

2.3. CD58 Expression Examined by Flow-Cytometry

1. Murine anti-human CD58mAb, clone TS2/9 (IgG1) (Ancell, Bayport, MN).
2. Stock solution of phorbol ester: 1 mg 12-myristate-13-acetate (PMA) in 1.6 mL of DMSO (keep it frozen at −20°C).
3. 0.5% BSA/PBS.
4. FITC-conjugated CD2 mAb: Rabbit anti-human CD2mAb (IgG) (Immunotech, Quebec, Canada).
5. 0.5% BSA/10 mM HEPES/PBS.
6. 1% Paraformaldehyde/PBS.
7. Flow Cytometer equipped with the Cell Quest software program.

2.4. Confocal Microscopy

1. Microscope chamber slides (8 chamber polystyrene vessel, BD falcon, BD Biosciences).
2. Blocking serum: 2% normal horse serum in PBS.
3. Blocking buffer: 1% BSA/PBS.
4. Washing buffer: PBS.
5. Fixing Buffer: 100% methanol kept at −20°C.
6. Fluorescence mounting medium with DAPI (Vector Laboratories, Burlingame, CA).
7. Confocal microscope.
8. 2.2×5.5 cm^2 Coverslips.
9. FITC-labeled CD58 antibody dilutions.

2.5. BCECF Labeling of Jurkat Cells

1. Bis-carboxyethyl-carboxyfluorescein,acetoxymethyl(BCECF-AM) (Invitrogen, Carlsbad, CA).
2. High-quality anhydrous DMSO.
3. PBS.

2.6. Cell–Cell Adhesion

1. Washing solution: MEM medium supplemented with 10% FBS.
2. Working solution: RPMI medium with 10% FBS.
3. Lysis solution: 2% Triton X-100 in 0.1 M NaOH.
4. Microplate reader with filter excitation 485 nm, emission 530 nm.

2.7. E-Rosetting Assay

1. Sheep red blood cells (SRBC) in Alsever's solution (Colorado Serum Company, Denver, CO).
2. PBS.
3. Complete RPMI medium.
4. FBS.
5. 2-Aminoethylisothiouronium bromide (AET) solution: Dissolve 0.5 g AET hydrobromide in 12.5 mL distilled water. Adjust to pH 9 with 4N NaOH. Filter sterilize through a 0.2-μm filter. Prepare fresh before use.
6. Sterile distilled water.
7. Beckman GPR centrifuge with GH-3.7 horizontal rotor (or equivalent temperature-controlled centrifuge).
8. 15 and 50-mL conical centrifuge tubes (e.g., Falcon).
9. Microscope with different magnification for counting and hemocytometer.

3. Methods

In this protocol, Jurkat cells (T lymphocytes) are conveniently labeled with nonpolar BCECF-AM before its usage in the attachment assay. BCECF (2′,7′-bis-(2-carboxyethyl)-5-(and-6)-carboxyfluorescein), introduced by Roger Tsien and coworkers in 1982 (17), is the most widely used fluorescent indicator for intracellular pH and also for various functional properties of cells including viability and cytotoxicity, apoptosis, adhesion, multidrug resistance, and chemotaxis. Most mammalian cells can be loaded without permeabilization by incubation with dilute aqueous dispersions of cell permeant BCECF-AM. Once within the cell, the AM derivatives of the nonfluorescent indicator BCECF are readily cleaved by high activity and large capacity cytoplasmic esterase into fluorescent, free acid form. Thus, only live cells can be stained by this dye. BCECF has 4–5 negative charges at pH 7–8, aiding intracellular retention. The low leakage rate of the polyanionic indicator and the small intracellular volume result in the final intracellular concentration being much higher than the external incubation concentration. In general, BCECF loaded via the AM ester method appears less susceptible to intracellular compartmentalization than calcium indicators such as Fura-2. In addition, most fluorimeters and fluorescence microscopes are equipped with a filter set for FITC, which can be used for detecting this dye.

A potential problem with BCECF-loaded cells is dye leakage from Jurkat cells and subsequent labeling of Caco-2 cells during adhesion assay (18). However, the epithelial cells investigated in our assay are human colonic adenocarcinoma cells, which stably express the human multidrug transporter, P-glycoprotein, in the plasma membrane. P-glycoprotein can actively extrude the hydrophobic AM form of the fluorescent indicator BCECF (19, 20). Moreover, since the hydrophilic free-acid form of BCECF is not membrane-permeant, Caco-2 cells will not be fluorescently labeled. In addition, BCECF release was found to be less than 3% after plated as a monolayer for 60 min (21). Therefore, the likelihood of BCECF leakage may be excluded under our adhesion assay conditions.

3.1. ELISA Assay for Detection of CD58 Expression on Caco-2 Cells

1. Plate Caco-2 cells at a density of 10^4cells/well in a 96-well tissue culture plate and incubate at 37°C with 5% CO_2 for about 72 h (see Notes 1 and 2). It is assumed that in the microplate, columns 1–8 and A–G are plated with cells.
2. Rinse the cells with 200 μL/well of 0.3% BSA/PBS and fix with 100 μL/well of 3% PFM/PBS for 15 min at room temperature (RT).
3. Wash the cells and block the cells for 20 min with 0.05 M Tris–HCl (pH 7.4).
4. Add 100 μL of a twofold dilution range of primary antibody CD58 (1:125–1:16,000) in a microplate column 1–8 using multichannel pipette. Add column 9 diluent only.
5. Incubate overnight at 4°C, and wash the cells three times with 0.3% BSA/PBS by flooding and emptying the wells. Then add 100 μL of a twofold dilution range of the anti-mouse Ig-HRP conjugate (1:125–1:8,000) from row A to row G. Add row H diluent only.
6. Incubate for 2 h at RT, wash the cells five times (0.3% BSA/PBS), and then incubate with substrate solution (ABTS) for 30 min at RT. Measure optical density readings at 430 nm using a fluorescent plate reader.
7. Plot a histogram of added antibody vs. optical density. Compare with blank and control (without the addition of antibody) to determine the binding of CD58 antibody to Caco-2 cells expressing CD58.

3.2. Sample Preparation for Flow-Cytometry

1. Plate appropriate number of Caco-2 cells in a 25 cm^2 flask and maintain the cells until 80% or more confluence is achieved.
2. Detach the cells to form single cells using 10 mM EDTA in HEPES/PBS for 30 min at 37°C, followed by washing with 1% BSA/PBS (see Note 3).
3. Incubate the cell pellet (1×10^6 cells) with FITC-CD58 for 1 h in the dark at 4°C.
4. Wash with BSA/PBS, resuspended the pellet in cold PBS.
5. Flow cytometry data from 1×10^4 cells were collected, and the fluorescence of each sample was measured and expressed as a percentage of the fluorescence of the respective control sample (without reaction with FITC-CD58).

3.3. Preparation of Microscopy Slides for Confirming the Expression of CD58 on Caco-2 Cell

1. Plate Caco-2 cells at a density of 20,000–40,000 cells/well in a multichamber slide and incubate at 37°C with 5% CO_2 for about 24 h for cell attachment. 200 μL of appropriate medium is added per well.
2. Gently rinse the cells, twice, with 200 μL/well of PBS and block the cells with 2% normal blocking serum solution for 30 min at RT.
3. Add 100–200 μL of FITC-CD58 antibody dilutions (dilutions were made in 2% normal blocking serum solution) and incubate the wells for 2 h at 37°C with 5% CO_2.
4. Wash the cells three times with PBS by flooding and emptying the wells and allow the wells to dry for about 2 min.
5. Fix the cells with 100 μL/well of 100% methanol at −20°C and incubate for about 5 min at RT before washing the wells with PBS and then drying it for about 2–3 min.
6. Add appropriate amount of DAPI stain and incubate for 10 min at RT.
7. Carefully remove the multichamber slide gasket (with a razor blade) and place the cover slip with the mounting medium.
8. Observe the images under a fluorescence microscope. Compare with blank and control (without the addition of antibody) to determine the binding of CD58 antibody to Caco-2 cells expressing CD58.

3.4. Expression of CD2 on Jurkat Cells by Fluorescence Microscopy

1. Aliquot 2×10^6 Jurkat cells in appropriate culture tubes and wash the aliquots twice with 1% BSA/PBS by centrifuging the floating cells.
2. Incubate overnight with 20 μL FITC-CD2 mAb at 4°C and in the dark.

3. Wash the cells with 1% BSA/PBS by centrifugation and fix the labeled cells with 1% PFA/PBS for about 10 min.
4. Wash the cells with 1% BSA/PBS and store it in the dark at 4°C before observing for fluorescence microscopy. As a negative control, cells incubated in the absence of mAb were used.

3.5. Cultivation of Caco-2 Cell Monolayers (Use 96 or 24-Well Plate)

Timing: start 3 days in advance of actual experiment.

1. Trypsinize Caco-2 cells from maximally (90%) confluent Caco-2 cultures. Remove the medium by aseptical decantation, rinse with prewarmed PBS (15 mL per 75 cm^2 flask) and decant; repeat for one more time; add the prewarmed trypsin/EDTA solution (5 mL per 75 cm^2 flask); rinse the cells and pour off the majority of the trypsin/EDTA so that only about 500 μL to 1 mL remains in the flask; the remaining trypsin must wet the entire cell layer. Incubate the flask (closed lid) at 37°C for 4–10 min (as shortest as possible) and check the detachment of the cells from the plastic surface by mildly knocking the sidewall of the flask with palm. As soon as the cells are detached, immediately stop trypsinization by resuspending the cells in 10 mL complete DMEM.
2. After mixing and resuspending the monolayer to single cells, take an aliquot and count the cells. The percentage of dead cells must not exceed 5%. This is assessed by counting the total number of cells as well as the number of nonviable cells. Living cells extrude the vital dye Trypan blue, whereas dead or dying cells with a compromised plasma membrane take up the dye and turn blue. The cells can be counted using a hemocytometer to give an estimate of the cell concentration and percentage viability.
3. Resuspend the cells in DMEM (at a concentration of 1×10^5 cells/mL).
4. Seed Caco-2 cells onto 96-well culture plates at approximately 4×10^4 cells/well and incubate at 37°C with 5% CO_2 for about 72 h. Avoid using the outer wells on a plate for epithelium cultures, as these are most subject to evaporation and temperature fluctuations over time. The outer wells can be filled with PBS. It has been reported that IFN-γ treatment can enhance the expression of adhesion molecules such as LFA-1 and ICAM-1. We have studied the effect of IFN-γ treatment on the regulation of CD58 expression but did not find any upregulation (Fig. 2); therefore, we recommend cultivating Caco-2 monolayer at least until 70% confluent in normal medium.
5. Change medium every 2 days or every day as required.

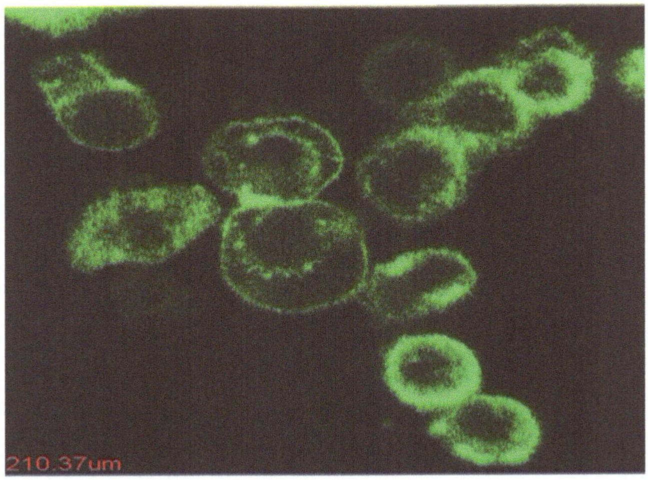

Fig. 2. Confocal microscopy of Caco-2 cells showing the expression of CD58 on Caco-2 cells.

3.6. Stimulation of Jurkat Cells with PMA

1. Maintain the culture between 1×10^5 and 1×10^6 cells/mL. Renew the medium every 3 days by taking out appropriate volume of medium containing Jurkat cells and adding 9 volumes of fresh medium.
2. Timing: start 2 days in advance of actual experiment.
3. Transfer the medium containing the cells into a suitable sterile centrifuge tube and centrifuge at $200 \times g$ for 5 min at RT. It should be noted that cells should be in log-phase and the cell viability for the assay should be greater than 95% (determined by trypan blue exclusion).
4. Carefully remove the medium without touching the cell pellet. Replace with fresh medium and adjust the cell concentration to 2×10^6cells/mL.
5. Add PMA solution into the cells to final concentration of 10 ng/mL in RPMI medium. We recommend stimulating Jurkat cells prior to the adhesion assay with PMA (at 10 ng/mL for 48 h) (see Note 4).

3.7. BCECF Labeling of Lymphocytes (Jurkat Cells)

Timing: ~1.5 h

1. Preparing BCECF AM.
2. Add 50 μL of dimethyl sulfoxide (DMSO) to the whole package (50 μg) (1–10 mM). Mix well to dissolve the entire contents of the package. Store frozen at -20°C. DMSO stock solutions should be stored desiccated at -20°C, and preferably used within a short period of time for one series of experiments. Stock solutions of BCECF AM should be stable for at least 6 months if prepared and stored as directed above. Solutions exhibiting strong fluorescence and coloration

(indicated by absorbance at >400 nm) probably contain a significant amount of hydrolyzed material and should be discarded. Dilute working solutions in aqueous media should be used immediately and should not be stored (see Notes 5 and 6).

3. Resuspend and wash the Jurkat cells twice with 0.5% BSA/PBS and aliquot the cell number to 3×10^6 cells/mL, for BCECF labeling. We recommend the cells be prepared in 5% BSA/PBS to improve the cell viability and loading efficiency.
4. Prepare an aqueous dilution of BCECF-AM. Mix an appropriate volume of the dilution with the Jurkat cell suspension to give a final concentration of 2 μM. The optimum labeling concentration of BCECF for Jurkat cells is determined previously. Although higher dose of BCECF-AM makes the cells more fluorescent (Fig. 3), the loading concentration should

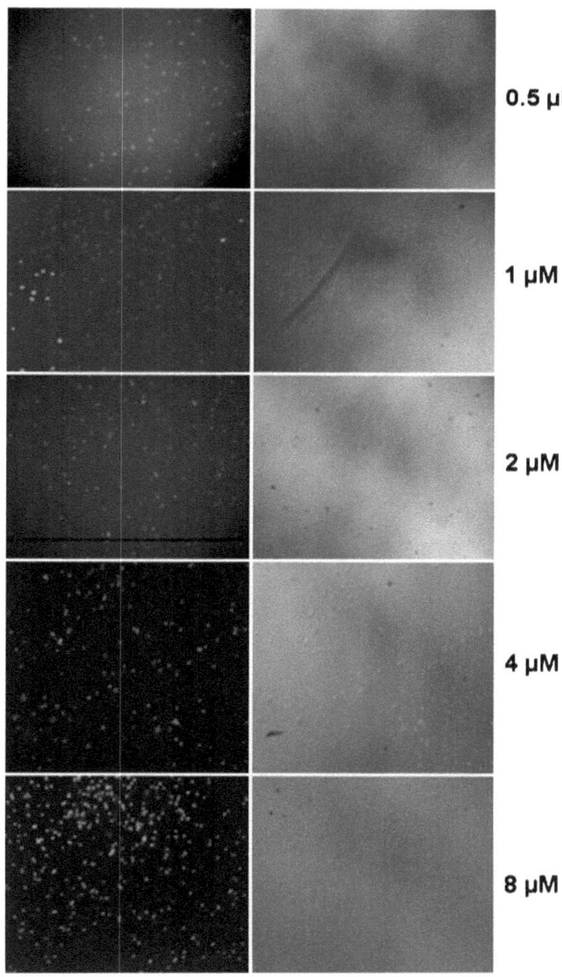

Fig. 3. Fluorescence microscopy examination of the BCECF-AM-labeled Jurkat cells at different concentration of BCECF-AM.

be kept as low as possible to minimize accumulation of the by-products of AM ester hydrolysis (formaldehyde and acetic acid). For example, 3×10^6/mL of Jurkat cells was labeled with 0.5–8 μM of BCECF-AM for 1 h and was examined for morphology by fluorescence microscopy and for fluorescence intensity by a fluorescence plate reader. Although a concentration of 4 μM BCECF-AM is close to the saturation level (Fig. 3), confocal microscopic observations revealed that the Jurkat cells labeled with 2 μM BCECF-AM exhibited a bright and uniform cytoplasmic staining pattern (Figs. 4 and 5) (see Note 6).

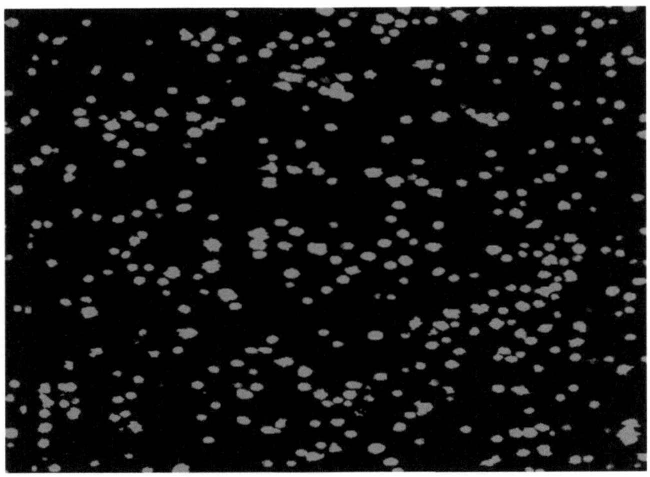

Fig. 4. Confocal microscopy of labeled Jurkat cells (3×10^6 cells/mL) loaded with 2 μM BCECF-AM for 60 min.

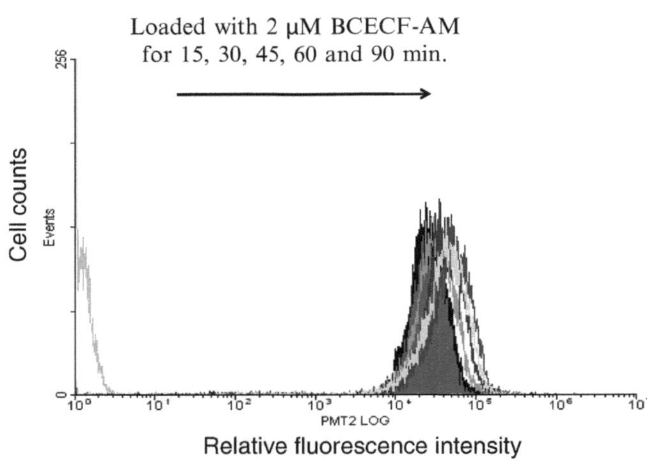

Fig. 5. Effect of labeling times on the uptake of BCECF assayed by flow cytometry. Results are shown as cell number (*y* axis) vs. log of fluorescence intensity (*x* axis).

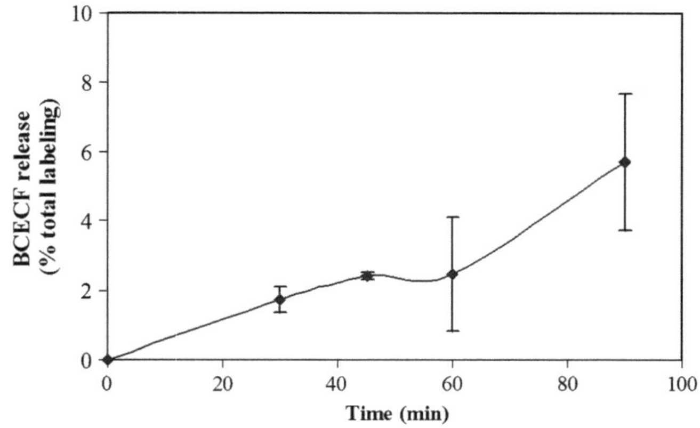

Fig. 6. Release of BCECF from labeled Jurkat cells incubated at various times (15–90 min). Mean values and S.D. of three separate measurements are plotted (reproduced with permission from Elsevier).

5. Thoroughly mix the BCECF solution with the cell suspension and incubate the cells for labeling for 45 min at 37°C with 5% CO_2, to achieve optimum labeling of the cells without affecting the cell viability (determined by trypan blue staining).
6. Resuspend the pellet with RPMI containing 1% FBS at 4°C with aliquots containing 2.5×10^6 labeled cells/mL. Fluorescence is not detected in the medium after plating, and less than 6% of BCECF is released under adhesion assay conditions (Fig. 6).

3.8. Cell–Cell Adhesion Assay

Timing: ~2 h

1. Gently rinse the Caco-2 confluent monolayer, three times, with prewarmed medium (MEM-α with 10% FBS).
2. Add 100 μL/well (400 μL for 24-well plate) of antibody or peptide dilutions in RPMI/FBS and incubate for 30 min at 37°C with 5% CO_2.
3. Add 100 μL/well of BCECF-labeled Jurkat cells (2.5×10^6 cells/mL). We add the given number of cells since our studies indicate that optimal number of Jurkat cells should be added per well for the necessary interaction with the Caco-2 monolayer. As shown in Fig. 5, fluorescence studies reveal that 2×10^5 Jurkat cells/well is close to the saturation level, and also exhibit a good linear relationship ($r^2 = 0.9972$, in the range of $0.5–2 \times 10^5$ cells/well) with the original cell concentration per well. Thus, we recommend a standard cell concentration of 2.5×10^5 cells/well for the assay.
4. Shake the plate gently and incubate for 45 min at 37°C with 5% CO_2. We have established the time required for Jurkat cells to attach to Caco-2 cells and have tested it at different

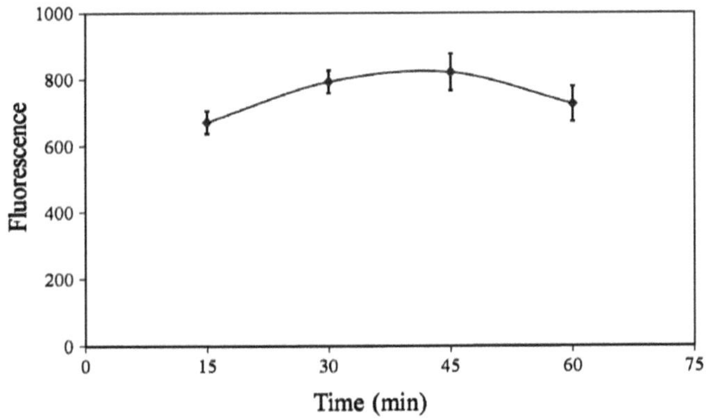

Fig. 7. The kinetics of Jurkat cell adhesion to Caco-2 monolayers. Add BCECF-loaded Jurkat cells to confluent Caco-2 monolayers, and allow adhering for various time periods at 37°C.

time intervals (Fig. 7). As shown in Fig. 7, no significant difference in fluorescence is observed at 15, 30, 45, and 60 min from the adherent Jurkat cells. Thus, the kinetics of Jurkat cell adhesion with the Caco-2 monolayers is rapid enough to be completed by 15 min. However, we still recommend incubating the monolayer for 45 min to ensure sufficient exchange time and adhesion (see Note 7).

5. Wash thrice with PBS to remove any traces of the nonadherent, labeled Jurkat cells.
6. Add 0.5 mL of 2% Triton X-100 in 0.1 M NaOH to the wells and incubate it for about 10 min to lyse the monolayer associated with the Jurkat cells.
7. Measure the fluorescence using a fluorescent plate reader. The excitation filter centered at 485 nm, while the emission filter centered at 535 nm, which corresponds well within BCECF's excitation maximum of 500 nm and emission maximum of 535 nm (see Note 8).
8. The data (results) of lymphocyte-epithelial adhesion by antibody or peptides/small molecules are presented as relative fluorescence or as percent of inhibition. Relative fluorescence (FL) intensity can be calculated by subtracting the values of fluorescence intensity corrected for the reading of background (cell monolayers only) (Fig. 8).

$$\text{Inhibition}(\%) = \{1 - (\text{FL}_{\text{treated cells}}) / (\text{FL}_{\text{nontreated cells}})\} \times 100$$

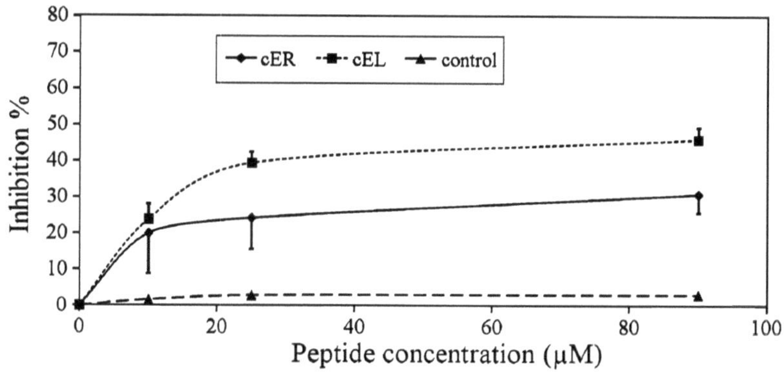

Fig. 8. Dose-response curves for the inhibitory activity of peptides cER and cEL by the lymphocyte-epithelial adhesion assay.

$FL_{treated\ cells}$ is fluorescence of cells treated with compounds or antibody.

$FL_{nontreated\ cells}$ is fluorescence of cells that are not treated with compounds or antibody.

3.9. E-Rosetting Assay

Timing: ~2 h

1. Place 15–25 mL of SRBCs in Alsever's solution in a 50-mL centrifuge tube. Fill the tube with PBS and centrifuge it at 10 min at 1,000 × *g* (~2,100 rpm).
2. Wash the cells by removing the supernatant, and using a pipet, resuspend the cells in PBS. Centrifuge for 10 min at 1,000 × *g*. Repeat the washing step (see Note 9).
3. Add 8 mL AET solution to 2 mL packed, washed SRBC in a 50-mL centrifuge tube. Incubate 20 min in a 37°C water bath (suspension should darken).
4. Fill the tube with cold PBS and centrifuge for 10 min at 400 × *g* (1,300 rpm). Remove supernatant, resuspend cells in PBS, and repeat the wash two times.
5. After the last wash, remove the supernatant and add 48 mL complete RPMI to the pelleted AET-treated SRBC (~2 mL). Store at 4°C. Final concentration of SRBC is 4% (v/v).
6. For each peptide/antibody sample, take 1 mL of the SRBC suspension and centrifuge 5 min at 400 × *g*. Carefully remove the entire medium and add 400 μL of dilutions of antibody or peptides in RPMI/FBS in the well. Gently tap to resuspend the cells in the peptide/antibody solution.
7. Incubate the cell mixture at 37°C for 30 min.
8. Prepare 10 mL of Jurkat cells (1×10^6 cells/mL) and centrifuge for 10 min at 400 × *g* (1,300 rpm). Remove supernatant

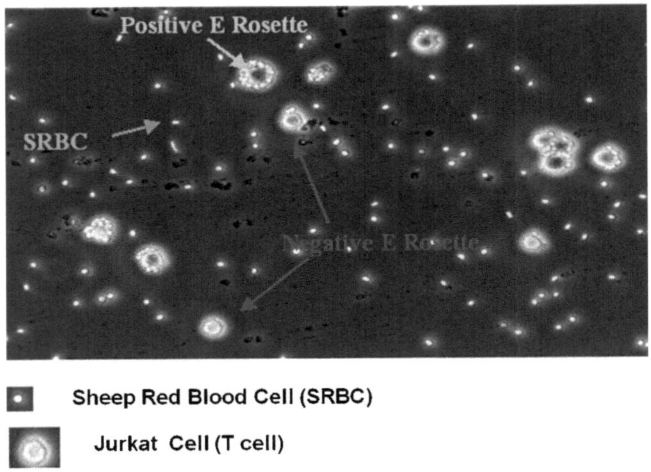

Fig. 9. E-rosette formation between T-cells and sheep red blood cells (SRBCs). Adhesion of five or more SRBCs is considered as positive E-rosette and less than five SRBCs is considered as negative E-rosette.

and resuspend pellet in complete RPMI to a final concentration of 2.5×10^6 cells/mL.

9. Add 100 μL of Jurkat cells to the preincubated SRBCs.
10. Roll slowly to mix and incubate the cell mixture for another 15 min.
11. Centrifuge ($400 \times g$) for 5 min at 4°C and incubate at 4°C for 1 h.
12. Using a pipette, remove ~3/4 of the upper layer (culture medium) from the centrifuged suspension.
13. Gently resuspend PBMC/peptide/SRBC mixture by rolling slowly.
14. Take a small aliquot from the pellet and count E-rosette in a hemocytometer. Rosettes containing less than five SRBCs were considered as non-E-rosette forming cells (non-E-RFC) (Fig. 9). Count at least 200 cells from each repeat. Repeat three times for each concentration of the compound added.
15. Calculate the percentage of inhibition of E-rosettes by the compound and control using the following formula

$$\text{Inhibition } (\%) = \{(A - B) / C\} \times 100$$

A = percentage of non-E-rosetteing forming cells treated with compound or antibody.

B = percentage of non-E-rosetting forming cells without compound.

C = percentage of E-rosettes formed in nontreated cells.

4. Notes

1. After thawing a vial of Caco-2 cells from the stock, cultivate the cells for two passages before plating the cells for the assay. It is recommended to use about ten passages. It is also advisable to use constant passage numbers every time the assay is performed, for example, passages 50–60, in order to get reproducible results. Following plating, incubate the cells for about 72 h for sufficient confluence.
2. It is critical that CD58 protein is constitutively expressed on the surface of Caco-2 monolayer for the assay. Therefore, we recommend cultivating Caco-2 monolayer until atleast 70% confluence for CD58 expression.
3. To avoid surface protein damage by trypsin, detach the Caco-2 monolayer by treating with 10 mM EDTA/2% HEPES/PBS at 37°C for 30 min, prior to their resuspension for the assay.
4. We have studied cytokine regulation of surface CD2 expression by flow cytometry. Downregulation of CD2 occurs due to (1) exposure to PHA (at 1, 2 μg/mL) for 24 h; (2) exposure to a combination of PHA (at 1, 2 μg/mL) and PMA (at 1, 2 ng/mL) for 24 h or; (3) exposure to PMA (at 25, 50 ng/mL) for 24 h. Enhancement of CD2 expression is not observed with a reduced dose treatment of PMA (at 10, 20 ng/mL) for 24 h. However, marginal upregulation of CD2 expression on Jurkat cells, after activation by 10 ng/mL of PMA for 48 h, and a considerable decrease in the CD2 expression levels following all the treatments on day 3 are observed. Thereby, it is recommended to stimulate the Jurkat cells prior to the assay with PMA (at 10 ng/mL for 48 h).
5. Preparing BCECF AM: DMSO stock solutions must be kept anhydrous, since the solvent readily takes up moisture, leading to decomposition of the dye. It is advisable to keep the AM ester heavily concentrated as a stock solution so that minimal amounts (ideally ≤0.1%) of DMSO are present in the loading solution.
6. BCECF will react quickly in aqueous solution. Thereby, it is critical that it is dispersed rapidly in the cell suspension and, that the cells are as close to a homogeneous suspension of single cells as possible, to ensure even labeling of lymphocytes.
7. It should be noted that upon labeling, BCECF becomes fluorescent and thereby prone to photo bleaching. As a protective measure, cover the flask/plate containing the BCECF-labeled Jurkat cells with an aluminum foil to avoid exposure to excessive light.

8. Since BCECF has higher emission efficiency in alkaline solution, we recommend lysing the attached Jurkat cells in NaOH solution. To test the stability of the fluorescence signal in alkaline solution, fluorescence was assessed immediately after lysis and after overnight incubation at RT. There was no detectable loss of fluorescence signal after the incubation period.
9. SRBC can be stored in Alsever's solution for 2–3 weeks. Washed SRBC can be stored 2–3 days in PBS before treatment with AET.

Acknowledgments

Ms. Sharon Ronald was supported by funding from Louisiana Biomedical Research Network grant (LBRN/INBRE Grant Number P20RR016456, Bioinformatics, Biostatistics and Computational Biology Core, from the National Center for Research Resources. The content is solely the responsibility of the authors and does not necessarily represent the official views of the National Center for Research Resources or the National Institutes of Health). Part of the work was supported by funding from Louisiana Board of Regents (LEQSF(2009-12)-RD-A-23) to SJ.

References

1. Davis, S.J., Ikemizu, S., Wild, M.K., van der Merwe, P.A. (1998) CD2 and the nature of protein interactions mediating cell-cell recognition. *Immunol Rev.* **163**: 217–236.
2. Van der Merwe, P.A., Davis, S.J. (2003) Molecular interactions mediating T cell antigen recognition. *Annu Rev Immunol.* **21**: 659–684.
3. Kim, M., Sun, Z.Y., Byron, O., Campbell, G., Wagner, G., Wang, J., Reinherz, E.L. (2001) Molecular dissection of the CD2-CD58 counter-receptor interface identifies CD2 Tyr86 and CD58 Lys34 residues as the functional "hot spot". *J Mol Biol.* **312**: 711–720.
4. Bachmann, M.F., Barner, M., Kopf, M. (1999) CD2 sets quantitative thresholds in T cell activation. *J Exp Med.* **190**: 1383–1391
5. Mojcik, C.F., Shevach, E. (1997) Adhesion molecules: a rheumatologic perspective. *Arthritis Rheum.* **6**: 991–1004.
6. Takahashi, H., Soderstrom, K., Nilsson, E., Kiessling, R., Patarroyo, M. (1992) Integrins and other adhesion molecules on lymphocytes from synovial fluid and peripheral blood of rheumatoid arthritis patients. *Eur J Immunol.* **22**: 2879–2885.
7. Qin, L.H., Chavin, K.D., Lin, J.X., Yagita, H., Bromberg, J.S. (1994) Anti-CD2 receptor and anti-CD2 ligand (CD48) antibodies synergize to prolong allograft survival. *J Exp Med.* **179**: 341–346.
8. Hirahara, H., Tsuchida, M., Wanatabe, T., Haga, M., Matsumoto, Y., Abo, T., Eguchi, S. (1995) Long-term survival of cardiac allografts in rats treated before and after surgery with monoclonal antibody to CD2. *Transplantation* **59**: 85–90.
9. Mrowietz, U. (2002) Treatment targeted to cell surface epitopes. *Clin Exp Derm.* 27: 591–596.
10. Braun, J., Sieper, J. (2003). Role of novel biological therapies in psoriatic arthritis: effects on joints and skin. *Biodrugs* **17**: 187–199.
11. Aruffo, A., Hollenbaugh, D. (2001) Therapeutic intervention with inhibitors of co-stimulatory pathways in autoimmune disease. *Curr Opin Immunol.* **13**: 683–686.
12. Wang, J., Smolyar, A., Tan, K., Liu, J., Kim, M., Sun, Z.J., Wagner, G., Reinherz, E.L.

(1999) Structure of a heterophilic adhesion complex between the human CD2 and CD58 (LFA-3) counterreceptors. *Cell* **97**: 791–803.

13. Branco, L., Barren, P., Mao, S.Y., Pfarr, D., Kaplon, R., Psotema, C., Langermann, S., Koenig, S., Johnson, S. (1999) Selective deletion of antigen-specific, activated T cells by a humanized mAb to CD2 (MEDI-507) is mediated by NK cells. *Transplantation* **68**: 1588–1596.
14. Hunig, T. (1985) The cell surface molecule recognized by the erythrocyte receptor of T lymphocytes identification and partial characterization using a monoclonal antibody. *J Exp Med.* **162**: 890–901.
15. Albert-Wolf, M., Meuer, S.C., Wallich, R. (1991) Dual function of recombinant human CD58: inhibition of T-cell adhesion and activation via the CD2 pathway. *Int Immunol.* **3**: 1335–1347.
16. Liu, J., Ying, J., Chow, V.T., Hruby, V.J., Satyanarayanajois, S.D. (2005). Structure-activity studies of peptides from the "hot spot" region of human CD2 protein: development of peptides for immunomodulation. *J Med Chem.* **48**: 6236–6249.
17. Rink, T.J., Tsien, R.Y., Pozzan, T. (1982) Cytoplasmic pH and free Mg^{2+} in lymphocytes. *J Cell Biol.* **95**: 189–196.
18. Hahn, W.C., Burakoff, S.J., Bierer, B.E. (1993) Signal transduction pathways involved in T cell receptor-induced regulation of CD2 avidity for CD58. *J Immunol.* **150**: 2607–2619.
19. Hollo, Z., Homolya, L., Davis, C.W., Sarkadi, B. (1994) Calcein accumulation as a fluorometric functional assay of the multidrug transporter. *Biochim Biophys Acta* **1191**: 384–388.
20. Homoloya, L., Hollo, Z., Germann, U.A., Pastan, I., Gottesmann, M.M., Sarkadi, B. (1993) Fluorescent cellular indicators are extruded by the multidrug resistance protein. *J Biol Chem.* **268**: 21493–21496.
21. Liu, J., Chow, V.T., Jois, S.D. (2004). A novel, rapid and sensitive heterotypic cell adhesion assay for CD2-CD58 interaction, and its application for testing inhibitory peptides. *J Immunol Methods* **291**: 39–49.

Chapter 15

Evaluation of Antibacterial Activity of Proteins and Peptides Using a Specific Animal Model for Wound Healing

Ramar Perumal Samy, Maung Maung Thwin, Vincent T.K. Chow, Ho Bow, and Ponnampalam Gopalakrishnakone

Abstract

Wound healing is a complex process involving the integrated actions of numerous cell types, soluble mediators, and extracellular matrix (ECM). In this study, phospholipase A_2 (PLA_2) purified from crotalid snake venom was found to express in vitro bactericidal activity against a group of clinical human pathogens. Based on the sequence homology of PLA_2, a series of peptides were derived from the C-terminal region of crotalid PLA_2. These short synthetic peptides were found to reproduce the bactericidal activity of its parent molecule. In vitro assays for bactericidal and cytolytic activities of these peptides showed very high microbicidal potency against Gram-negative and Gram-positive (*Staphylococcus aureus*) bacteria. Variants of the peptides showed reduced toxicity toward normal human cells, while retaining high bactericidal potency. Here we describe the protocol for evaluating the wound healing process by antibacterial peptides. We evaluated the biological roles of the candidate peptides in skin wound healing, using a specific BALB/c mice model. Peptide-treated animals showed accelerated healing of full-thickness skin wounds, with increased reepithelialization, collagen synthesis, and angiogenesis observed during the healing process. Healing wounds in protein/peptide-treated mice had higher densities of neutrophils, macrophages, and fibrocytes. Along with increased leukocyte infiltration, levels of macrophage-derived chemokine expression were also upregulated. These results demonstrate that the protein/peptide derived from snake venoms promotes healing of skin wounds. The primary mechanism seems to be an increase in leukocyte infiltration, leading to locally elevated synthesis and release of collagen and growth factors.

Key words: Antimicrobial protein, Membrane damaging, Peptides, Snake venom, Wounds

1. Introduction

Wound healing involves several overlapping phases including inflammation, cell proliferation, migration, angiogenesis, and production of extracellular matrix (ECM) molecules (1, 2). It is a

Seetharama D. Satyanarayanajois (ed.), *Drug Design and Discovery: Methods and Protocols*,
Methods in Molecular Biology, vol. 716, DOI 10.1007/978-1-61779-012-6_15,

dynamic, complex process involving the integrated action of numerous cell types, extracellular matrices, and soluble mediators. A hallmark of the inflammatory phase is the recruitment of neutrophils and macrophages into the injury (3). In the proliferative phase, the migration and proliferation of keratinocytes, fibroblasts, and endothelial cells result in reepithelialization and tissue granulation. During the remodeling phase, excess collagen in the wound is degraded by proteolytic enzymes leading to the completion of tissue repair (1). A newly identified fibrocyte cell type has recently been reported to contribute to wound healing (4, 5). However, the aerobic or facultative pathogens such as *Staphylococcus aureus*, *Pseudomonas aeruginosa*, and beta-hemolytic streptococci are the primary causes of delayed wound healing and infection in both acute and chronic wounds. *S. aureus* is a leading cause of bloodstream, skin, soft tissue, and lower respiratory tract infections worldwide (6, 7). Patients with infection of such pathogen suffer increased trauma due to wound infection. Despite the large numbers of antibiotics currently available (8), antibiotic resistance, resulting from an extensive clinical use of classical antibiotics (9–11), has been a great concern during the last decades. Recently, a number of cationic and amphipathic peptides that essentially modulate immune responses, have been shown to display a variety of host defense functions against microbial cells (12, 13). By contrast, the mammalian group IIA myotoxic secretory phospholipase A_2s (sPLA_2s) isolated from the venom of the snake *Bothrops asper* was shown to directly kill both Gram-positive and Gram-negative bacteria (14). One of them, *B. asper* myotoxin II, is a catalytically inactive Lys49 PLA_2 (15), thus demonstrating the first catalytic independent bactericidal mechanism exerted by a sPLA_2 homolog (14). Furthermore, bactericidal action was reproduced by a synthetic peptide (14) derived from the short sequence of the protein corresponding to residues 115–129 of its cytolytic C-terminal region (16). The majority of peptides that exhibit broad-spectrum antimicrobial activity (17) are relatively small, cationic, amphipathic molecules, having variable length, sequence, and structure. Because of the increasing concern on antibiotic resistance, a new strategy is required for the development of novel chemotherapeutic agents for the prevention of *S. aureus* infections. The antimicrobial peptides hold promise as chemotherapeutic agents due not only to their antibacterial activity against *S. aureus* but also because of their ability to activate the innate immune responses. So far, the interaction of *S. aureus* with antimicrobial peptides is only partially understood. Here we describe the protocol for evaluating the wound healing process by antibacterial peptides.

2. Materials

2.1. Buffer Solutions

1. Tris–HCl buffer: 50 mM Tris–HCl, pH 7.4; stored at room temperature.
2. Acetonitrile: (80% acetonitrile in 0.1% TFA), 800 mL of acetonitrile from 1 L HPLC analytical grade is dissolved in 200 mL sterile double distilled water and store at room temperature.
3. Trifloroacetic acid solution: 1 mL of TFA (99% in 100 mL HPLC analytical grade) in 999 mL sterile double distilled water.
4. Separating buffer (4×): 1.5 M Tris–HCl (pH 8.7), 0.4% SDS.
5. Stacking buffer (4×): 0.5 M Tris–HCl (pH 6.8), 0.4% SDS solution (Biotechnological grade) and store at 18–26°C.
6. Running buffer (5×): 125 mM Tris, 960 mM glycine, 0.5% (w/v) SDS and store at room temperature (Bio-Rad, Hercules, CA, USA).
7. Perfusion fixation: Perfuse the animal initially with a warm (37°C) buffered salt solution (saline or Ringer's solution with an anticoagulant) to clear the blood from the vessels. Then use freshly prepared fixative mixture in a buffer system appropriate for the tissue for 15 min. After the tissues are removed and cut into small pieces of 1 mm, immerse in the same fixative for 4 h at 4°C.
8. Phosphate Buffer (PB): 78 g of 0.5 M of monobasic sodium phosphate dissolved in 1,000 mL of water and stored at room temperature.
9. Phosphate Buffer Saline (PBS): 8.00 g of sodium chloride (NaCl), 0.20 g of potassium chloride (KCl), 1.15 g of disodium hydrogen phosphate (Na_2HPO_4), and 0.20 g of potassium dihydrogen phosphate (KH_2PO_4). Dissolve in 1,000 mL deionized water and adjust pH to 7.2.

2.2. Purification and Characterization of Venom

1. High performance liquid chromatography (HPLC).
2. Columns for HPLC (1.6×40 cm) HPLC column (Superdex G-75 column, 30 pg), (Amersham Pharmacia Biotech AB, Uppsala, Sweden).
3. Reversed-phase HPLC column C18, (250×4.6 mm, 300 A), C8 column (250×4.60 mm, 5 μm, 100 A, Phenomenexr®).
4. Mobile phase: Acetonitrile/water 50:50, flow rate 1 mL per min, injection volume 5 μL, ambient temperature, detection UV range at 254 nm.

5. UNO™ Q & S Cation Exchange columns, 7 mm ID × 35 mm L, S-1 or Q-1 flow rate 1 mL per min.
6. Buffer A: 20 mM Tris, pH 8.2
7. Buffer B: 20 mM Tris + 1 M NaCl (pH 8.2).
8. Matrix-assisted laser desorption/ionization-time of fight (MALDI-TOF) mass spectrophotometer (Framingham, MA, USA).
9. Calibration sample: The mass spectra are calibrated using the sequazyme peptide mass standards kit (Perspective Biosystems, Framingham, MA).

2.3. SDS: Polyacrylamide Gel Electrophoresis (SDS: PAGE)

1. 30% Acrylamide/bis solution (37.5:1 with 2.6% C) and *N,N,N′,N′*-tetramethyl-ethane-1,2-diamine (TEMED).
2. 10% Ammonium persulfate solution: in water and immediately freeze in single use (200 μL) aliquots at −20°C.
3. Water-saturated isobutanol: Shake equal volumes of water and isobutanol in a glass bottle and allow separating. Use the top layer and store at room temperature.
4. Prestained molecular weight markers (Bio-Rad, Hercules, CA, USA).
5. Model GS-710 Gel calibration imaging densitometer (Bio-Rad).

2.4. Antimicrobial Assay

1. BBL™ Mueller Hinton II Agar and Mueller Hinton (MH) broth. Store at 4°C.
2. MH agar: 17.5 g of casein acid hydrolysate, 2 g of beef extract, 1.5 g of starch, 17 g of agar, and 21 g of MH powder are dissolved in 1,000 mL of double deionized water with thorough mixing (final pH 7.3 ± 0.1 at 25°C).
3. Sterilization: Steam sterilization is for elimination of bacteria, viruses, and all transmissible agents from the surface of instruments. Autoclave is mainly used to sterilize media and glasswares with high-pressure steam at 121°C for 15–20 min depending upon the size of the content.
4. 0.22 μm membrane filter (Millipore, Billerica, MA, USA).
5. BD Sensi-Disc™ Blank disc (vial of 50 disks, pack of 6): used for in vitro susceptibility testing.
6. Antibiotic disk (Becton Dickinson Biosciences, Sparks MD, 21152, USA).
   (a) 10 μg of Ampicillin (50 disk, pack)
   (b) 30 μg of Cefoxitin (10 packs)
   (c) 30 μg of Chloramphenicol (50 disk, pack)
   (d) 10 μg of Streptomycin (50 disk, pack)

(e) 30 μg of Vancomycin (50 disk, pack)

(f) Microwell 96F, (Nunc A/S, Roskilde, Denmark).

7. Sterile 96-well plates and reader (example: Benchmark plus Spectrophotometer, Bio-Rad, CA, USA).
8. Cotton swabs 6 cm lengths, one bud, wood stick foam tip.
9. Streaking loop: The loop is resterilized and dragged across the inoculated quadrant of the streak plate and is used to collect some bacteria on the loop.
10. Storage: Store the solid MH agar plates in the dark 2–8°C, avoid freezing and overheating. Do not open the plates until ready to use. Allow the plate-containing medium to warm in room temperature before inoculation.

2.4.1. Scanning Electron Microscopy (SEM)

1. Osmium tetroxide (OsO_4): OsO_4 is a widely used staining agent used in transmission electron microscopy (TEM) to provide contrast to the image. It is also useful in SEM as an alternative to sputter coating.
2. OsO_4: Ferrocyanide solution: mixed with equal volumes of 2% osmium tetroxide and 2.5% potassium ferrocyanide. The final solution consisting of 1% osmium tetroxide and 1.25% of potassium ferrocyanide appears brown in color.
3. Paraformaldehyde (PF): 2 g of PF dissolve in 20 mL of deionized water and mixed with 16.2 mL of 0.5 M dibasic sodium phosphate solution (Na_2HPO_4), and the solution kept at 60°C until the PF is dissolved. Cool the solution at room temperature. Add 12 mL of 25% glutaraldehyde (GA) and dilute to about 80 mL with deionized water. Filter the solution (Nunc, USA) and use.

2.4.2. Transmission Electron Microscopy (TEM)

1. 2% PF + 2.5% glutaraldehyde.
2. Ethanol.
3. Vibratome.

2.5. Mouse Model of Skin Infection

1. Ketamine hydrochloride: used as human anesthetic and as general anesthetic in veterinary medicine.
2. Medetomidine hydrochloride: synthetic drug used as surgical anesthetic and analgesic.
3. 2% Fucidin^R 5 g ointment (Antibiotic) contains 20 mg/g of sodium fusidate. Store at controlled room temperature 15–25°C (LEO-Pharmaceutical Products, Ballerup, Denmark).
4. Latex free syringe 5 mL, nonpyrogenic (Becton Dickinson, Singapore).
5. Sterile needle 07 × 19 mm.
6. Eight weeks-old BALB/c female mice (body weight 25–30 g).

7. Anesthesia: 0.2 mL of ketamine + medetomidine injected intraperitoneally (i.p).
8. Mid-logarithmic growth phase of *S. aureus* (5×10^7 CFU/mL).
9. Aqueous cream contains chlorocresol 0.1% w/w no fragrance, used as a vehicle control.
10. 2% Fusidic acid (LEO-Pharmaceutical Products, Ballerup, Denmark): used as reference drug.
11. Mueller Hinton (MH) agar (Oxoid, Basingstoke, UK).

2.6. Hematoxylin and Eosin (H & E) Staining

1. Polysine[R] slides ($25 \times 75 \times 1.0$ mm), (Menzel Gmbtl, Germany).
2. Reagents for Haematoxylin solution: 5 g of haematoxylin, 50 g of aluminum ammonium sulfate, 1 g of sodium iodate, 20 mL of acetic acid, 270 mL glycerol, 10 mL of ethanol, 700 mL of distilled water.
3. Eosin: 40 mL of 1% eosin, 40 mL of 1% aqueous phloxine, 6 mL of 95% alcohol, 14 mL of glacial acetic acid mix the above reagents, stir and store the stock solutions at room temperature.
4. 0.3% acid alcohol: 52 mL of ethanol, 24 mL of distilled water, and 24 mL of concentrated hydrochloric acid.
5. Scott's tap water substitute: 2 g of sodium hydrogen carbonate, 20 g of magnesium sulfate dissolved in 1,000 mL of distilled water.
6. CO_2 inhalation.
7. 10% formalin used for fixative.
8. Ethyl alcohol (99% absolute alcohol) used in dehydration series (50–100%).
9. Paraffin (Paraplast™ resin).
10. Light microscope.

2.7. Masson's Trichrome (MT) Stain for Collagen

1. Fixation: 10% formalin or Bouin's solution (paraffin sections at 5 μm).
2. Bouin's Solution: 75 mL of saturated picric acid, 20 mL of formaldehyde (37%) mixed well with 5 mL of glacial acetic acid used for tissue fixation. This solution will improve Masson Trichrome (MT) staining quality.
3. Weigert's Iron Hematoxylin solution: Stock solution A: 1 g of hematoxylin dissolve in 100 mL of 95% alcohol; Stock solution B: 4 ml of 29% ferric chloride in water, 95 mL of distilled water (H_2O), 1 mL of concentrated hydrochloric acid (HCL). Mix equal parts of stock solution A and B and this Weigert's Iron Hematoxylin working solution is stable for 3 months (90 days).

4. Biebrich Scarlet-Acid Fuchsin solution: 90 mL of Biebrich scarlet, 10 mL of 1% aqueous of acid fuchsin, 1 mL of 1% aqueous glacial acetic acid dissolve in double distilled water for washing.
5. Phosphomolybdic-Phosphotungstic Acid solution: 25 mL of 5% phosphomolybdic acid, 25 mL of 5% phosphotungstic acid store at room temperature.
6. Aniline Blue solution: 2.5 g of aniline blue, 2 mL of glacial acetic acid dissolve in 100 mL of distilled water.
7. 1% Acetic Acid solution: 1 mL of glacial acetic acid solution dissolves in 99 mL of distilled water and store at room temperature.

2.8. Double Immunofluorescence Labeling

1. Primary antibodies type I collagen (PanCytokeratin).
2. TNF-α (PanCytokeratin), COX-2 (PanCytokeratin) diluted 1:500 in phosphate buffer saline (pH 7.4) containing 1% BSA (SantaCruz Biotechnology, CA, USA).
3. Secondary antibody (polyclonal antirabbit IgG HRP) 1:5,000 diluted in PBS with 12% BSA.
4. PBS containing 0.1% Tween-20, prior to mounting in 0.5 μg/mL of DAPI (Sigma, St Louis, MO).
5. Olympus fluorescence microscope equipped with a broad range of visible lasers, including the Argon (458, 488, 515 nm), Green Helium Neon (543 nm), Yellow Krypton (568 nm), and Red Helium Neon (633 nm). XY scanning is used to capture a single confocal optical image at 360° image rotation (supplied by Olympus America, Inc.,).
6. FluoView 300 software (Olympus America Inc., Center Valley, PA).

2.9. Enzyme-Linked Immunosorbent Assay (ELISA)

1. Tissue homogenizer.
2. 5% Trichloroacetic acid.
3. Centrifuged.
4. Type I collagen, commercial ELISA kits (BioSource, Inc., Camarillo, CA).

3. Methods

3.1. Purification of Phospholipase A_2 Enzymes

1. 250 mg of snake venom is dispersed into 10 mL of 50 mM Tris–hydrochloric acid (Tris–HCl) buffer (pH 7.4), and the suspension centrifuged at 500×g at 4°C for 10 min (see Note 1).
2. The yellowish clear venom sample is applied on a Superdex G-75 column (1.6×40 cm) equilibrated and eluted with 50 mM Tris–HCl buffer (pH 7.4) (see Note 2).

3. Gel-filtration fractions are collected at a flow rate of 15 mL/h. Absorbance of the entire fractions monitored at 280 nm.
4. Total fractions collected from the single pool of venom separated from the Superdex column, and aliquots used for testing biochemical activities and protein measurement.
5. The fraction showing highest antibacterial activity is further separated by reversed-phase (RP)-high performance liquid chromatography (HPLC) on C18 column. Fractions are monitored at 215 nm.
6. The most active fraction is further purified by a C8 column (250×4.60 mm, 5 μm, 100 A,) in 0.1% aqueous trifluoroacetic acid (TFA), and eluted with a linear gradient of 80% acetonitrile (ACN) in 0.1% TFA. All steps of the purification procedure are carried out at room temperature (25°C) (see Notes 3 & 4).
7. The solid venom and final pure protein are analyzed by sodium dodecyl sulfate polyacrylamide gel electrophoresis (SDS-PAGE) according to Laemmli (18), and the protein estimation is done by Bradford method (19) (see Notes 5 & 6).
8. Separating gels containing 15% acrylamide and stacking gels of 4.5% acrylamide are used.
9. The protein is diluted (1:1) with sample buffer (0.12 M Tris–HCl, pH 6.8 containing 2% SDS, 5% 2-mercaptoethanol, 10% glycerol, 0.02% bromophenol blue) and heated for 5 min in a boiling water bath.
10. Electrophoresis is carried out at a constant current of 20 mA for 2.5 h.
11. The gel is fixed with 5% acetic acid overnight and stained for 2 h in 0.1% Coomassie blue R-250 in 5% acetic acid (see Note 7).
12. Destaining is carried out in a solution containing 35% methanol and 7% acetic acid until the background becomes clear.
13. The molecular weights of protein bands were determined using standard markers.
14. Mass spectrometry is done using a matrix-assisted laser desorption ionization-time of flight (MALDI-TOF) Voyager-DE mass spectrometer operated in delayed extraction mode.
15. The sample is analyzed using a saturated solution of α-cyano-4-hydroxycinnamic acid in acetone containing 1% TFA, the mass elected in the range of 1–30 kDa.
16. The mass spectra are calibrated using calibration mixture of the sequazyme peptide mass standards kit.
17. N-terminal sequencing is subjected to Edman degradation using an Applied Biosystems 494 pulsed liquid-phase sequencer equipped with an online 120 A PTH-amino acid analyzer (see Note 4).

18. The amino acid (AA) sequences are subjected to protein BLAST (Basic Local Alignment Search Tool) for similarity searches with the reported snake venom PLA_{2s}.

3.2. In Vitro Assay for Antibacterial Evaluation

Mueller Hinton (MH) agar is recommended for antimicrobial disk diffusion susceptibility testing of common, rapidly growing bacteria by Bauer–Kirby method as standardized by Clinical and Laboratory Standards Institute (CLSI).

Antimicrobials are usually regarded as bactericidal. The minimum inhibitory concentrations (MICs) are determined by the broth microdilution susceptibility test following the National Committee for Clinical Laboratory Standards (20, 21) guidelines (NCCLS).

1. In brief, fresh overnight culture (*Escherichia coli*, *Enterobacter aerogenes*, *Proteus vulgaris*, *Proteus mirabilis*, *Pseudomonas aeruginosa*, and *Staphylococcus aureus*) is inoculated to a turbidity of 0.5–1.2 McFarland units.
2. Diluted bacterial suspensions in Mueller Hinton (MH) broth are incubated for another 5 h to reach exponential phase. The diluted bacterial suspensions are added ($0.5 \times 10^5 - 1.2 \times 10^6$ colony forming units, CFU/mL) to wells containing serial dilutions of protein samples prepared (at final concentrations) in microtiter trays with MH broth.
3. Wells containing bacteria with sterile phosphate buffer saline (pH 7.4) are used as control.
4. Fucidic acid ointment (FAO) and streptomycin commercial antibiotics are used as reference controls. Adjusted bacterial inoculums of 10^6 CFU/mL are added to each well with 50 μL of protein sample (at a known concentration).
5. The 96-well plates are incubated at 37°C for 24 h, and the inhibition of bacterial growth is determined by measuring the absorbance at 560 nm.
6. The MICs are recorded as the lowest concentration of protein that inhibited the growth of bacteria. The results are repeated as the mean values of three independent determinations ($n = 3$).
7. The minimum bactericidal concentration (MBC) is the lowest concentration of protein or peptide in μg/mL required to kill an organism (99.9%). It is determined from broth dilution MIC tests by subculturing to agar media without antibiotics. Examples of antimicrobial activity are shown in Figs. 1 and 2.

3.3. Scanning Electron Microscopy (SEM)

The damage to cell membranes caused by snake venom proteins/peptides is studied. In this protocol, we attempt to summarize the electron microscopy data for understanding the modes of

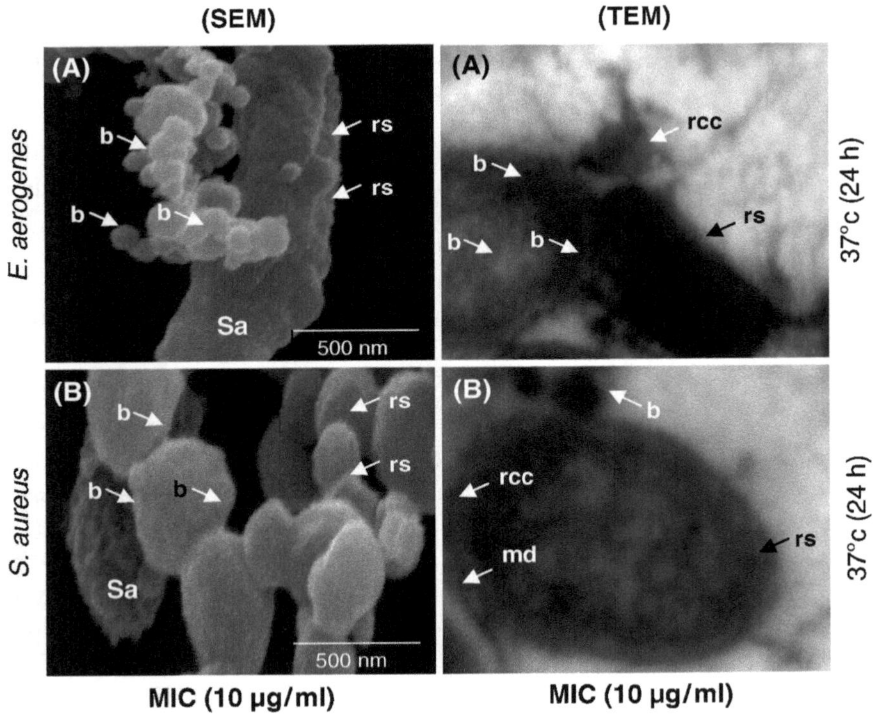

Fig. 1. Antimicrobial activity of purified protein from *C. adamanteus* venom was tested in a disk-diffusion assay for antibacterial effects against Gram-positive and Gram-negative bacteria. The protein gave a zone of inhibition against human skin-infection causing pathogens, *Enterobacteraerogenes* and *Staphylococcus aureus*. The bactericidal activity of the protein is more effective than the standard antibiotic fucidine. It inhibits bacterial growth at same MIC (10 μg/mL), but shows different mode of mechanistic action against the two pathogens. (**a**, **b**) The electron micrograph images (TEM and SEM) of *S. aureus* and *E. aeroginosa* treated with the bactericidal protein showing pore-formation and outer membrane damage at the indicated concentrations (*b* blebs, *rs* rough surface, *rcc* release cellular content, *md* membrane damaging).

action of pore forming and membrane damaging effects. The characterization of the membrane damage induced by the protein on Gram-negative and Gram-positive is studied using SEM and TEM as described earlier (22).

1. Protein/peptide treated samples that contained bacterial cells (3.2×10^6 CFU/mL) in MH broth are preincubated for 24 h at 37°C.
2. The control contains an equivalent volume (100 μL) of MH broth containing bacteria.
3. The bacterial cells are centrifuged for 10 min at $2,800 \times g$. Each pellet is resuspended and fixed with an equal volume of 2.5% glutaraldehyde in 1 mM phosphate buffer (pH 7.4) for 1 h.
4. The cells are postfixed for 1 h with 1% osmium tetroxide (OsO_4 is a widely used staining agent for TEM to provide

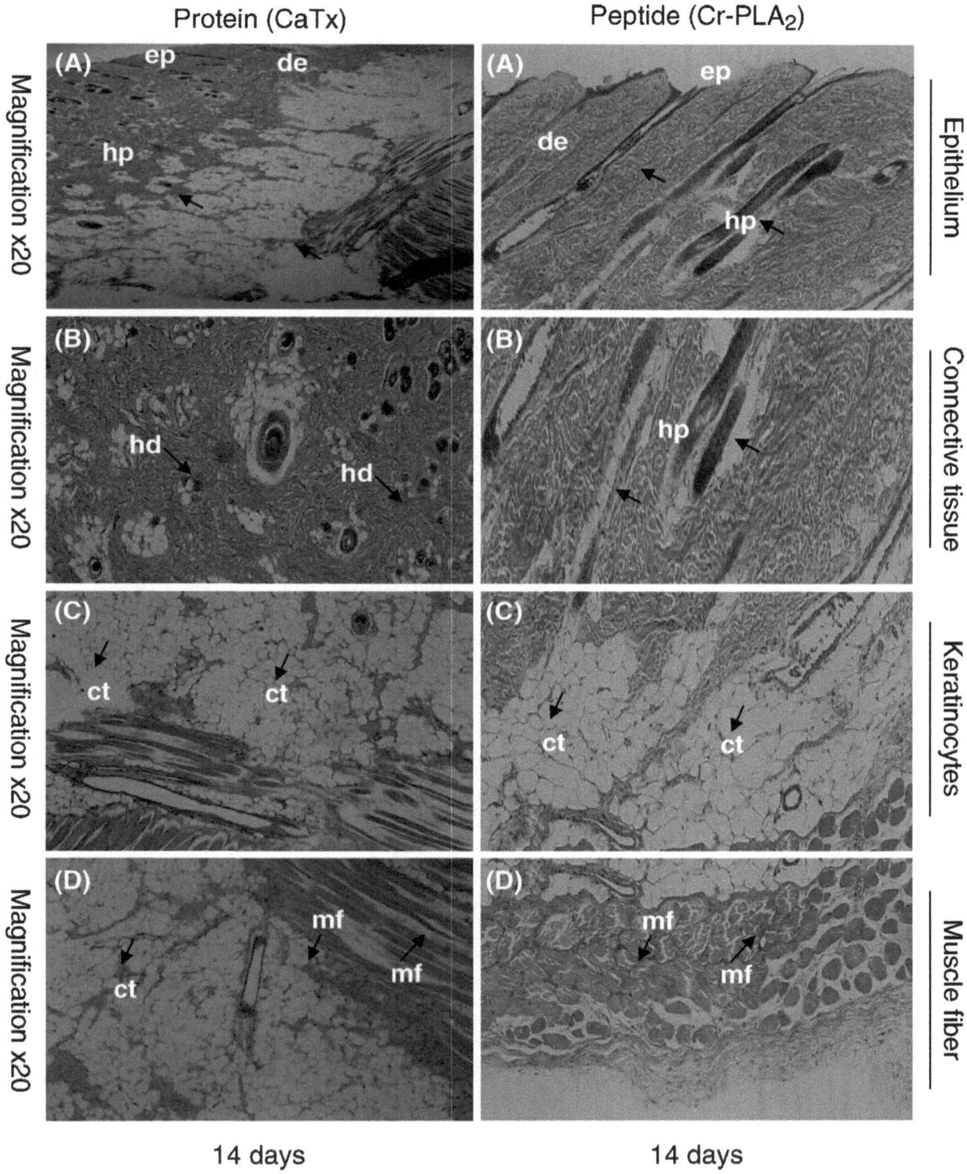

Fig. 2. (**a**–**d**) Antimicrobial peptides (effectors of pathogen clearance) modify host cell behaviors to promote wound repair. The microbial killing activity of protein/peptides were analyzed and correlated with the ability to influence wound repair in mice. (**a**–**d**) The antimicrobial peptides showed up to 64% improvement in wound repair compared to PLA2 protein, an effect comparable to that obtained with 2% Fucidin (antibiotic) treatment. Wounds treated with peptide showed keratinocyte hyperplasia and increased leukocyte infiltration. The peptide stimulated the formation of endothelial cells, an effect that may explain the increase in leukocyte migration. These findings confirm that antimicrobial peptides can function as effectors of cutaneous wound repair. This study furthers our understanding of antimicrobial peptides by showing that their wound repair properties can be independent of antimicrobial function (*ep* epidermis, *de* dermise, *hf* hair folicle, *ct* connective tissue, *mf* muscle fiber, *hd* hypodermis).

contrast to the image) in PBS and 1 μL of cells pipetted on a sterile cover glass coated with poly-L lysine. Sections are dehydrated by a series of alcohol (25–100%).

5. The samples in 100% ethanol are transferred to a critical point dryer, and dried using carbon dioxide (CO_2) as the transition solvent.
6. The samples are mounted on aluminum specimen supports with carbon adhesive tabs, and coated with 15-nm thick gold-palladium metal (60:40 alloy) using a Hummer X sputter coater SC D005.
7. Samples are examined with a Philips XL 30 FEG scanning electron microscope (SEM) using an accelerating voltage of 5–10 kV.

3.4. Transmission Electron Microscopy (TEM)

The structural changes induced by protein on bacteria are studied using TEM (23).

1. Bacterial cells are suspended in 10 mM phosphate buffer (pH 7.4) and fixed with an equal volume of 2.5% glutaraldehyde in 10 mM phosphate buffer, pH 7.4 for 1 h.
2. The bacteria were washed with distilled water 3 times.
3. Then the bacterial samples were postfixed in 1% OsO_4 (pH 7.4) for 1 h at room temperature at 4°C in the fixative.
4. The excess OsO_4 was discarded after the stained bacteria exposed to OsO_4 for a minute.
5. The postfixed cells are rinsed with 10 mM phosphate buffer for 5–10 min – two changes at room temperature.
6. Dehydrate through a graded series of ethanol series at room temperature.

   25% Ethanol – 5 min

   50% Ethanol – 10 min

   75% Ethanol – 10 min

   95% Ethanol – 10 min

   100% Ethanol – 10 min

   100% Ethanol – 10 min
7. During the entire filtration, rinsing, and dehydration process, cells are kept covered with fluid to prevent air-drying.
8. Polymerization was done with pure epoxy resin in the embedding oven at 75°C for 2 h and 90°C for another 2 h.
9. The bacteria infiltrated by a mixture of acetone and epoxy resin as follows:
   (a) 100% acetone: resin (1:1) for 30 min at room temperature.
   (b) 100% acetone: resin (1:6) for overnight at room temperature.

(c) First change of fresh resin – 20 min at room temperature then transfer to 40°C for 30 min.

(d) Second change of fresh resin – 1 h at 45°C.

(e) Third change of fresh resin – 1 h at 50°C.

10. The bacterial sample blocks were trimmed and cut to 90 nm ultra thin sections and mounted on 200 mesh thin bar copper grids.

11. The sections were stained with Uranyl acetate for 1 min. Each section was examined at 30,000 magnification by using TEM (JEF 2220) at an accelerating voltage of 5–10 kV.

3.5. In Vivo Mouse Model for Wound Healing

Wounds of rodents or small mammals have emerged as the model of choice for many researchers. This type of study is beneficial to wound research for mutable reasons. Small animals usually have accelerated modes of healing compared to humans. Invasiveness of mouse skin is established by modification of previously described infection model (24–26). Procedures to be approved by the Institutional Animal Care and Use Committee (IACUC) on animal studies (see Note 8).

1. Eight weeks-old BALB/c female mice (body weight 25–30 g) are divided into four groups ($n = 5$ mice per group).
2. The hairs on the back are shaved and full thickness of wounds (0.5×0.4 mm (20 mm^2)) created on the skin after giving 0.2 mL of ketamine + medetomidine anesthesia by intraperitoneal injection (i.p).
3. A mid-logarithmic growth phase of Gram-positive *S. aureus* (5×10^7 CFU/mL) 50 μL is applied topically on the wound site to maximize the wound.
4. Group I wound control (WCtrl) receives phosphate buffered saline (PBS); G (II) mice are treated with an aqueous gel to serve as a vehicle control (VCtrl); G (III) received bactericidal protein mixed with gel (10 mg/kg), and G (IV) are treated with 2% Fusidic acid ointment (μg/mouse) as reference drug (27, 28).
5. Wound reduction is monitored, and lesion sizes measured daily up to 14 days. Statistical significance between groups is evaluated by one-way ANOVA and student's *t*-test.
6. Changes in wound areas are expressed as percentage of the wound (closure) reduction.
7. At the predetermined experimental end points (1–14 days), all the animals are killed by excess CO_2, and the wound skin in the healed area is removed by a sterile surgical blade.
8. The collected tissues are weighed, homogenized using tissue extraction buffer (T-PER), and the samples assayed.

9. Bacterial counts are determined from the wound of skin tissues (10 mm) corresponding to the inoculation sites. The tissues are homogenized and suspended in 2 mL sterile phosphate buffered saline (pH 7.4) for counting.
10. Bacterial suspensions are plated in appropriate dilutions on Mueller Hinton (MH) agar and incubated at 37°C for 24 h in ambient air.
11. Bacterial counts are expressed as number of *S. aureus* colony forming units per gram (cfu/g) of tissue (25).

3.6. Histopathological Examinations

1. Mice are sacrificed by excess CO_2 inhalation, and the skin around the wound area incised (approximately 6 mm diameter) from both the treated and control animals at 14 days posttreatment.
2. Wound tissues are fixed in 10% formalin, processed for dehydration through alcohol series (50–100%), and embedded in paraffin (see Notes 9 & 10).
3. Thin sections (8 μm) are taken from the embedded wounds and the nuclei stained with Hematoxylin (29, 30) (see Notes 11 & 12).
4. The sections were rinsed in running tap water for 3 s.
5. Differentiate with 0.3% acid alcohol and rinsed in running tap water for 3 s.
6. Rinse in Scott's tap water substitute for 2 s.
7. Specimens are stained with eosin for 2 min.
8. Dehydrate in alcohol series (50–100%), clear and mount on the slides.
9. The sections are examined under a light microscope for pathological evaluation.

3.7. Masson's Trichrome (MT) Stain for Collagen

MT staining technique is used for the selective detection of collagen fibers in mouse skin tissue sections harvested from treated and untreated wounds following formalin fixation and paraffin embedding. The collagen fibers are stained in blue, and the nuclei stained in black, while the muscle, cytoplasm, and keratin are stained in red.

1. Formalin fixed tissue is refixed in Bouin's solution for 1 h at room temperature.
2. Sections are rinsed in running tap water for 5 min to remove the yellow color.
3. Deparaffinize and rehydrate through 100, 95, 70, and 50% alcohols and wash in distilled water.
4. After deparaffinization, all the skin sections are stained in Weigert's iron hematoxylin working solution for 3 min.
5. Rinse in running warm tap water for 3 min.

6. Stain in Biebrich scarlet-acid fuchsin solution for 5 min, and wash in distilled water.
7. Differentiate in phosphomolybdic-phosphotungstic acid solution for 10 min or until collagen is not red.
8. Transfer sections directly (without rinsing) to aniline blue solution and stain for 5 min.
9. Rinse the sections briefly in distilled water and differentiate in 1% acetic acid solution for 2–5 min prior to washing in distilled water.
10. Dehydrate very quickly through 50–100% ethyl alcohol, absolute ethyl alcohol (these step will wipe off Biebrich scarlet-acid fuchsin staining) and clear in xylene.
11. Mount the slides with resinous mounting medium for examination of collagens under light microscope (31).
12. Examples of wound healing are shown in Figs. 3 and 4.

3.8. Double Immunofluorescence Labeling

Assessment of immunostaining (32).

1. The following groups are used: – G (I) WCtrl, G (II) VCtrl, G (III) infected wound treated with CaTx (5 mg/kg, b.w), G (IV) wound treated with 2% FAO (5 mg/kg, b.w) as a reference drug. Mice were sacrificed and skin tissues excised and fixed in 30% Bouin's solution for 1 h at room temperature to improve staining quality.
2. Paraffin sections (7 μm) from controls and wound treated mouse skin sections are rinsed in running tap water for 5 min to remove the yellow color.
3. Deparaffinize and rehydrate through 100, 95, 70, and 50% alcohols, and wash in distilled water.
4. Blocking step: incubate sections with 10% serum for 30 min to block nonspecific binding of the antibodies (alternatively 1% BSA is used for blocking) at room temperature.
5. Incubate the sections with the primary antibodies for type I collagen (PanCytokeratin), TNF-α (PanCytokeratin), and COX-2 (PanCytokeratin). The antibody solutions are diluted 1:500 in phosphate buffered saline (pH 7.4) containing 1% BSA, or 1% PBST in a humidified chamber for 1 h incubation at room temperature or over night at 4°C, depending on the concentration of antibody (see Note 13).
6. Discard the primary antibody solutions and wash the sections three times (3×) in PBS for 5 min each wash.
7. Incubate sections in the dark with secondary antibody (polyclonal antirabbit IgG HRP diluted 1:5,000 in PBST-1% BSA buffer for 1 h at room temperature).
8. Discard the secondary antibody solutions and wash the sections three times (3×) in PBS for 5 min per wash.

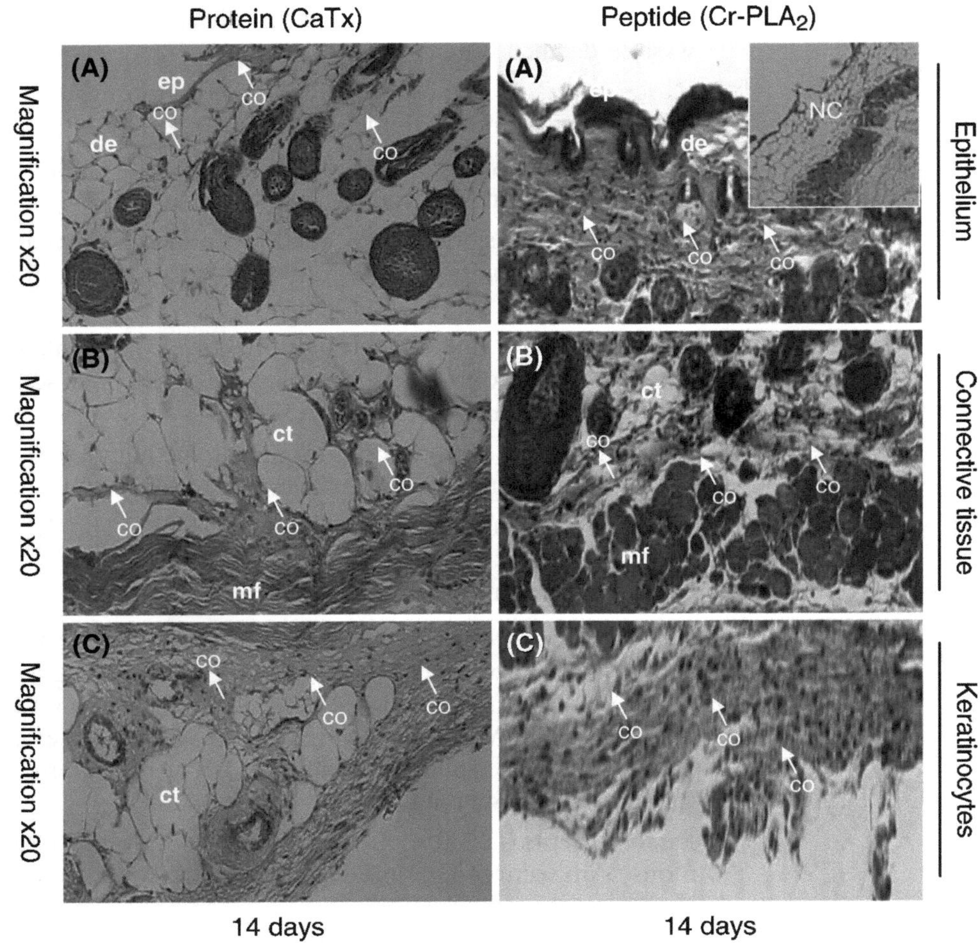

Fig. 3. Skin samples from the wound of the animals were excised and processed for histology with Masson's trichrome staining. Histologic sections of the wound (at 14th day) showing collagen synthesis after treatment with snake venom proteins and peptides. MT staining shows collagen in *blue* and endothelial cells in *red*. (NC) Low magnification view of a control wound treated with saline showing absence of collagen expression. (**a**–**c**): photomicrographs showing the induced collagen expression after 2 weeks. *Arrows* indicate the edges of the original wound at higher magnification showing baseline collagen; (co) accumulation. Wounds of mice topically treated with protein and peptides resulted in enhanced collagen production/accumulation compared to wounds treated with saline. The wound penetrates the epidermis (*ep*) and dermis (*de*) and is in contact with the fat (*f*) and muscle (*mf*) layer. The re-epithelialization (gap) and contraction of dermis (width) are measured to calculate wound closure.

9. Subsequently, sections are rinsed with PBS (in dark) containing 0.1% Tween-20 before counter staining in 0.5 μg/mL of DAPI and photographing on an Olympus fluorescence microscope.
10. All sections are mounted on 13 mm cover slips with a drop of mounting medium, and the mounted sections left for 30 min at room temperature for drying, before being stored in dark at 4°C (see Note 14).

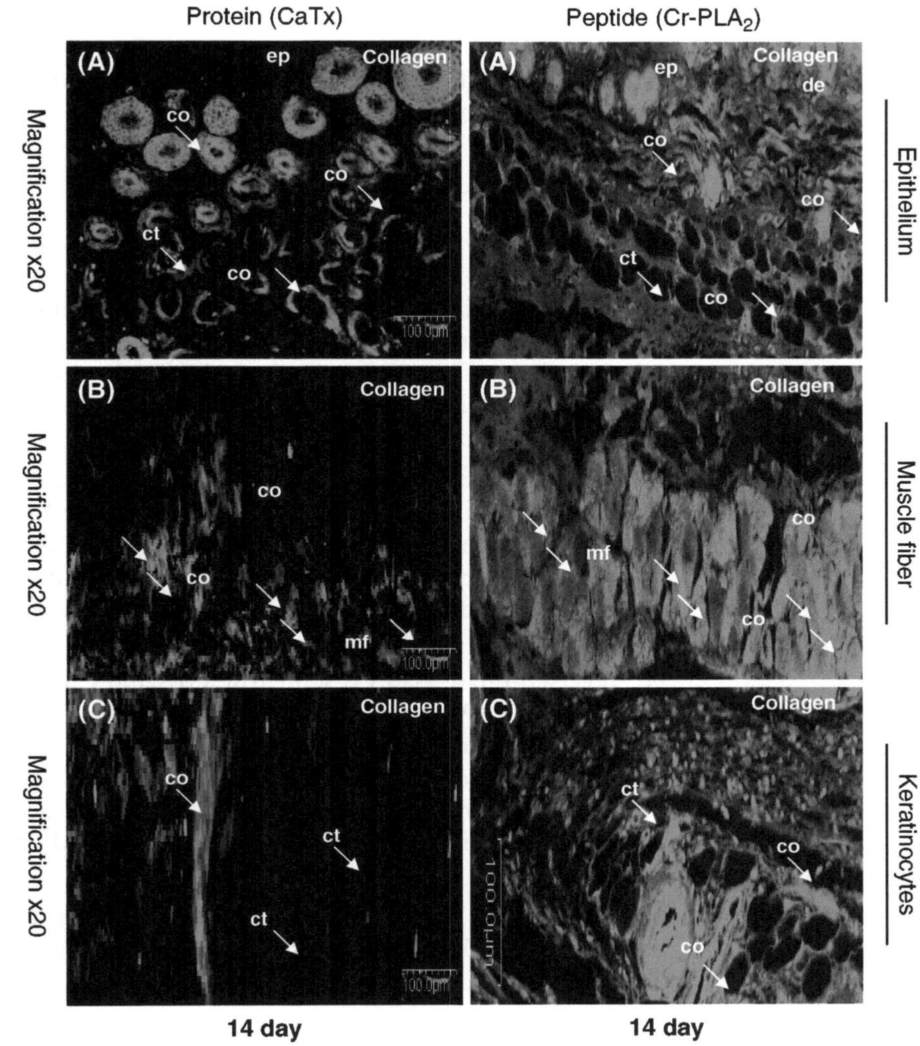

Fig. 4. (**a**–**c**) Peptide-treated wound showed very strong intensity of staining for collagen than the protein-received mice. Subcellular localization of collagen and keratinocytes was examined by immunofluorescence microscopy of mice skin wound. Results revealed specific labeling of collagen in granules, some of which displayed a characteristic lamellar structure (*co* collagen, *ep* epidermis, *de* dermis, *ct* connective tissue, *mf* muscle fiber).

3.9. Enzyme-Linked Immunosorbent Assay (ELISA)

1. Wound tissues are excised with a punch biopsy (8 mm) and homogenized with 300 μL of 5% trichloroacetic acid. The homogenates are centrifuged at 15,000 × *g* for 15 min.
2. The supernatant is applied to ELISA. Type I collagen protein levels are measured with commercial ELISA kits according to the manufacturers' recommendations.
3. Total protein in the supernatant is measured with a commercial kit. The data are expressed as cytokines (pg/mL)/total protein (mg/mL) for each sample.

4. For statistical analysis, the results are presented as mean ± standard deviation (S.D.) of five replicates. Statistical significance is evaluated using Student's *t*-test. The value of $p > 0.05$ is considered significant.

4. Notes

1. Sample preparation: venom sample contains mixture of all other components and is therefore very viscous (viscosity) in solution form. The sample (1:5 or 1:10 w/v) should be diluted as much as possible before centrifugation to prevent clogging of columns during chromatography.
2. HPLC purification: 50 mM Tris–HCl buffer pH is essential for gel-filtration chromatography (Superdex column 1.6 × 60), which was optimized for the AKTA explorer machine. The buffer system varies depending on the type of column used, and the prepared buffer can be stored for 1 week at room temperature.
3. For reversed-phase HPLC (Sepharose C18 and C8 column): solvent system (A) – 80% acetonitrile is prepared (inside the fume hood) in double distilled water (H_2O). Solvent system (B) 0.1% trifluoroacetic acid (TFA) in H_2O can be stored at room temperature for 1 month. All the solutions should be prepared in MilliQ water (H_2O), as specified in the protocols.
4. This purification protocol can be adapted for several types of natural venoms. Purified proteins should be kept in small aliquots at −20°C for in vitro antimicrobial assays and treatment procedures on mice skin.
5. TEMED is stored in desiccators at room temperature (26–31°C). Longer storage time after opening the bottle will reduce the reagent's potency (i.e., gels will take longer to polymerize etc.)
6. Freshly prepared running buffer is more suitable for gel-electrophoresis (SDS-PAGE). The buffer may be used for 3–4 times provided that the voltage is maintained constant for each consecutive run.
7. We used GS-710 calibrated imaging densitometer for analysis of the gel data, provided that special care is taken to ensure that the gel is free from air bubbles and is not damaged during the transfer. The gel picture may be acquired either in gray scale or in blue color that is matched to the Coomassie Brilliant blue (R-250) stain.

8. Evaluation of wound healing potential using antimicrobial protein and peptides on mice model should be carried out in the bio-safety level 3 (BSL-3) cabinets, with special precautions taken for handling class II human pathogen (*S. aureus*).
9. Fixative is toxic to most commonly used bacteria. In this protocol, 2.5% glutaraldehyde is suitable for the scanning (SEM) and transmission electron microscopic (TEM) studies. The chemical fixative alters the cells on a molecular level to increase their mechanical strength or stability.
10. Osmium tetroxide (OsO_4) is often used as a secondary fixative for bacterial cells. It is a widely used staining agent in SEM and TEM to provide contrast to the image. It is highly toxic to humans, and special care should be taken while handling.
11. For the skin tissues, we used 10% neutral buffered formalin containing 3.7% formaldehyde in phosphate buffered saline (PBS).
12. For Haematoxylin and eosin staining, dewaxing is one of the important steps followed in this protocol to remove the excess wax on the tissues embedded in the paraffin sections before staining. The staining exposure timing is 3 min for 7 μm thin tissues section. Exposure time exceeding the staining of the section will be dark and very hard to distinguish the details under microscope.
13. Several solvents, reagents, and antibodies (markers) are available from different commercial sources. However, we found that the following antibodies such as ant-collagen, anti-panCytokeratin, TNF-alpha, COX-2 antibody extremely good for both western blotting and double immunofluorescence staining, respectively.
14. Mounting: slow and careful application of the top layer minimizes the appearance of air bubbles in the mounting medium. Mounting can be applied in the dark to prevent fainting of bright color during storage.

Acknowledgments

The authors thank the Academic Research Fund (ARF, NUS), Singapore for financial support (Grant R-181 000 078 112) to carry out this investigation.

References

1. Martin, P. (1997) Wound healing-aiming for perfect skin regeneration. *Science* **276**: 75–81.
2. Auguste, P., Vincent, F., Gabbiani, G., Desmoulière, A. (2008) The fibroblast and myofibroblast in inflammatory angiogenesis. In: Seed MP and Walsh DA (eds) Progress in Inflammation Research- Angiogenesis in Inflammation: Mechanisms and Clinical Correlates, Birkhäuser Basel, Springer pp 59–82.
3. Martin, P., Leibovich, S. J. (2005) Inflammatory cells during wound repair: the good, the bad and the ugly. *Trends Cell Biol.* **15**: 599–607.
4. Abe, R., Donnelly, S. C., Peng, T., Bucala, R., Metz, C. N. (2001) Peripheral blood fibrocytes: differentiation pathway and migration to wound sites. *J Immunol.* **166**: 7556–7562.
5. Quan, T. E., Cowper, S., Wu, S. P., Bockenstedt, L. K., Bucala, R. (2004) Circulating fibrocytes: collagen-secreting cells of the peripheral blood. *Int J Biochem Cell Biol.* **36**: 598–606.
6. Diekema, D. J., Pfaller, M. A., Schmitz, F. J., Smayevsky, J., Bell, J., Jones, R. N., Beach, M. (2001) Survey of infections due to *Staphylococcus* species: frequency of occurrence and antimicrobial susceptibility of isolates collected in the United States, Canada, Latin America, Europe, and the Western Pacific region for the SENTRY Antimicrobial Surveillance Program, 1997-1999. *Clin Infect Dis.* **32**: S114–S132.
7. Komatsuzawa, H., Ouhara, K., Yamada, S., Fujiwara, T., Sayama, K., Koji Hashimoto, K., Motoyuki Sugai, M. (2006) Innate defences against methicillin-resistant *Staphylococcus aureus* (MRSA) infection. *J Pathol.* **208**: 249–260.
8. Zähner, H., Fiedler. H. P. (1995) The need for new antibiotics: possible ways forward. In: Hunter P. A., Darby G. K., Russell N. J. (eds.) Fifty years of antimicrobials: past perspectives and future trends. Cambridge University Press, Cambridge, England, pp 67–85.
9. Bonomo, R. A. (2000) Multiple antibiotic-resistant bacteria in long-term-care facilities: an emerging problem in the practice of infectious diseases. *Clin Infect Dis.* **31**: 1414–1422.
10. Wong, A. H., Wenzel, R. P., Edmond. M. B. (2000) Epidemiology of bacteriuria caused by vancomycin-resistant enterococci-a retrospective study. *Am J Infect Control.* **28**: 277–281.
11. Williams, J. D. (2001) Antibiotic resistance in hospital pathogens-acquisition or spread?. *Int J Antimicrob Agents.* **18**: 295–298.
12. Gennaro, R., Zanetti, M. (2000) Structural features and biological activities of the cathelicidin-derived antimicrobial peptides. *Biopolymers.* **55**: 31–49.
13. Zanetti M. (2004) Cathelicidins, multifunctional peptides of the innate immunity. *J Leukoc Biol.* **75**: 39–48.
14. Paramo, L., Lomonte, B., Pizarro-Cerda, J., Bengoechea, J. A., Gorvel, J. P., Moreno, E. (1998) Bactericidal activity of Lys49 and Asp49 myotoxic phospholipases A_2 from *Bothrops asper* snake venom: synthetic Lys49 myotoxin II-(115–129)- peptide identifies its bactericidal region. *Eur J Biochem.* **253**: 452–461.
15. Lomonte, B., Angulo, Y., Calderon, L. (2003) An overview of Lysine-49 phospholipase A_2 myotoxins from crotalid snake venoms and their structural determinants of myotoxic action. *Toxicon.* **42**: 885–901.
16. Lomonte, B., Moreno, E., Tarkowski, A., Hanson, L. A., Maccarana, M. (1994) Neutralizing interaction between heparins and myotoxin II, a Lys-49 phospholipase A_2 from *Bothrops asper* snake venom. *J Biol Chem.* **269**: 29867–29873.
17. Zhang, L., Falla, T.J. (2010) Potential therapeutic application of host defense peptides. *Methods Mol Biol.* **618**: 303–327.
18. Laemmli, U.K. (1970). Cleavage of structural proteins during the assembly of the head of bacteriophage. *Nature* **227**: 680–685.
19. Bradford, M. M. (1976) A rapid and sensitive method for the quantitation of microgram quantities of protein utilizing the principle of protein-dye binding. *Ann Biochem.* **72**: 248–254.
20. Hancock, R. E., Fall, T., Brown, M. (1995). Cationic bactericidal peptides. *Advance Microb Physiol.* **37**: 135–175.
21. National Committee for Clinical Laboratory Standards. (1997). Methods for Dilution Antimicrobial Susceptibility Tests for Bacteria that Grow Aerobically. Approved Standard M7-A4. National Committee for Clinical Standards, Wayne, Pennsyvania, USA.
22. Matsuzaki, K. (1999) Why and how peptide-lipid interactions utilized for self-defense?. Magainins and tachyplesins as archetypes. *Biochim Biophys Acta* **1442**: 1–10.
23. Yenugu, S., Hamil, K. G., Radhakrishnan, Y., French, F. S., Hall, S. H. (2004) The androgen

regulated epididymal sperm-binding protein, ESC42, Is an antimicrobial beta-defensin. *Endocrinol.* **145**: 3165–3173.

24. Kugelberg, E., Norstrom, T., Petersen, T. K., Duvold, T., Andersson, D. I., Hughes, D. (2005) Establishment of a superficial skin infection model in mice by using *Staphylococcus aureus* and *Streptococcus pyogenes*. *Antimicrob Agents Chemother.* **49**: 3435–3441.
25. Nizet, V., Ohtake, T., Lauth, X., Trowbridge, J., Rudisill, J., Dorschner, R.A. (2001) Innate antimicrobial peptide protects the skin from invasive bacterial infection. *Nature* **414**: 454–457.
26. Godin, B., Touitou, E., Rubinstein, E., Athamna, A., Athamna, M. (2005) A new approach for treatment of deep skin infections by an ethosomal antibiotic preparation: an in vivo study. *J Antimicrob Chemother.* **55**: 989–994.
27. Faber, M., Rosdahl, V.T. (1990) Susceptibility to fusidic acid among Danish *Staphylococcus aureus* strains and fusidic add consumption. *J Antimicrob Chemother* **25**: 7–14.
28. Koning, S., van Suijlekom-Smit, L. W. A., Nouwen, J. L., Verduin, C. M., Bernsen, R. M. D., Oranje, A. P., Thomas, S., van der Wouden, J. C. (2002) Fusidic acid cream in the treatment of impetigo in general practice: double blind randomized placebo controlled trial. *BMJ.* **324**: 203–206.
29. Rodrigues, V. M., Soares, A. M., Andriao-Escarso, S. H., Franceschi, A. M., Rucavado, A., Gutierrez, J. M. (2001) Pathological alterations induced by neuwiedase, a metalloproteinase isolated from *Bothrops neuwiedi* snake venom. *Biochimie.* **83**: 471–479.
30. D'Suzea, G., Salazarb, V., Dıaza, P., Sevcika, C., Azpuruac, H., Bracho, N. (2004) Histophatological changes and inflammatory response induced by *Tityus discrepans* scorpion venom in rams. *Toxicon.* **44**: 851–860.
31. Pache, M., Meyer, P. (2006) Morphological changes of the retrobulbar optic nerve and its meningeal sheaths in glaucoma. *Opthalmologica.* **220**: 393–396.
32. Egging, D. F., van Vlijmen-Willems, I., Choi, J., Peeters, A. C. T. M., van Rens, D., Veit, G., Koch, M., Davis, E. C., Schalkwijk, J. (2008) Analysis of obstetric complications and uterine connective tissue in tenascin-X-deficient humans and mice. *Cell Tissue Res.* **332**: 523–532.

Chapter 16

In Vitro Immunogenicity Risk Assessment of Therapeutic Proteins in Preclinical Setting

Puneet Gaitonde and Sathy V. Balu-Iyer

Abstract

Immunogenicity against therapeutic proteins is a clinical problem in the successful treatment of many diseases and, as such, immunogenicity risk assessment in preclinical setting would be useful to improve safety and efficacy of protein-based therapeutics in the product development stages. Here, we attempted a mechanism-based *in vitro* study as screening tool to capture clinically observed antibody-based immune response against two representative therapeutic proteins: recombinant human Erythropoietin-alpha (rHuEPO)and recombinant Factor VIII (rFVIII). Flow-cytometry was used to determine the maturation level of dendritic cells (DCs), a primary initiator of T-cell responses. Studies to capture T-lymphocyte proliferation upon challenge with free rFVIII were performed and secretion of immunomodulatory cytokines was analyzed by ELISA assay. These *in vitro* techniques could be used as risk assessment tool to determine the immunogenic potential of formulations of recombinant proteins in preclinical setting.

Key words: Cytokine, Dendritic cell, ELISA, Erythropoietin, Factor VIII, Flow-cytometry, Immunogenicity, Recombinant protein, T-cell proliferation

1. Introduction

With the advent of recombinant DNA technology, tremendous breakthrough is achieved in developing therapeutic proteins for the treatment of many severe diseases. Unfortunately, many untoward effects were observed in patients including the development of clinical immune responses against the therapeutic proteins. It is recognized that the immune response towards recombinant proteins is a complex interplay (Fig. 1) between antigen presenting cells (APCs), T-lymphocytes, and B-lymphocytes. The proposed steps that are involved in the immunological cascade were illustrated by Chirino et al. (1) wherein, (a) the exogenously administered protein is taken up,

Seetharama D. Satyanarayanajois (ed.), *Drug Design and Discovery: Methods and Protocols*, Methods in Molecular Biology, vol. 716, DOI 10.1007/978-1-61779-012-6_16,

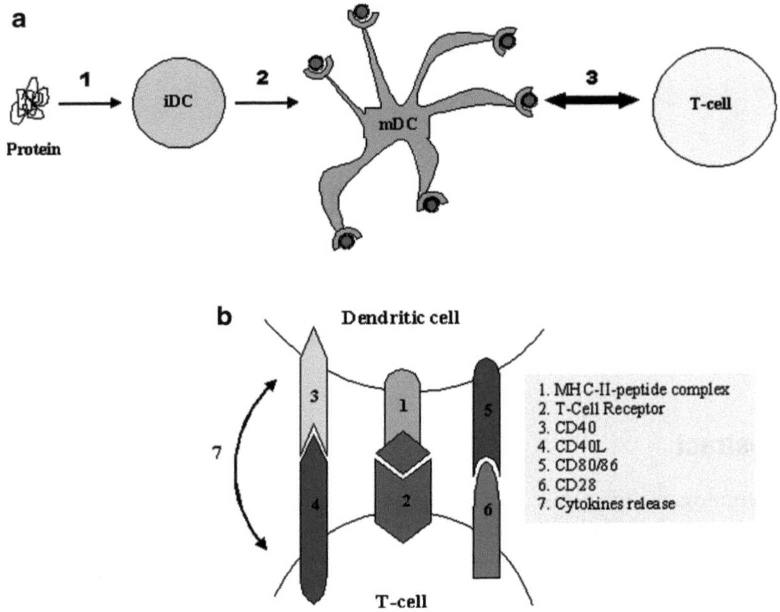

Fig. 1. Protein immunogenicity and cell interaction: (**a**) Initial steps involved in protein immunogenicity: *Step 1*: Protein uptake and processing by immature dendritic cell (iDC), *step 2*: Maturation of dendritic cell (mDC), and *step 3*: Interaction between mDC and T-cell. (**b**) Signaling between mDC and T-cell: *1, 2*: peptide-MHC-II and TCR signal, *3–6*: costimulation, *7*: release of immunomodulatory cytokines by mDC and activated T-cell.

processed, and the immunogenic epitopes are presented by APC in the context of major histocompatibility complex (MHC), (b) APC-T-cell interaction, (c) interaction between T-cell and B-cell, and (d) differentiation of B-cells into antibody secreting plasma cells. Thus, *ex vivo/in vitro* antigen presentation and cell interaction studies could be useful to gauge the immunogenicity risk against a therapeutic protein. Here, we have used two recombinant proteins, viz., Erythropoietin-alpha and factor VIII (rFVIII), as representative therapeutic proteins and determined their influence on APCs and T-cells, respectively.

Flow-cytometry is a well-established technique that was used to determine differences in the expression level of APC-surface molecules *in vitro*. The activation and proliferation of T-cells in the presence of antigen was studied by performing *in vitro* by using ^{3}H-Thymidine-based T-cell proliferation studies. It has been demonstrated that cytokines play a critical role in directing the immune response either towards immunity or regulation. TGF-β (2) and IL-10 (3) are two important cytokines that are known to induce the generation of regulatory T-lymphocytes, whereas cytokines such as IFN-γ, IL-6, IL-17, and IL-23 are known to contribute to the immunity arm of the immune response.

Pertinently, the level of immunomodulatory cytokines can be characterized by an ELISA assay. The use of such techniques as well as development of other *in vitro*-based techniques, e.g., B-cell-based assays, will enhance the early assessment of immunogenicity of the next generation of therapeutic proteins.

2. Materials

Factor-VIII knockout mice, which bear a targeted deletion in exon 16 of the FVIII gene, was established using breeding pairs provided by Drs. Kazazian and Sarkar from the University of Pennsylvania, PA. Normal mice were used for Erythropoietin studies. All animal studies were preapproved by the Institutional Animal Care and Use Committee of the University at Buffalo.

2.1. Cell culture

1. RPMI-1640 medium: with L-glutamine and without calcium or magnesium (GIBCO, Carlsbad, CA). Supplemented with Penicillin (100 U/mL) and Streptomycin (100 μg/mL).
2. 2-Mercaptoethanol (see Note 1).
3. Heat-inactivated and sterile-filtered premium fetal bovine serum (Lonza Inc., Walkersville, MD) (see Note 2).
4. Recombinant murine Granulocyte Macrophage Colony Stimulating Factor (rmGMCSF, 200 U/mL) (Peprotech Inc., Rocky Hill, NJ) (see Note 3).
5. 0.4% Trypan blue dye.
6. Neubauer Chamber (Hemocytometer).
7. Sterile tissue-culture dishes (100 × 20 mm).
8. Sterile phosphate-buffered saline: (10× PBS) and DNase-RNase-free distil water. The sterile 10× PBS is diluted 10× with the distilled water and pH adjusted to 7.2 and sterile-filtered via 0.22-μm filter. The solution is stored at 4°C.
9. 25-Gauge sterile hypodermic needle (25 gauge): 10 mL sterile syringe and sterile cell-strainer with 100-μm pore-size.
10. Sterilized 15 and 50 mL centrifuge tubes, sterilized 0.22 μm bottle-top filter.
11. 10 mL Serological pipettes.
12. Aerrane™ isoflurane (Henry Schein Inc., Melville, NY): used as a mixture with oxygen to anesthetize the animals.
13. Centrifuge: which can hold 15 and 50 mL centrifuge tubes and run at 4°C for 10 min and centrifugal speed of up to 1,000 × g is required.
14. Cell-culture incubator.

2.2. DC Maturation Study

1. Albumin-free recombinant human erythropoietin-alpha (rHuEPO; Prospec-Tany TechnoGene Ltd.). Reconstitute and store at −80°C.
2. Fc-Block®, FITC-anti-MHC-II, FITC-anti-CD11c, PE-anti-CD40, PE-anti-CD80, PE-anti-CD86, and corresponding isotype controls (BD Biosciences and eBioscience Inc., San Diego, CA).
3. 10% Ultrapure paraformaldehyde (diluted to 2 X with sterile and ice-cold 1× PBS as required).
4. Calibrite® calibration kit, FACS cleaning solution, and Sheath fluid.
5. FACS Calibur Flow-cytometer.
6. CellQuest software (BD Biosciences).

2.3. T-Cell Proliferation and Cytokine Analysis

1. Full-length, excipients-free recombinant Factor VIII (rFVIII) (store at −80°C).
2. 0.5-mL sterile syringe with 29-gauge hypodermic needle (used to administer formulation to the animals).
3. Sterilized, flat-bottom glass pestle.
4. Dynal® $CD8^+$ (Lyt 2) T-cell depletion kit and Dynal® magnet (Invitrogen). The kit is stored at 4°C.
5. 30% sterile-filtered Bovine serum albumin (BSA).
6. Sterile 96-Well flat-bottom plates with lids.
7. Concanavalin A (Con A; Sigma-Aldrich).
8. ^{3}H-Thymidine (6.7 Ci/mmol), (Perkin Elmer, Waltham, MA) is stored at −20°C in a freezer which is distinctly labeled and used for storing radioactive materials.
9. Unifilter-G 96-well plate, Scintillation "O" fluid, and plate seals.
10. Cell-dyn®-1700 cell counter (Abbott labs, Abbott Park, IL).
11. Plate harvester, plate sealer, and Top-count™ scintillation counter (Perkin Elmer).

2.4. Cytokine Analysis

1. Duoset® ELISA development kit for Transforming growth factor-beta (TGF-β), Interleukin (IL)-2, 6, 10, 17, 23, and Interferon-γ (R&D systems, Minnesota, MN). Store at 4°C (see Note 4).
2. NUNC maxisorp 96-well flat-bottom plates with lids.
3. Wash buffer: 0.1% Tween-20 in PBS, pH 7.0 and 0.22 μm filtered. Prepare fresh and store at room temperature.
4. Stop solution: 2 N Sulfuric acid.
5. Plate washer (Tecan US, Inc., Durham, NC).

3. Methods

3.1. Dendritic Cell Culture

Murine bone marrow isolation and dendritic cell (DC) culturing method was followed using the procedure of Lutz et al. (4).

1. Use naïve normal mice aged between 8 and 12 weeks old for the bone marrow isolation.
2. Transfer the animal to a chamber that has an inlet and outlet for a constant flow of oxygen and isoflurane. Anesthetize the animal and verify complete anesthesia by the lack of righting reflex of the animal as well as by monitoring the slowness of breathing.
3. Take the animal out of the chamber and place on a surgery board covered with cotton-lined underpad. Keep the animal under anesthesia using a nose-cone which is constantly supplied with isoflurane and oxygen. Keep monitoring the breathing of the animal. If the animal starts to gasp, reduce the flow of isoflurane accordingly.
4. To verify that the animal is completely anesthetized, press the paws of the hind limbs as a form of stimuli. Mice paws are very sensitive to stimuli, and hence, a lack of "twitching" reflex action will indicate that the animal has been completely subdued.
5. Lay the animal on its dorsal side with its forelimbs and hind limbs stretched and fastened using a fastening tape to keep the limbs from interfering with the surgery.
6. Spray 70% alcohol using a squirt bottle onto the chest, abdomen, and hind limbs of the animal to disinfect. Alcohol also wets the skin hairs and makes it easier to do incisions without loose hair contaminating the procedure.
7. With the help of a pair of sterilized forceps and scissors, make an incision in the skin near the abdomen area and slowly cut the skin up to the sternum. Then, carefully cut the diaphragm and sacrifice the animal by cardiac puncture.
8. Upon sacrifice, turn off the flow of isoflurane and oxygen.
9. Make two skin incisions on the two hind limbs starting from the pelvic region till the ankle.
10. Then, carefully clear the muscle surrounding the proximal region of the femur near the pelvic joint by scraping using the pair of scissors. One can also make use of wet alcohol wipes or 2 in. × 2 in. cotton gauze to remove the muscle tissue by hand.
11. Cut the pelvic bone so as not to damage the head of the femur. Keep the ball-and-socket joint intact.

12. Once the two hind limbs are isolated, clear the muscle attaching to the bones by carefully scraping it using a pair of scissors. Take care not to break or cut the bones. Discard the fibula, part of the pelvic bone, and the feet. Collect only the femurs and tibiae.
13. Put the femurs and tibiae in a 15-mL centrifuge tube containing 70% alcohol for 2–3 min to disinfect.
14. Turn on the centrifuge and let the temperature come down to 4°C.
15. All of the following steps involving cells must be carried out in a cell-culture hood with laminar airflow and HEPA filters. The hood should be sterilized by turning on the UV light for 30 min. All the material that is moved into the hood must be wiped with 70% alcohol to maintain sterile conditions inside the hood.
16. Also, keep a pair of sterilized forceps and scissors, two sterilized 50 mL tubes, a cell-strainer, 10 mL syringe with a 25 gauge needle, a serological 10 mL pipette and sterile, ice-cold PBS into the hood.
17. Transfer the bones along with the alcohol into a sterilized Petri dish.
18. Then immediately take the bones out of the alcohol with forceps and place them in another Petri dish. This step is required to make sure the alcohol does not come in contact with the bone marrow; otherwise, the bone marrow cells will die in presence of alcohol.
19. Transfer approximately 40 mL of PBS to one of the 50 mL tube and aspirate 10 mL of it using the 10-mL syringe with an attached needle.
20. With a sterile pair of scissors, cut both the ends of the bones, thus making a open-ended cylinder with the bone marrow inside it.
21. Flush the bone marrow using the PBS-filled syringe into an empty Petri dish. All the bones are flushed in a similar manner till all the bone marrow is collected in the Petri dish.
22. Place the cell-strainer atop the second empty 50 mL tube.
23. Using a serological pipette, disperse any cell clumps present in the flushed cell suspension and transfer the cell suspension to the tube via the cell-strainer.
24. Centrifuge the tube at 300 × *g* for 10 min at 4°C.
25. After the centrifugation, discard the supernatant and resuspend the cell pellet in 2 mL of sterile RPMI-1640 media and mix thoroughly.
26. Take 50 μL of the cell suspension into a 1.5-mL microcentrifuge tube containing an equivalent volume of 0.4% Trypan

blue dye (1:1 dilution, i.e., dilution factor of 2) and mix thoroughly.

27. Load approximately 15 μL (or an appropriate volume to cover the entire counting area of the slide) of the mixture onto a Hemocytometer (Neubauer chamber) and place under a light microscope for cell counting.
28. There will usually be two types of cells visible under the microscope, transparent and blue-colored cells. Transparent cells are the ones which have not taken up the dye and are viable cells, whereas the cells that have taken up the dye are dead cells. Count only the transparent cells.
29. The viable cell count is done manually by counting the cells present in the five squares on the hemocytometer grid as described in Fig. 2.
30. Calculate the concentration of viable cells/mL present in the reconstituted cell suspension as per the following formula:

$$\text{Viable cells/mL of suspension} = (\text{Cell count in five squares}/5) \times \text{dil. factor} \times 10^4$$

where;

dil.factor = 2 (50 μL of cell + 50 μL of Trypan blue),

10^4 = Dilution factor of the hemocytometer as directed by the manufacturer.

31. Accordingly, add 10 mL of DC media (RPMI-1640 containing Penicillin/streptomycin and 2-mercaptoethanol and 0.22 μm filtered) containing 2×10^6 viable cells, 1 mL (10%) heat-inactivated FBS, and 200 U/mL of rmGMCSF to sterile

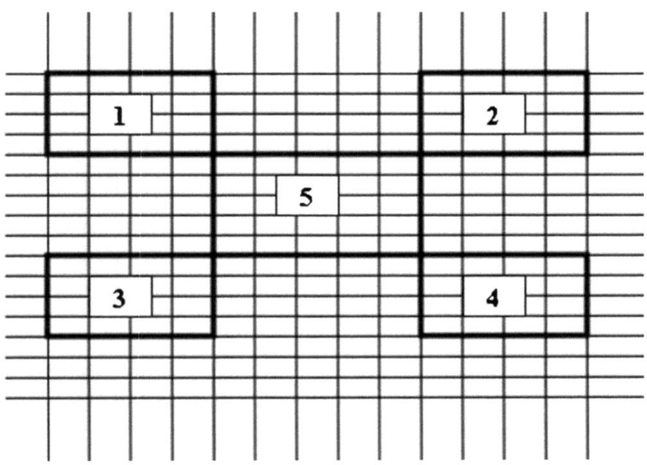

Fig. 2. Diagram of a hemocytometer: All the five large squares (as denoted by numbers *1–5*, consisting of 16 smaller squares or 25 smaller squares for the center square) are counted and the average count is determined.

100 × 20 mm Petri dishes. This day is considered as "Day 0." Incubate the plates in a humidified cell-culture incubator at 37°C and 5% CO_2.

32. Add 10 mL of fresh DC media (containing 10% FBS and rmGMCSF) slowly to each of the plates on day 3 without disturbing the basal cell layer.
33. On day 6 and 8, aspirate half of the supernatant from each plate (approximately 10 mL) and add to 15-mL centrifuge tubes. Centrifuge the tubes at 300 × *g* for 10 min at 4°C. Discard the supernatant and resuspend the cell pellet in 10 mL of fresh DC media (containing 10% FBS and rmGMCSF).
34. Carefully add the resuspended cell suspension back to the plates without disturbing the basal cell layer.
35. On day 9, harvest the loosely attached cells from the plates without scraping the plates and collect in 50-mL centrifuge tubes. Centrifuge the tubes at 300 × *g* for 10 min at 4°C and discard the supernatant.
36. Resuspend the cell pellet in 5 mL of sterile and ice-cold 1× PBS.
37. Determine the concentration of viable cells as described in steps 25–29.
38. Characterize the DCs by determining the cell-surface expression level of key molecules such as MHC-II, CD11c (a marker of DC), CD86, CD80, and CD40 (for detailed flow-cytometry sample preparation look at section 3.2. DC Maturation Study).
39. Based on our numerous flow-cytometric analyses, it was found that the cell suspension contains approximately 80% of DCs.

3.2. DC Maturation Study

1. On day 9 of DC culture, harvest the cells and count viable cells as described previously.
2. Take a 24-well sterile tissue-culture plate with lid and plate 2×10^6 DCs/well in DC media.
3. Thereafter, add 2 μg/mL of free rHuEPO to each of the wells and mix well. Keep four wells untreated to serve as negative control. Incubate the plate at 37°C and 5% CO_2 for 24 h.
4. After 24 h of incubation, harvest the DCs from each well and transfer to appropriately labeled 15 mL centrifuge tubes. Centrifuge the tubes at 300 × *g* for 10 min at 4°C.
5. Discard the supernatant and resuspend the pellet in another 10 mL of RPMI-1640 media. Centrifuge the cells for a second time and discard the supernatant.

6. Resuspend the resulting cell pellet in 2 mL of sterile, ice-cold 1× PBS and count viable cells by Trypan blue exclusion method as described earlier.
7. Accordingly, transfer 1×10^6 viable cells to appropriately labeled microcentrifuge tubes such that each treatment group has two tubes. One tube will be used for analyzing the cell-surface expression, whereas the other tube will serve as isotype control. If the cell volume is greater than 500 μL, use 5 mL flow-cytometry tubes instead of microcentrifuge tubes.
8. Add PBS to fill the tubes and centrifuge the tubes at $300 \times g$ for 10 min at 4°C.
9. Discard the supernatant carefully and resuspend the cell pellet in residual volume (100 μL) and keep on ice.
10. Add 3 μL of Fc-Block® antibody to each of the tubes, mix well, and let tubes incubate for 15 min on ice (see Note 5).
11. Add 5 μL of either FITC-anti-MHC-II or PE-anti-CD86 or PE-anti-CD40 antibody to one of the two tubes from each group. Add 5 μL of the corresponding isotype control to the other tube from each group (see Note 5). Mix the tubes well and incubate the tubes on ice for 30 min in dark.
12. Add PBS to fill the tubes and centrifuge the tubes at $1{,}000 \times g$ for 5 min at 4°C and discard the supernatant. This step will remove any unbound antibodies.
13. Resuspend the cell pellet in 0.5 mL of ice-cold and ultrapure 2% Paraformaldehyde to fix the cells and keep the tubes on ice. The cells are now ready to be analyzed using flow-cytometry.
14. Flush the flow-cytometer with the manufacturer-provided cleaning solution or 10% filtered bleach for 10 min. Then run distil water for 10–15 min.
15. Connect the flow-cytometer to the computer and start the FACScomp software. Calibrate the machine using the Calibrite® calibration kit and follow the manufacturer's protocol.
16. Upon calibration, start the CellQuest program for analyzing the samples.
17. Create a template with four plots: (a) SSC vs. FSC, (b) cell count vs. FL1 (FITC), (c) cell count vs. FL2 (PE), and (d) FL1 vs. FL2.
18. Run the autofluorescence tube for optimizing the settings such that all the cells show up on the plot A and observe peak in plot B and C; and the peak is towards the left of the plot, and most of the cells are present in the lower left quadrant of plot D. This can be optimized using "Detection & Threshold" window which can be selected from the "Cytometer" tab.

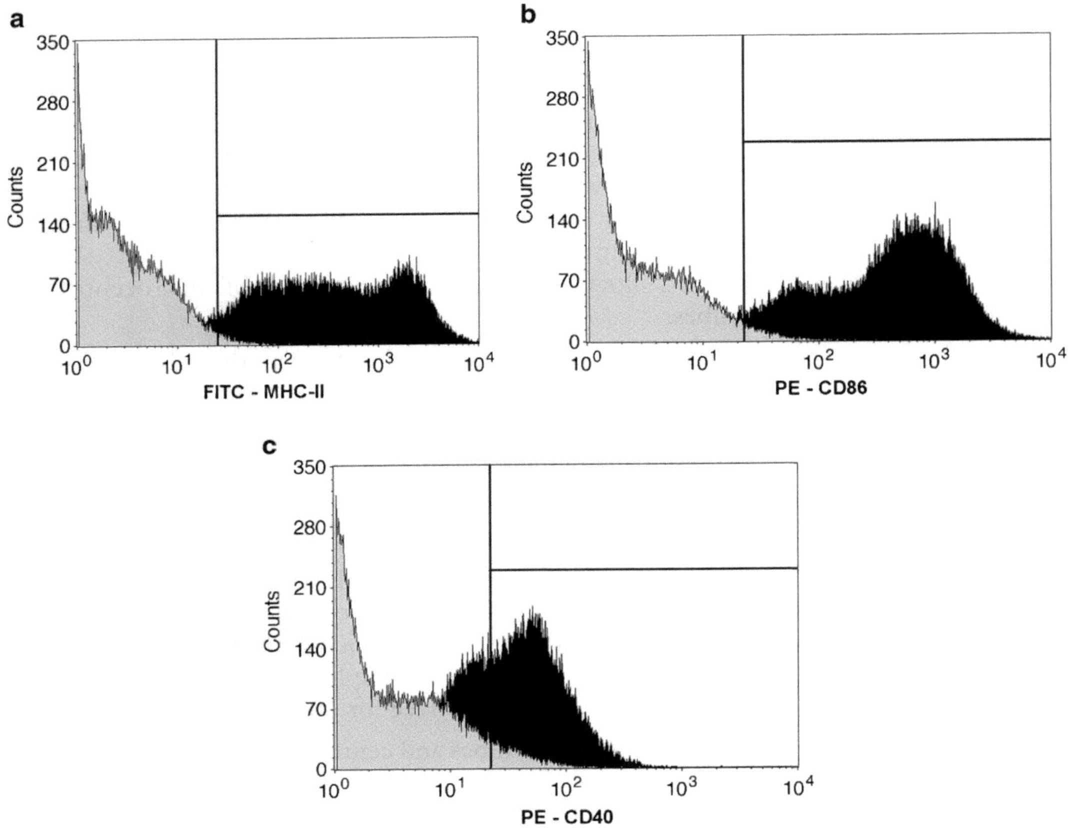

Fig. 3. DC maturation study: Dendritic cell-surface expression level (**a**) MHC-II, (**b**) CD86, (**c**) CD40 as determined by using flow-cytometric analysis upon cell exposure to free rHuEPO.

19. Once the optimization is complete, run the samples in order to capture 50,000 events.
20. After completion of analysis, follow step 14 before turning the flow-cytometer off. The results of the study are shown in Fig. 3a–c.

3.3. T-Cell Proliferation Study

1. Divide naïve FVIII-knockout mice into two groups. Immunize one group of animals with 2 μg of free rFVIII in 100 μL of total injection volume using 29-gauge sterile needle and 0.5 mL syringe via the subcutaneous route of administration once a week for 2 consecutive weeks. It has been shown that this immunization protocol is able to prime the immune system in these animals towards rFVIII (5, 6). The other group will serve as control.
2. On the third day after second weekly immunization, sacrifice all mice by cardiac puncture and collect the individual spleens in 10 mL of sterile and ice-cold RPMI-1640 media in 15-mL centrifuge tubes.

3. Transfer the spleen into a Petri dish inside the sterilized cell-culture hood.
4. Homogenize the spleen using a sterile flat-bottom glass pestle.
5. Disperse any cell clumps using a 10 mL serological pipette.
6. Pass the cell suspension through sterile 100 μm cell-strainer three times to remove debris.
7. Transfer the filtered cell suspension into a sterile 15-mL centrifuge tube and centrifuge the tube at 200 × *g* for 10 min at 4°C.
8. Discard the supernatant and resuspend the cell pellet in 3 mL of sterile and ice-cold 1× PBS.
9. After thorough mixing, add 80 μL of the cell suspension to a microcentrifuge tube and determine lymphocyte count using Cell-Dyn®-1700 instrument.
10. Upon determination of total lymphocyte concentration in the sample, take 1×10^7 total lymphocytes for use with Dynal $CD8^+$ (Lyt 2) T-lymphocyte depletion kit and follow the manufacturer's protocol to enrich $CD4^+$ T-lymphocytes.
11. At the end of the $CD4^+$ T-cell enrichment, count the cells as described in step 9.
12. Accordingly, add 2×10^5/well of $CD4^+$ T-lymphocytes in quadruplicate wells to a sterile tissue-culture 96-well plate with lid. Make up the volume in each cell to 200 μL by adding T-cell media (RPMI-1640, Penicillin–Streptomycin, Sodium pyruvate, Polymyxin-B and 10% FBS, 0.22 μm filtered).
13. Challenge the T-cells from immunized animals with 1,000 ng/mL of free rFVIII.
14. Use T-cells from untreated animals as the negative control.
15. Add 125 ng/mL of Concanavalin A (Con A) to another four wells of untreated T-cells to serve as the positive control.
16. Incubate the plates in a humidified cell-culture incubator at 37°C for 72 h.
17. After 72 h, add 1 μCi/10 μL of ^{3}H-Thymidine (6.7 Ci/mmol) to each well and incubate the plate for an additional 16 h in a "radioactive materials only"-labeled humidified cell-culture incubator at 37°C and 5% CO_2.
18. After the incubation, mount the plate on a plate harvester and harvest the cells onto a Unifilter membrane-backed 96-well plate (see Note 6).
19. Add 30 μL of scintillation "O" fluid to each of the wells of the Unifilter plate and the plate is sealed using a plate sealer.

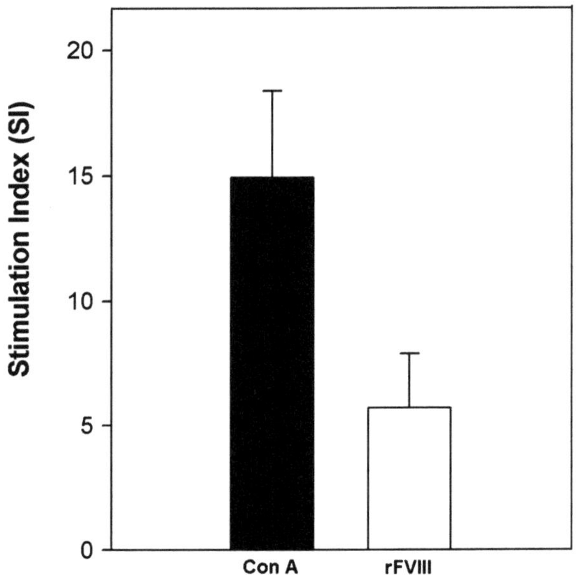

Fig. 4. T-cell proliferation study: Performed by the incorporation of ^{3}H-Thymidine into the cells and measuring the indirect cell count by radioactivity counts.

20. Analyze the plate for radioactivity (counts per minute, cpm) in each well by using a Top-count scintillation counter.
21. Calculate the average count of the quadruplicate wells for each group and, accordingly, determine the stimulation index (SI) for each individual group as per the following formula:

SI = Average count of sample/average count of negative control.

22. The results are shown in Fig. 4.

3.4. Cytokine Analysis by ELISA

1. Follow steps described in Subheading 3.3, steps 1–14.
2. After 72 h, centrifuge the plate at 300 × *g* for 10 min at 4°C.
3. Carefully aspirate the supernatant from each of the quadruplicate wells and pool them in a 1.5-mL microcentrifuge tube and keep on ice.
4. Store the tubes at −80°C until further analysis.
5. Perform cytokine analysis for TFG-β, IL-2, IL-6, IL-10, IL-17, IL-23, and IFN-γ using the Duoset ELISA kit (R&D systems, MN).

4. Notes

1. Penicillin–Streptomycin is aliquoted and stored at −20°C. 2-mercaptoethanol is stored at 4°C and away from light.
2. The frozen bottle is thawed by initially keeping it at 4°C for 24 h and later thawing at room temperature. It is advisable not to thaw FBS by directly keeping the bottle at 37°C atmosphere. Upon complete thawing, the bottle is opened in aseptic condition in a sterilized cell-culture hood and aliquoted into sterilized 50 mL conical tubes. The tubes are then stored at −20°C.
3. The lyophilized powder is reconstituted with the manufacturer's recommended reconstitution buffer or with sterile water for injection. The reconstituted protein is aliquoted into microcentrifuge tubes as a single-use volume and stored at −20°C.

   Do not use any stocks which are more than 6 months old, as it has been observed that the activity of reconstituted rmG-MCSF decreases significantly over time.
4. The ELISA standards and antibodies are aliquoted as per the manufacturer's instructions and stored in microcentrifuge tubes at −80°C.
5. Prior titration of the antibodies with the cells is required in order to add optimum concentration of the antibodies to all the respective binding sites.
6. Make sure to scrape the bottom of the plate with the harvesting probes in order to deposit as many cells as possible onto the membrane of Unifilter plate. Rinse the plate with water sufficiently to flush any radioactive material. Take appropriate steps to ensure safe disposal of radioactive material.

Acknowledgment

This work is supported by a grant from the National Institutes of Health (R01 HL-70227) to SVB. We thank Dr. William Jusko, Department of Pharmaceutical Sciences, University at Buffalo, for letting us to use the flow-cytometer (FACSCalibur), Cell-Dyn-1700®, Plate harvester, and Top-count scintillation counter instruments available in his lab. We are grateful to Drs. Kazazian and Sarkar of the University of Pennsylvania for providing the rFVIII knockout mice model, and to Dr. Zale Bernstein of Western New York Hemophilia Foundation for providing albumin-free recombinant Factor VIII.

References

1. Chirino, A. J., Ary, M. L., and Marshall, S. A. (2004) Minimizing the immunogenicity of protein therapeutics. *Drug Discov Today* **9**: 82–90.
2. Zheng, S. G. (2008) The critical role of TGF-beta1 in the development of induced Foxp3+ regulatory T cells. *Int J Clin Exp* Med. **1**: 192–202.
3. Hara, M., Kingsley, C. I., Niimi, M., Read, S., Turvey, S. E., Bushell, A. R., Morris, P. J., Powrie, F., and Wood, K. J. (2001) IL-10 is required for regulatory T cells to mediate tolerance to alloantigens in vivo. *J Immunol.* **166**: 3789–3796.
4. Lutz, M. B., Kukutsch, N., Ogilvie, A. L., Rossner, S., Koch, F., Romani, N., and Schuler, G. (1999) An advanced culture method for generating large quantities of highly pure dendritic cells from mouse bone marrow. *J Immunol Methods* **223**: 77–92.
5. Ramani, K., Miclea, R. D., Purohit, V. S., Mager, D. E., Straubinger, R. M., and Balu-Iyer, S. V. (2008) Phosphatidylserine containing liposomes reduce immunogenicity of recombinant human factor VIII (rFVIII) in a murine model of hemophilia A. *J Pharm Sci.* **97**: 1386–1398.
6. Purohit, V. S., Ramani, K., Sarkar, R., Kazazian, H. H., Jr., and Balasubramanian, S. V. (2005) Lower inhibitor development in hemophilia-A mice following administration of recombinant factor VIII-O-phospho-L-serine complex. *J Biol Chem.* **280**: 17593–17600.

INDEX

Seetharama D. Satyanarayanajois (ed.), *Drug Design and Discovery: Methods and Protocols*,
Methods in Molecular Biology, vol. 716, DOI 10.1007/978-1-61779-012-6,

J

K

L

M

N

O

P

MIX
Papier aus verantwortungsvollen Quellen
Paper from responsible sources
FSC® C105338

If you have any concerns about our products,
you can contact us on
ProductSafety@springernature.com

In case Publisher is established outside the EU,
the EU authorized representative is:
Springer Nature Customer Service Center GmbH
Europaplatz 3, 69115 Heidelberg, Germany

Printed by Libri Plureos GmbH
in Hamburg, Germany